Psychopathology and Function

THIRD EDITION

Psychopathology and Function

THIRD EDITION

Bette R. Bonder, PhD, OTR/L, FAOTA

Professor
Departments of Health Sciences and Psychology
Cleveland State University
Cleveland, Ohio

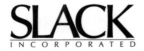

SLACK
INCORPORATED

An innovative information, education, and management company
6900 Grove Road • Thorofare, NJ 08086

Bonder, Bette.
  Psychopathology and function / Bette R. Bonder.-- 3rd ed.
      p. ; cm.
  Includes bibliographical references and index.
  ISBN 1-55642-627-5 (alk. paper)
  1. Psychology, Pathological. 2. Occupational therapists.
  [DNLM: 1. Mental Disorders--diagnosis. 2. Mental
Disorders--classification. 3. Mental Disorders--therapy. 4.
Occupational Therapy--methods. WM 141 B711p 2003] I. Title.
RC454.B5765 2003
616.89--dc22
                                        2003021459

Printed in the United States of America.

Published by: SLACK Incorporated
                     6900 Grove Road
                     Thorofare, NJ 08086 USA
                     Telephone: 856-848-1000
                     Fax: 856-853-5991
                     www.slackbooks.com

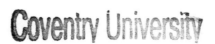

DEDICATION

For my aunts, Vivian Braun and Betty Schwartz, with love.

CONTENTS

Dedication . . . . *v*

Acknowledgments . . . . *ix*

About the Author. . . . . *xi*

Introduction . . . . *xiii*

Chapter 1   Psychiatric Diagnosis and the Classification System 1

Chapter 2   DSM-IV and Occupational Therapy 17

Chapter 3   Disorders of Infancy, Childhood, and Adolescence 35

Chapter 4   Delirium, Dementia, Amnestic, and Other Cognitive Disorders . . . 65

Chapter 5   Substance-Related Disorders 77

Chapter 6   Schizophrenia and Other Psychotic Disorders 95

Chapter 7   Mood Disorders 109

Chapter 8   Anxiety Disorders 127

Chapter 9   Personality Disorders 141

Chapter 10   Other Disorders 159

Chapter 11   Psychopharmacology 175
               Darrell Hulisz, PharmD and Phillip J. Fischer, MD

Glossary 207

Appendix A   DSM-IV-TR Classification. 213

Appendix B   An Overview of the International Classification of Function 233

Index 235

ACKNOWLEDGMENTS

This book is the result of the efforts of many individuals. I am grateful to my students over the years for their critical review of material, and to Karen Bradley and Susan Stupp for their clerical assistance. I am particularly appreciative of the efforts of my colleagues Phillip Fischer and Darrell Hulisz in ensuring that the psychopharmacology chapter is accurate and up-to-date.

Many individuals at SLACK Incorporated have been supportive of my projects over the years. In particular, I thank Amy McShane—who has shepherded this edition, like those before it into production. Debra Toulson, Lauren Biddle Plummer, Michelle Gatt, April Billick, and Jim Pennewill have also provided assistance in bringing this project to fruition and making sure people know about it. The reviewers provided extremely useful input that has enhanced the final product. John Bond has provided invaluable assistance through our many years of association.

As always, my family—Patrick, Aaron, and Jordan Bray—deserves thanks and recognition. They tolerated many fast-food dinners and weekends of fending for themselves while this book was in process. They provided moral support throughout this effort. For this and for many other reasons, they have my profound gratitude.

About the Author

Bette R. Bonder, PhD, OTR/L, FAOTA, professor of health sciences and psychology at Cleveland State University in Cleveland, Ohio, is an occupational therapist and psychologist with experience working with individuals from diverse backgrounds in mental health, gerontology, and developmental disabilities. She is currently engaged in a study of the meaning of occupation for older adults.

INTRODUCTION

Rapid changes in health care in the past several decades have had a disproportionate impact on mental health services. Lack of clarity about what constitutes a psychiatric illness and uncertainty about effective treatment have resulted in dilemmas regarding methods for providing and paying for care (Murphy, 1998). This has caused considerable turmoil in mental health care reflective of, but perhaps more profound than, the turmoil in health care generally.

That turmoil has had several sources. On the positive side of the equation, scientific knowledge is expanding rapidly. Experimentally validated information about etiology and treatment of psychiatric disorders has increased greatly, allowing for more effective intervention and, in many instances, a more positive prognosis. An example is the improvement in imaging techniques that allow researchers to see what is happening in the brain when individuals are experiencing hallucinations, anxiety, or other symptoms of psychiatric disorder (Epstein, Isenberg, Stern, & Silbersweig, 2002).

Interest in science has led to a push for evidence-based practice or EPB (i.e., development of intervention strategies based on careful review of relevant research findings) (Law, 2002). A problem with EBP is the possibility that individual differences may be overlooked. This dilemma is addressed through a growing emphasis on client-centered care (Gage, 1993), a concept that encourages collaboration with the client in structuring treatment goals and methods.

A more problematic consequence of the upheaval in health care is the fact that systems for delivery of care, as well as treatment options, have become increasingly complex. Patients, their families, third-party payers, and health care providers all struggle with issues about quality of care, cost, and the rights of the various interested parties. Occupational therapists, like other health care professionals, have had to cope with these increasing complexities to continue to provide high quality care.

Occupational therapy as a profession originated in mental health (Bruce & Borg, 1987). The earliest therapists provided activities that were thought "useful" and "healthful" to divert patients from their problems, as "moral treatment" emerged as a theory for intervention. Meyer (1922/1977), a founder of occupational therapy, believed mental illness to be a "problem of living," suggesting that a balance of work, leisure, and rest would restore health.

The emerging beliefs of occupational therapy fit within the two primary forms of treatment employed by physicians and other mental health care providers at that time (for an excellent brief history of psychiatric treatment, see Healy, 2002). For individuals who were psychotic (i.e., severely disturbed and out of contact with reality), removal from the environment and placement in an institution was the norm. It was felt that these disorders were largely intractable, and little could be done except to relieve the families of the burden for caring for their bizarre relatives. There was some suspicion that such illnesses had a physical component, as a result of which insulin shock, psychosurgery, and, later, electroshock treatments were employed. For those who were "neurotic" (i.e., emotionally disturbed but in contact with reality), psychoanalysis or other verbal therapies were implemented, usually while the patient continued to reside at home. This form of treatment often meant years of intensive verbal therapy focused on discussion of experiences that might have molded maladaptive emotional reactions.

A revolution in mental health care occurred with the discovery of a variety of psychopharmacological agents in the middle of the last century. These drugs made it possible, albeit with many unpleasant side effects, to control some psychotic symptoms as well as depression and anxiety. At the same time, a variety of new theories about behavior increased the range of psychosocial therapies from which treatment choices were made. Behavior therapy, cognitive therapy, and family therapies are among the alternatives that emerged. Such interventions have been investigated for effectiveness through a variety of research methods.

Current mental health care centers around several primary strategies. Most notable of these is drug treatment. Since the discovery of the potential for psychopharmacological agents, new kinds of medications have been developed, many of them more effective than earlier versions, and with fewer undesirable effects. Some can be taken for years, allowing for acceptable control of an array of symptoms.

Psychotropic medications, however, remain imperfect (Healy, 2002). Difficulties determining the right medication and dose and the continuing problems of unacceptable side effects mean that these drugs may not entirely resolve psychological problems. Other interventions, the vast majority now provided in the community, are common. Many of the new therapies are brief, often designed to last a few days to a few weeks. Most are provided outside of institutional settings, in out-patient mental health centers, day treatment centers, or other community-based facilities. The shift away from institutional care has many positive consequences, although it has also contributed to dilemmas as a result of the discharge from long-term in-patient care of many individuals who are ill-equipped to manage in the community (Austad & Morgan, 1998).

Occupational therapists work in all of these mental health settings, but their approach to psychiatric disorders differs from other professionals. In the provision of occupational therapy services, the presenting problem may, in fact, not be an identified psychiatric disorder, but rather a problem with daily function. Difficulties in performance of important activities can be caused by, or can affect, psychological state, but the two are not synonymous.

Many of the psychosocial issues treated by occupational therapists emerge during the course of treatment for a "physical" disorder. Some psychosocial problems, including depression and anxiety for example, emerge as a result of onset of physical disability (Lisspers, Nygren, & Soderman, 1998; Livneh & Antonak, 1994; Owen, Koutsakis, & Bennett, 2001). Family issues may be exacerbated by the need for care following accident or illness.

To function effectively in providing mental health services, occupational therapists must have a clear understanding of the needs of the individual, the system in which they are providing care, the roles of other professionals, and their own potential contributions to treatment. They must examine payment sources because payment for services is almost always provided, at least in part, by someone other than the identified patient. This may be an insurance company, the government, or an employer; someone whose interests may be different from those of the patient. They are interested in service that is effective but is within reasonable cost limits.

Because they work within the mental health system, occupational therapists must understand the diagnostic structure used by their professional colleagues and be able to communicate effectively across disciplinary lines. This book is designed to guide occupational therapists in understanding their clients, communicating with other professionals, and providing care to individuals in real life situations, assuring that quality of life is maintained or enhanced for those being served. The text is not intended to provide comprehensive coverage of the occupational therapy process in mental health. Many other books discuss that subject from a variety of perspectives. Rather, it is designed as an overview of the kinds of clients with whom occupational therapists and other health care providers are likely to work to give therapists an understanding of the ways in which other mental health professionals view these individuals. Understanding the context for service and the diagnostic conceptualizations of other professionals enables occupational therapists to enhance their interventions and define their unique contribution to mental health.

REFERENCES

Austad, C.S., & Morgan, T.C. (1998). Toward a social ethic of mental health care: Long-term therapy, short-term therapy, and managed health care. In R.F. Small & L.R. Barnhill (Eds.), *Practicing in the new mental health marketplace: Ethical, legal, and moral issues* (pp. 103-120). Washington, DC: American Psychological Association.

Bruce, M.A., & Borg, B. (1987). *Frames of reference in psychosocial occupational therapy.* Thorofare, NJ: SLACK Incorporated.

Epstein, J., Isenberg, N., Stern, E., & Silbersweig, D. (2002). Toward a neuroanatomical understanding of psychiatric illness: The role of functional imaging. In J.E. Helzer & J.J. Hudak, (Eds.), *Defining psychopathology in the 21st century: DSM-V and beyond* (pp. 57-70). Washington, DC: American Psychiatric Association.

Gage, M. (1993). Reengineering of health care: Opportunity or threat for occupational therapists? *Canadian Journal of Occupational Therapy, 62,* 197-207.

Healy, D. (2002). *The creation of psychopharmacology.* Cambridge, MA: Harvard University Press.

Law, M. (Ed.). (2002). *Evidence-based practice in rehabilitation: A guide to practice.* Thorofare, NJ: SLACK Incorporated.

Lisspers, J., Nygren, A., & Soderman, E. (1998). Psychological patterns in patients with coronary heart disease, chronic pain, and respiratory disorder. *Scandinavian Journal of Caring Sciences, 12,* 25-31.

Livneh, H., & Antonak, R. (1994). Psychosocial reactions to disability: A review and critique of the literature. *Physical and Rehabilitation Medicine, 6,* 1-100.

Meyer, A. (1922/1977). The philosophy of occupation therapy. *American Journal of Occupational Therapy, 31,* 639-642.

Murphy, M.J. (1998). Evolution of practice and values of professional psychology. In R.F. Small & L.R. Barnhill (Eds.), *Practicing in the new mental health marketplace: Ethical, legal, and moral issues* (pp. 37-52) Washington, DC: American Psychological Association.

Owen, R.L., Koutsakis, S., & Bennett, P.D. (2001). Post-traumatic stress disorder as a consequence of acute myocardial infarction: An overlooked psychosocial disability. *Coronary Health Care, 5,* 9-15.

Chapter 1

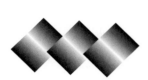

Psychiatric Diagnosis
and the
Classification System

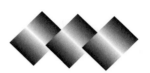

There are numerous theories about psychiatric disorders with varying implications for intervention. Biological, behavioral, analytical, developmental, and neuropsychological approaches differ greatly in terms of their postulates about the origins of psychiatric disorder, methods for intervening, and language for describing the disorders and their treatment. This variation creates a dilemma for service providers. Without a common ground for understanding, communication among professionals becomes impossible. The resolution of the dilemma has been the development of a widely-used system of classification, the *Diagnostic and Statistical Manual* (DSM). Since its appearance in 1952, it has undergone repeated revisions, the current version being the *Diagnostic and Statistical Manual of Mental Disorders, Fourth Edition, Text Revision* (DSM-IV-TR) (American Psychiatric Association [APA], 2000a). The purpose of such a diagnostic system is to provide "a common language with which to communicate about the types of psychological problems for which they assume professional responsibility. A diagnosis is simply a way of summarizing a large amount of information into a shorthand term" (Spitzer, Skodol, Gibbon, & Williams, 1983, p. xvi).

Communication is a vital function of a classification system, but there are others. According to Williams (1988), such a system provides a guide to cause and, by extension, assessment and treatment. Description of the characteristics of each disorder is vital to efforts to distinguish among diagnoses and improve diagnostic reliability (Kendall, 2002). Blacker and Tsuang (1999) note further that "how one defines disorder becomes important because of the critical role it plays in insurance reimbursement, disability, and forensic settings" (pp. 65-66). In addition, classification assists in research to further examine causes and treatment of mental disturbance. Without a shared system for identification of distinct disorders, such research would not be possible, as diagnostic criteria assists in distinguishing specific groups of individuals to be studied, behaviors to be examined, and outcomes of interest. If research findings reveal that categories do not provide accurate distinction, the diagnostic structure must be revised (Blacker & Tsuang, 1999).

EMERGENCE OF THE DSM

In 1840, the United States had a one-category classification system for mental illness: "idiocy" (Williams, 1988). By 1880, the system had increased to eight categories. As understanding and awareness increased over time, the classification system was refined, eventually formalized as a chapter in the *International Classification of Diseases* (ICD), now in its 10th edition (World Health Organization [WHO], 1992), and as the DSM.

The *Diagnostic and Statistical Manual, Mental Disorders*, later to be known as DSM-I, was published in 1952 by the APA (APA, 1952). It was a major breakthrough for the field of mental health, as it provided the first comprehensive volume describing a range of mental disorders. The descriptions were quite general, however, making diagnosis unreliable. As psychiatric knowledge grew, it became clear that a revision was needed.

DSM-II appeared in 1968, following 3 years of work by the APA (APA, 1968). It coincided with the eighth revision of the ICD. The differences between DSM-I and DSM-II were minor, with some changes in the names of syndromes and minor modifications in descriptive language. Like DSM-I, though, descriptions were general and often vague. A major criticism of both DSM-I and DSM-II was the poor reliability of diagnosis. Professionals were unable to consistently identify the same disorder in a specific patient (Klerman, 1988), or the diagnosis might change over time even if nothing had happened to change the behavior or symptoms of the individual.

DSM-III represented a major change in the nature of the diagnostic process (Blacker & Tsuang, 1999). As with DSM-II, its development coincided with a revision of the ICD. American psychiatrists and other mental health care providers were concerned that the ICD lacked many specific diagnoses that were well-accepted in the United States on the basis of research data. There was also concern that the glossary was inadequate in the area of mental health (Williams, 1988).

Furthermore, in the 1960s and '70s, there was heated debate about the nature, and even the existence, of mental illness. Szasz (1974) argued that mental illness was a societal phenomenon rather than a disease. He suggested that mental illness was used as a label to explain deviant, and therefore socially unacceptable, behavior, and that the purpose of the label was to provide an excuse to control such behavior. The poor reliability of diagnoses supported his contention. If two professionals were unlikely to make the same diagnosis, Szasz argued, perhaps it was because they were responding to societal expectations about proper behavior rather than to any real problem with the individual's health.

The 1970s saw several advances that contributed to the discussion. Foremost among these was the vastly increased knowledge about psychopharmacology and biology. For the first time, biological factors in mental disturbance could be identified, both in terms of genetic and biochemical characteristics. Research capabilities were enhanced through development of new methodologies and clinical instruments that were found to be reliable (Klerman, 1988). This meant that, based on better categorization of disorders and improved training, professionals became more consistent in their views of specific patients, and that diagnoses were more stable over time if the patient did not change. One of these instruments was the Research Diagnostic Criteria (RDC) (Spitzer, Endicott, & Robins, 1975). The emergence of this measure and others (for example, the Diagnostic Interview Schedule and Structured Clinical Interview for the DSM-III-R [Taylor & Jason, 1998]) demonstrated that it was possible to provide clear, consistent guidelines to allow discrimination among symptom constellations.

In 1974, the APA appointed a committee to begin development of DSM-III, a task that ultimately took 6 years. Both the process of development and the product were novel, representing a significant departure from DSM-II. The process involved not only a great deal of committee work to develop descriptions and diagnostic criteria, but also a major research effort to validate diagnoses and determine reliability in a systematic fashion. During the research phase, more than 12,000 individuals were evaluated (Spitzer, Forman, & Nee, 1979). Clinicians around the United States completed reports and commented on any difficulties they had while using the system.

Interrater reliability studies involved 796 patients, each of whom was evaluated by two clinicians. Because these were field studies, some variables were poorly controlled, but even so the new classification system had reliability coefficients in the range of 0.7 (Axis I) to 0.6 (Axis II) (Williams, 1985). This means, roughly, that professionals agreed 60% to 70% of the time. The attempt to confirm reliability was itself novel, even though some studies have found lower reliability, especially for Axis II (Mellsop, Varghese, Joshua, & Hicks, 1982).

The product was notably different from DSM-II. First of all, the number of diagnoses was expanded to more than 150. In addition, descriptions were designed to be as specific and concrete as possible, with criteria about constellations of symptoms, onset of the disorder, duration, and probable course. This was the first classification to provide operational criteria as a means to assure reliability (Klerman, 1988). Operational criteria are specific, observable characteristics that describe a particular syndrome or disorder. It is also noteworthy that the DSM-III provided descriptive psychopathology rather than inferred etiology. In other words, the guide described what clinicians saw, not what caused it. In addition, descriptions were intended to be atheoretical (i.e., without reference to particular theories or points of view). The intent was to make the product an effective mechanism for communication among therapists subscribing to divergent philosophies about cause and treatment (Williams, 1988).

DSM-III (APA, 1980) also reflected a realization that diagnosis alone might not provide sufficient data to implement treatment. As a result, several new categories were developed to provide additional information, making it the first multiaxial classification system for psychiatric disorders (Klerman, 1988). These axes made it possible not only to name a syndrome, but also to identify disordered personality characteristics, accompanying medical conditions of significance to treatment and prognosis, levels of stress encountered by the individual, and recent level of function.

Inclusion of this last axis is of particular importance to occupational therapists, as it represented an acknowledgment that diagnosis alone does not adequately describe a person's ability to accomplish daily tasks. It is also noteworthy that Axis V (level of function) appeared to be the most reliable of the axes, with a correlation coefficient between 0.7 and 0.8 (Williams, 1988).

In DSM-III, categories were hierarchical, based on the assumption that disorders higher on the hierarchy had symptoms found in those lower but not the opposite. Later research challenged this assumption (Boyd, Burke, Grundberg, Holzer, & Rae, 1984), one of the many findings that led to the almost immediate effort to revise DSM-III. DSM-III-R was published in 1987 and reflected advances in scientific knowledge at that time. One change was the deletion of the assumption of hierarchies (Williams, 1988). While changes were minor, they reflected an effort to resolve problems with DSM-III and to disseminate new knowledge as quickly as possible.

Before DSM-III-R was completed, discussion had turned to the development of DSM-IV (APA, 1994). As with other editions of DSM, this revision was timed to coincide with a revision of the IDC (Kendall, 1991). The 10th edition of that volume appeared in 1992, by which time DSM-IV was nearing completion.

The process by which DSM-IV (APA, 1994) was developed was intended to be a careful, thoughtful, largely empirical one. Task groups of experts for each existing and proposed diagnostic category began by undertaking massive reviews of research literature (Widiger, Frances, Pincus, & Davis, 1990). These reviews were to serve as meta-analyses to guide the working groups about whether or not to include each diagnosis and what criteria would be listed. A series of field trials of the proposed criteria was also undertaken (APA, 1994). Twelve trials including more than 6,000 research participants were designed to examine the reliability and clinical utility of the proposed categories.

Decisions were ultimately guided by a set of standards that the development committee had agreed to in advance. Criteria for the addition of a new category or exclusion of an existing category were to be more stringent than those to retain what existed (APA, 1994). This was done to avoid unnecessary changes that would confuse practitioners and reduce researchers' ability to track long-term consequences of mental disorder and treatment. In addition, an effort was made, where possible, to conform categories to those in ICD-10 (WHO, 1992), which was completed just prior to publication of DSM-IV (Kendall, 1991).

The best possible scientific evidence was used in developing criteria (Frances et al., 1991). Issues of reliability, validity, and utility were considered with an eye to assuring the highest possible standards.

Several new factors were included in DSM-IV. Among these was recognition of cultural differences in psychiatric constructs (Fabrega, 1992). DSM-IV (APA, 1994) includes an appendix listing terms that are applied to mental disorders in other cultures that might be encountered by practitioners in the United States. For example, "nervios" and "zar" are briefly explained in their cultural context. Another factor newly considered was recognition of the relationship between spiritual difficulties and mental disorders (APA, 1994).

The development of DSM-IV (APA, 1994) was a political, as well as scientific, process with numerous and sometimes heated arguments about inclusion and exclusion of categories (Caplan, 1991). One dispute, for example, related to the inclusion of a diagnosis of "self-defeating personality disorder (SDPD)" which had been listed in the appendices of DSM-III-R (APA, 1987) as a potential diagnosis requiring more study. Feminists argued that this validated the tendency of the legal system to "blame the victim" for crimes committed against him or her (e.g., suggesting that battered wives brought their problems upon themselves). A proposal to add a category for "delusional dominating personality disorder" (Caplan, 1991), which was to be applied to the batterer to counterbalance SDPD, was rejected by the task force examining the issue to the dismay of those proposing it. Among other potential diagnoses considered were caffeine abuse (Hughes, Oliveto, Helzer, Higgins, & Bickel, 1992) and psychotic major depression (Schatzberg & Rothschild, 1992). Those involved in the development of DSM-IV indicated that while scientific criteria should be primary and the burden of proof higher when changing a category, the issue of potentially stigmatizing the individual or, alternatively, excusing behavior because of psychiatric disorder was important to consider in decision making (Pincus, Frances, Davis, First, & Widiger, 1992).

Some disputes raged around criteria for existing categories. For example, the committee on gender identity disorders expressed concern that criteria could not be applied equally to males and females because of cultural differences in acceptability of behaviors (Bradley et al., 1991). King and Strain (1992) indicated that there were significant problems in the category of somatoform pain disorder because of the difficulties of clearly differentiating between normal and abnormal reactions to pain. In fact, the whole issue of organic versus nonorganic (i.e., the result of a known "physical" agent like a bacterium or the result of some unknown "nonphysical" agent) was a heated one (Spitzer, Williams, First, & Kendler, 1989).

These political disputes reflect the reality that "acceptance of the person into (or exclusion from) the mental health system invariably involves ethical and political judgments" (Horsfall, 2001, p. 425). Such judgments may lead to overdiagnosis for those who do not conform to societal expectations or to medicalization of problems that could also be considered simply problems of living. Underdiagnosis can likewise result from decisions to include or exclude particular factors from the diagnostic structure. Decisions about spending for mental health care may well be based on the view of a psychiatric disorder as either serious and enduring or less serious and more temporary depending on criteria in the diagnostic guide rather than on the subjective experience of the individual (Perkins & Repper, 1998).

Another dispute was based in theory. DSM-IV purports to be atheoretical (Busfield, 1996), but there has been some concern that this led to elimination of important constructs. Psychoanalysts and other dynamically oriented therapists, for example, wanted to see defense mechanisms added as a sixth axis (Skodol & Perry, 1993). This issue was addressed by the inclusion of these terms in an extensive glossary. Debate about how many axes and what dimensions they should reflect were numerous (Schacht, 1993). Family therapists believed that because so many problems center around family interactions, a new axis should be added to reflect family circumstances (Lange, Schaap, & von Widenfelt, 1993). Ultimately, these arguments were rejected in favor of minimizing the complexity of the model. The result is that many believe that DSM is excessively focused on biologically-based explanations of disorder (Rogers, 2000).

Concern was also expressed that the committees developing DSM-IV (APA, 1994) were comprised almost entirely of physicians, another factor contributing to a perceived tilt in the content toward a medical model (DeAngelis, 1991). Pressure from psychologists, social workers, and other mental health professionals resulted in their inclusion in the process, but physicians still dominated the deliberations. Many other relevant disciplines, including occupational therapy, were not involved in the development process.

Some felt that the development of DSM-IV was premature (Zimmerman, Jampala, Sierles, & Taylor, 1991). Critics suggested that although the DSM-III and DSM-III-R were gaining acceptance, they were not yet fully implemented in clinical settings (Maser, Kaelber, & Weise, 1991) and that change would be resisted (Morey & Ochoa, 1989; Smith & Kraft, 1989). These critics also suggested that rapid change in diagnostic categories would reduce the ability of researchers to follow outcomes longitudinally or to compare research results for a specific disorder. Certainly, these criticisms have been reflected in the long wait for DSM-V.

The working groups for DSM-IV fully recognized such dilemmas (Frances et al., 1991), noting that "the Task Force has not resolved fully, or indeed expects to resolve fully, any of these issues. Instead, the Task Force is attempting to find balanced, if imperfect, solutions to reflect the best available knowledge (p. 407)."

Because of the difficulties inherent in the development of DSM-IV and of concerns about excessively rapid change in the diagnostic structure, publication of DSM-V, originally planned for 2006, has been delayed. Now expected no earlier than 2010 (APA, 2000b), the next guide is being developed through a process similar to that used for DSM-IV. Committees have begun the work required to review literature and conduct relevant field studies of diagnoses, preparatory to discussion of inclusion, exclusion, and change for the guide. Research questions have been proposed (Kupfer, First, & Regier, 2002) and exploration of an array of issues will continue through the decade (APA, 2000b)

As a temporizing measure to bridge the time gap between editions, a text revision of DSM-IV was published in 2000. DSM-IV-TR (APA, 2000a) did not alter any of the diagnostic criteria. Rather, it provided an update of epidemiological and other information designed to clarify understanding of each category. So, for example, in the discussion of Asperger's Syndrome a newly included category in DSM-IV, information about specific examples of behavior that would assist in diagnosis, clarification of the possibility of communication deficits, and other relevant information has been added to the text even though the criteria themselves remain unchanged (see Chapter 3 for more information about Asperger's Syndrome).

Clearly, the development of the classification system is a complex scientific and political process that has involved physicians, psychologists, social workers, and some political or special interest groups. While final decisions about DSM-IV were based primarily on consensus of authorities (Spitzer, 1991) and while it remains an imperfect system, DSM-IV is, for better or for worse, the system by which professionals now communicate.

TOWARD DSM-V

There is general agreement that no new classification system should be published unless it improves on the existing one (Kendall, 2002). Each new version brings both improvements and problems, and the former must outweigh the latter if the change is to be worthwhile. Some of the dilemmas of change have already been discussed, including the disruption of longitudinal and replication research studies that have the potential to improve outcomes.

Kendall (2002, p. 3) has proposed five criteria by which a new taxonomy would be improved. He suggests that it should:

1. Be more comprehensive
2. Be easier to use
3. Deal better with the issue of "clinical significance"
4. Have higher reliability
5. Have higher validity.

However, he makes clear that users with different agendas (e.g., researchers and clinicians) will have differing views about what improves the system, based on their particular needs and interests.

Several specific issues have already emerged that will need to be addressed in a new taxonomy. One of these, as indicated by Kendall (2002), is clinical significance. Epidemiological studies suggest very high rates of psychiatric disorder, a finding not in keeping with the proportion of the population that appears to be managing daily life. The suggestion has been made that psychiatric symptoms, such as mood alterations and anxiety, may not in and of themselves impair performance to a degree that suggests that they should be identified as disordered. This suggests that some percentage of individuals diagnosed represent "false positives" (i.e., people who may have some symptoms but should not be classified as having psychiatric conditions).

Use of different instruments yields different estimates of disorder as well (Taylor & Jason, 1998). Wakefield (1992) suggested that disease or disorder actually has two components, a biological dysfunction (the failure of an internal mechanism) and evidence of participation, "involvement in a life situation" as defined by the WHO (2001, p. 10). This distinction between dysfunction, which Wakefield believes to be a value- and context-free term, and participation, an environmentally related construct, might lead to enhanced diagnosis, assuming that clinicians agreed that both must be present in order for a diagnosis to be made.

Another strategy for dealing with the issue of clinical significance would be to alter definitions of disorders to make sure that the constellation of symptoms required for diagnosis would be sufficiently extensive and severe to guarantee a substantial impairment in performance, or to add a criterion that excludes reaction to specific stresses of life (Spitzer & Wakefield, 1999). Including this stipulation for each diagnosis would add to the size and complexity of the taxonomy, however. A third suggestion, that disability be considered a separate dimension (Wakefield & Spitzer, 2002), would also add to the complexity of the classification system. This discussion is of particular importance to occupational therapists because their concern is with the extent to which psychiatric disorders impair performance of daily activities.

A second concern regarding the development of DSM-V is the increasing biomedicalization of the taxonomy. Researchers have argued that genetic and imaging studies have the potential to "erode, if not eradicate, the classification of mind/brain disorders as either psychiatric or neurologic" (Epstein, Isenberg, Stern, & Silbersweig, 2002, p. 57). If this argument is accepted, the idea that DSM is atheoretical must be discarded, a stance that is unlikely to be acceptable to some audiences for the taxonomy. It also increases the dilemma of diagnoses that describe problems that have no biological finding, at least at the present, or that may reflect problems of living that require intervention. Adjustment disorder is an example of this type of label as it represents a relatively short-term, situationally related constellation of symptoms, not a neurological or biological disease. Additional research may resolve this concern, but at present, science is far from providing clear biological findings that parallel those of diabetes or cancer, for example. An individual may carry a gene strongly associated with schizophrenia but not show signs of the disorder (Kendall, 2002). Schizophrenia as currently defined is also difficult to distinguish from a group of other diagnoses, schizoaffective disorder and schizotypal personality disorder among them. A diagnosis of schizotaxia has been recommended to cover the spectrum of schizophrenia-like disorders (Tsuang, Stone, & Faraone, 2000).

Another concern is the issue of comorbidity (Krueger, 2002). Many psychiatric diagnoses coexist in a single individual. In addition to so called "dual diagnoses" most often associated with substance abuse and one other psychiatric disorder, Krueger estimates that 14% of the US population has a lifetime history of three or more psychiatric disorders. As an example, it is common to find affective, anxiety, and substance abuse disorders concomitant in an individual. Some drugs (e.g., the selective serotonin reuptake inhibitors [SSRIs], such as Prozac) seem effective for multiple disorders (Dunner, 1998) including both anxiety and affective disorders. Similarly, the gene known to be associated with schizophrenia may be found in an individual with one of the forms of that disorder, with schizoaffective disorder, or with some other form of psychotic disorder (Merikangas, 2002). This high rate of comorbidity may mean that diagnoses currently described as separate phenomena may, in fact, be overlapping or the same disorder with differing manifestations (Krueger, 2002). If this is the case, substantial alteration of the diagnostic system would be required.

Finally, the issue of cultural variation in psychiatric disorder is one that the DSM has only begun to address. Cultural factors clearly influence both the kinds of symptoms an individual may experience and their help-seeking behavior (Herrick & Brown, 1999). Examples abound of misunderstanding caused by misinterpretation of such culturally mediated syndromes. An individual from a culture holding a belief in the spirit world might find him- or herself diagnosed with schizophrenia. An individual from a culture that prescribes reticence and avoidance of eye-contact might be diagnosed with depression. The simple problem of language difference can lead to misunderstanding and inappropriate diagnosis (see Bonder, Martin, & Miracle, 2002 for a comprehensive discussion of cultural factors in health care). The current strategy of using an appendix to briefly summarize the best identified of these syndromes works less well as the United States becomes more culturally diverse. It also suggests that somehow the syndromes presented in the main body of DSM are not culturally mediated, an assumption that can certainly be questioned. In a multicultural society, the assumption that one set of culturally mediated syndromes is "real" while another is an artifact of group values sets up the potential for conflict between care providers and clients and between institutions and the communities they wish to serve.

It is not yet possible this early in the development of DSM-V to see how these dilemmas will be resolved. Nor is it possible to know what other dilemmas may emerge. It is evident, however, that diagnostic categorization and description are not simple matters, and that in addition to science, culture, politics, and personal values, play important roles.

For now, care providers must use the best available system. At the moment, in the United States, that system is DSM-IV. We will now turn our attention to a description of the structure of that guide.

Table 1-1	
Axes in DSM-IV	
Axis I	Clinical disorders Other conditions that may be a focus of clinical attention
Axis II	Personality disorders Mental retardation
Axis III	General medical conditions
Axis IV	Psychosocial and environmental problems
Axis V	Global assessment of functioning

Reproduced with permission from American Psychiatric Association. (2000). *Diagnostic and statistical manual of mental disorders* (4th ed., text revision, p. 27). Washington, DC: Author.

FORMAT OF DSM-IV-TR

As noted, DSM-IV-TR (APA, 2000a) is a multiaxial classification system comprised of five axes (Table 1-1). Axis I lists psychiatric diagnosis; Axis II, personality disorders and mental retardation; Axis III, significant accompanying medical conditions; Axis IV, degree of stress within the 12 months preceding diagnosis; and Axis V, level of function. On this last Axis, two numbers can be listed: current level of function and/or highest level of function within the past 12 months. Diagnosis on all five axes is designed to provide maximal information about the individual's condition.

Appendix A contains the summary pages from DSM-IV-TR. The categories listed there are discussed in detail in the body of the DSM, with clarifying examples of behavior and specific symptoms that must be present to support a given diagnosis. Each description includes considerations such as duration of symptoms and course of the disorder.

Axis I lists diagnoses of specific psychiatric syndromes or disorders. Each category includes a description of major features of the disorder, the symptoms that must be present to warrant the diagnosis, and a discussion of accompanying features that may or may not be present. Typical age of onset and course of the disorder are described, as are predisposing factors, prevalence, and familial pattern. A section on impairment briefly discusses the social and occupational implications of the disorder. Complications that may occur are included. Finally, a discussion of differential diagnosis provides a summary of the characteristics that distinguish the disorder from others and a list of other diagnoses to consider if the criteria do not fit the presenting picture.

Axis II includes mental retardation and personality disorders, which persist throughout life (Blacker & Tsuang, 1999). Individuals may have psychiatric diagnoses without personality disorders, or vice versa, but they often accompany each other. A distinguishing characteristic of a personality disorder is its usually negative effect on those around the individual (Klerman, 1988), frequently resulting in a disordered social system. Mental retardation is included on this axis because, like personality disorders, it is defined as a condition that emerges early and continues throughout life, sometimes underlying or accompanying an Axis I condition. This definition of Axis II is somewhat different from DSM-III-R, in which several other conditions were included on this dimension. There had been controversy about making Axis I/Axis II distinctions (Widiger & Shea, 1991), but given the criteria for deciding on change in the DSM, the axis was retained. No decision has yet been made for DSM-V.

Axis III allows for diagnosis of coexisting medical conditions, coded according to the ICD-10 (WHO, 1992) categories. Medical conditions that might affect the course of the psychiatric disorder or the types of treatments to be implemented are noted on this axis, as are those that might have an impact on overall function.

Axis IV describes psychosocial and environmental problems. Among the factors that might be noted on this axis are educational and housing difficulties and problems with access to health care. This represents a change from DSM-III-R (APA, 1987) in which Axis IV was for noting level and source of stress. This change was due to dissatisfaction of clinicians using the axis, as well as disappointing results from the limited research data about its reliability (Skodol, 1991).

Axis V reflects the individual's highest level of function within the 12 months preceding diagnosis, as well as current level of function. Psychological, social, and vocational functioning are rated on a 0 to 90 point scale, with general descriptions of each 10 point range to provide guidance in making an assessment. An individual with a rating of 100 on this Global Assessment of Functioning Scale (GAF) (APA, 2000a) would be considered as having "superior functioning in a wide range of activities, life's problems never seem to get out of hand, is sought out by others because of his or her many positive qualities" (APA, 2000a, p. 34). Someone with a score of 60 would have functioning reflective of "serious symptoms (e.g., flat affect and circumstantial speech, occasional panic attacks) or moderate difficulty in social, occupational, or school functioning (e.g., few friends, conflicts with peers or coworkers)" (APA, 2000a, p. 34). This is, at present, the most subjective of the axes, as specific behaviors are not included. However, a moderate correlation has been noted between severity of symptoms and function (Klerman, 1988) (i.e., there is a moderate relationship between the degree of psychological impairment and performance). This axis was included in an attempt to acknowledge strengths of the client, as well as deficits (thus, highest, rather than average, level of function). In general, clinicians reported being satisfied with Axis V (Skodol, 1991). Further, no better measures of function were found (Goldman, Skodol, & Lave, 1992), so the axis remains unchanged from earlier versions of the DSM.

Not all axes are used by all clinicians. It is most typical that diagnoses will be made on axes I and II, and often Axis III diagnoses are included when there is a significant medical condition. However, axes IV and V are often omitted, a problem for occupational and other therapists who may be greatly concerned with function.

Table 1-2 provides the description of one common diagnosis, dysthymic disorder, as it appeared in DSM-I, DSM-II, DSM-III, DSM-III-R, and as it is seen now in DSM-IV and DSM-IV-TR. Among the obvious differences is the change in name from depressive neurosis. Increasing specificity can be noted in each revision, increasing the probability of reliable diagnosis, and thus, the clarity of therapeutic choice.

What follows in this text is a discussion of the relationship of diagnosis to occupational therapy and consideration of major diagnostic categories, with emphasis on what is known or theorized about etiology and course of the disorders, the types of treatments currently being employed, and the efficacy of those treatments. That information is linked to probable effects on the occupational performance of the individual and recommendations about potential occupational therapy interventions.

Table 1-2

Changes in the Diagnosis of Depression: DSM-I to DSM-IV-TR

DSM-I   000-x06 Depressive Reaction

The anxiety in this reaction is allayed, and hence partially relieved, by depression and self-depreciation. The reaction is precipitated by a current situation, frequently by some loss sustained by the patient, and is often associated with a feeling of guilt for past failures or deeds. The degree of the reaction in such cases is dependent upon the intensity of the patient's ambivalent feeling toward his loss (love, possession) as well as upon the realistic circumstances of the loss.

The term is synonymous with "reactive depression" and is to be differentiated from the corresponding psychotic reaction. In this differentiation, points to be considered are (1) life history of patient, with special reference to mood swings (suggestive of psychotic reaction), to the personality structure (neurotic or cyclothymic) and to precipitating environmental factors and (2) absence of malignant symptoms (hypochondrical preoccupation, agitation, delusions, particularly somatic, hallucinations, severe guilt feelings, intractable insomnia, suicidal ruminations, severe psychomotor retardation, profound retardation of thought, stupor).

DSM-II   300.4 Depressive Neurosis

This disorder is manifested by an excessive reaction of depression due to an internal conflict or to an identifiable event such as the loss of a love object or cherished possession. It is to be distinguished from Involutional melancholia (q.v.) and Manic-depressive illness (q.v.). Reactive depressions or Depressive reactions are to be classified here.

DSM-III   Diagnostic Criteria for Dysthymic Disorder

A. During the past two years (or one year for children and adolescents) the individual has been bothered most or all of the time by symptoms characteristic of the depressive syndrome but that are not of sufficient severity and duration to meet the criteria for a major depressive episode (although a major depressive episode may be superimposed on Dysthymic Disorder).

B. The manifestations of the depressive syndrome may be relatively persistent or separated by periods of normal mood lasting a few days to a few weeks, but no more than a few months at a time.

C. During the depressive periods there is either prominent depressed mood (e.g., sad, blue, down in the dumps, low) or marked loss of interest or pleasure in all, or almost all, usual activities and pastimes.

(continued)

REFERENCES

American Psychiatric Association, Task Force on Nomenclature. (1952). *Diagnostic and statistical manual of mental disorders* (1st ed.). Washington, DC: American Psychiatric Association.

American Psychiatric Association, Task Force on Nomenclature. (1968). *Diagnostic and statistical manual of mental disorders* (2nd ed.). Washington, DC: American Psychiatric Association.

American Psychiatric Association, Task Force on Nomenclature. (1980). *Diagnostic and statistical manual of mental disorders* (3rd ed.). Washington, DC: American Psychiatric Association.

Table 1-2 (Continued)

D. During the depressive period at least three of the following symptoms are present:
   1. insomnia or hypersomnia
   2. low energy level or chronic tiredness
   3. feelings of inadequacy, loss of self-esteem, or self-deprecation
   4. decreased effectiveness or productivity at school, work, or home
   5. decreased attention, concentration, or ability to think clearly
   6. social withdrawal
   7. loss of interest in or enjoyment of pleasurable activities
   8. irritability or excessive anger (in children, expressed toward parents or caretakers)
   9. inability to respond with apparent pleasure to praise or rewards
   10. less active or talkative than usual, or feels slowed down or restless
   11. pessimistic attitude toward the future, brooding about past events, or feeling sorry for self
   12. tearfulness or crying
   13. recurrent thoughts of death or suicide
E. Absence of psychotic features, such as delusions, hallucinations, or incoherence, or loosening of associations.
F. If the disturbance is superimposed on a preexisting mental disorder, such as Obsessive Compulsive Disorder or Alcohol Dependence, the depressed mood, by virtue of its intensity or effect on functioning, can be clearly distinguished from the individual's usual mood.

DSM-III-R   Diagnostic Criteria for 300.4: Dysthymic Disorder

A. Depressed mood for most of the day, for more days than not, as indicated either by subjective account or observation by others, for at least 2 years. Note: In children and adolescents, mood can be irritable and duration must be at least 1 year.
B. Presence, while depressed, of two (or more) of the following:
   1. poor appetite or overeating
   2. insomnia or hypersomnia
   3. low energy or fatigue
   4. low self-esteem
   5. poor concentration or difficulty making decisions
   6. feelings of hopelessness
C. During the 2-year period (1 year for children or adolescents) of the disturbance, the person has never been without the symptoms in Criteria A and B for more than 2 months at a time.
D. No Major Depressive Episode has been present during the first 2 years of the disturbance (1 year for children and adolescence); i.e., the disturbance is not better accounted for by chronic Major Depressive Disorder, or Major Depressive Disorder, In Partial Remission.
   Note: There may have been a previous Major Depressive Episode provided there was a full remission (no significant signs or symptoms for 2 months) before development of the Dysthymic Disorder. In addition, after the initial 2 years (1 year in children or adolescents) of Dysthymic Disorder, there may be superimposed episodes of Major Depressive Disorder, in which case both diagnoses may be given when the criteria are met for a Major Depressive Episode.
E. There has never been a Manic Episode, a Mixed Episode, or a Hypomanic Episode, and criteria have never been met for Cyclothymic Disorder.
F. The disturbance does not occur exclusively during the course of a chronic Psychotic Disorder, such as Schizophrenia or Delusional Disorder.   *(continued)*

Table 1-2 (Continued)

G. The symptoms are not due to the direct physiological effects of a substance (e.g., a drug of abuse, a medication) or a general medical condition (e.g., hypothyroidism).

H. The symptoms cause clinically significant distress or impairment in social, occupational, or other important areas of functioning.

Specify if:

Early Onset: if onset is before age 21 years

Late Onset: if onset is age 21 years or older

Specify (for most recent 2 years of Dysthymic Disorder):

With Atypical Features

DSM-IV and IV-TR   Diagnostic Criteria for 300.4 Dysthymic Disorder

A. Depressed mood for most of the day, for more days than not, as indicated either by subjective account or observation by others, for at least 2 years. Note: In children and adolescents, mood can be irritable and duration must be at least 1 year.

B. Presence, while depressed, of two (or more) of the following:
   1. poor appetite or overeating
   2. insomnia or hypersomnia
   3. low energy or fatigue
   4. low self-esteem
   5. poor concentration or difficulty making decisions
   6. feelings of hopelessness

C. During the 2-year period (1 year for children or adolescents) of the disturbance, the person has never been without the symptoms in Criteria A and B for more than 2 months at a time.

D. No Major Depressive Episode has been present during the first 2 years of the disturbance (1 year for children and adolescents); i.e., the disturbance is not better accounted for by chronic Major Depressive Disorder, or Major Depressive Disorder, In Partial Remission. **Note:** There may have been a previous Major Depressive Episode provided there was a full remission (no significant signs or symptoms for 2 months) before development of the Dysthymic Disorder. In addition, after the initial 2 years (1 year in children or adolescents) of Dysthymic Disorder, there may be superimposed episodes of Major Depressive Disorder, in which case both diagnoses may be given when the criteria are met for Major Depressive Episode.

E. There has never been a Manic Episode, a Mixed Episode, or a Hypomanic Episode, and criteria have never been met for Cyclothymic Disorder.

F. The disturbance does not occur exclusively during the course of a chronic Psychotic Disorder, such as Schizophrenia or Delusional Disorder.

G. The symptoms are not due to the direct physiological effects of a substance (e.g., a drug of abuse, a medication) or a general medical condition (e.g., hypothyroidism).

H. The symptoms cause clinically significant distress or impairment in social, occupational, or other important areas of functioning.

Specify if:

Early Onset: if onset is before age 21 years

Late Onset: If onset is age 21 years or older

Specify (for most recent 2 years of Dysthymic Disorder):

With Atypical Features

Reprinted with permission from American Psychiatric Association, Task Force on Nomenclature. (1952). *Diagnostic and statistical manual of mental disorders* (1st ed.). Washington, DC: American Psychiatric Association; American Psychiatric Association, Task Force on Nomenclature. (1968). *Diagnostic and statistical manual of mental disorders* (2nd ed.). Washington, DC: American Psychiatric Association; American Psychiatric Association, Task Force on Nomenclature. (1980). *Diagnostic and statistical manual of mental disorders* (3rd ed.). Washington, DC: American Psychiatric Association; American Psychiatric Association, Task Force on Nomenclature. (1987). *Diagnostic and statistical manual of mental disorders* (3rd ed., revised). Washington, DC: American Psychiatric Association; American Psychiatric Association, Task Force on Nomenclature. (1994). *Diagnostic and statistical manual of mental disorders* (4th ed.). Washington, DC: American Psychiatric Association.

American Psychiatric Association, Task Force on Nomenclature. (1987). *Diagnostic and statistical manual of mental disorders* (3rd ed., revised). Washington, DC: American Psychiatric Association.

American Psychiatric Association, Task Force on Nomenclature. (1994). *Diagnostic and statistical manual of mental disorders* (4th ed.). Washington, DC: American Psychiatric Association.

American Psychiatric Association, Task Force on Nomenclature. (2000a). *Diagnostic and statistical manual of mental disorders* (4th edition, text revision.). Washington, DC: American Psychiatric Association.

American Psychiatric Association (2002b). *Current DSM activities: Diagnostic and statistical manual of mental disorders*. Retrieved July 10, 2002, from http://www.psych.org/clin_res/dsm/currentactivities81301.cfm.

Blacker, D., & Tsuang, M.T. (1999). Classification and DSM-IV. In A. M. Nicholi (Ed.), *The Harvard guide to psychiatry* (3rd ed., pp. 65-73). Cambridge, MA: Harvard University Press.

Bonder, B.R., Martin, L., & Miracle, A.W. (2002). *Culture in clinical care*. Thorofare, NJ: SLACK Incorporated.

Boyd, J.H., Burke, J.D., Grundberg, E., Holzer, C.E., & Rae, D.S. (1984). Exclusion criteria of DSM-III: A study of co-occurrence of hierarchy-free syndromes. *Archives of General Psychiatry, 41*, 983-989.

Bradley, S.J., Blanchard, R., Coates, S., Green, R., Levine, S., Meyer-Bahlburg, H.F., et al. (1991). Interim report of the DSM-IV subcommittee on gender identity disorders. *Archives of Sexual Behavior, 20*, 333-343.

Busfield, J. (1996). *Men, women and madness. Understanding gender and mental disorder*. London: Macmillan.

Caplan, P.J. (1991). How do they decide who is normal? The bizarre, but true, tale of the DSM process. *Canadian Psychology, 32*, 162-170.

DeAngelis, T. (1991). DSM being revised, but problems remain. *American Psychological Association Monitor, 22*, 12-13.

Dunner, D.L. (1998). The issue of comorbidity in the treatment of panic. *International Journal of Clinical Psychopharmacology, 13*, S19-S24.

Epstein, J., Isenberg, N., Stern, E., & Silbersweig, D. (2002). Toward a neuroanatomical understanding of psychiatric illness: The role of functional imaging. In J.E. Helzer & J.J. Hudak (Eds.), *Defining psychopathology in the 21st century: DSM-V and beyond* (pp. 57-70). Washington, DC: American Psychiatric Association.

Fabrega, H. (1992). Diagnosis interminable: Toward a culturally sensitive DSM-IV. *The Journal of Nervous and Mental Disease, 180*, 5-7.

Frances, A.J., First, M.B., Widiger, T.A., Miele, G.M., Tilly, S.M., Davis, W.W., et al. (1991). An A to Z guide to DSM-IV conundrums. *Journal of Abnormal Psychology, 100*, 407-412.

Goldman, H.H., Skodol, A.E., & Lave, T.R. (1992). Revising Axis V for DSM-IV: A review of measures of social functioning. *The American Journal of Psychiatry, 149*, 1148-1156.

Herrick, C., & Brown, H.N. (1999). Mental disorders and syndromes found among Asians residing in the United States. *Issues in Mental Health Nursing, 20*, 275-296.

Horsfall, J. (2001). Gender and mental illness: An Australian overview. *Issues in Mental Health Nursing, 22*, 421-438.

Hughes, J.R., Oliveto, A.H., Helzer, J.E., Higgins, S.T., & Bickel, W.K. (1992). Should caffeine abuse, dependence, or withdrawal be added to DSM-IV and ICD-10? *The American Journal of Psychiatry, 149*, 33-40.

Kendall, R.E. (1991). Relationship between the DSM-IV and the ICD-10. *Journal of Abnormal Psychology, 100*, 297-301.

Kendall, R.E. (2002). Five criteria for an improved taxonomy of mental disorders. In J.E. Helzer & J.J. Hudak (Eds.), *Defining psychopathology in the 21st century: DSM-V and beyond* (pp. 3-18). Washington, DC: American Psychiatric Association.

King, S.A., & Strain, J.J. (1992). Revising the category of somatoform pain disorder. *Hospital and Community Psychiatry, 43*, 217-219.

Klerman, G.L. (1988). Classification and DSM-III-R. In A.M. Nicholi (Ed.), *The new Harvard guide to psychiatry* (pp. 70-87). Cambridge, MA: Belknap Press.

Krueger, R.F. (2002). Psychometric perspectives on comorbidity. In J.E. Helzer & J.J. Hudak (Eds.) *Defining psychopathology in the 21st century: DSM-V and beyond* (pp. 41-56). Washington, DC: American Psychiatric Association.

Kupfer, D.J., First, M.B., & Regier, D.A. (2002). *A research agenda for DSM-V*. Washington, DC: American Psychiatric Press.

Lange, A., Schaap, C., & von Widenfelt, B. (1993). Family therapy and psychopathology: Developments in research and approaches to treatment. *Journal of Family Therapy, 15*, 113-146.

Maser, J.D., Kaelber, C., & Weise, R.E. (1991). International use and attitudes toward DSM-III and DSM-III-R: Growing consensus in psychiatric classification. *Journal of Abnormal Psychology, 100*, 271-279.

Mellsop, G., Varghese, F., Joshua, S., & Hicks, A. (1982). The reliability of Axis II of DSM-III. *The American Journal of Psychiatry, 139*, 1360-1361.

Merikangas, K.R. (2002). Implications of genetic epidemiology for classification. In J.E. Helzer & J.J. Hudak (Eds.), *Defining psychopathology in the 21st century: DSM-V and beyond* (pp. 195-210). Washington, DC: American Psychiatric Association.

Morey, L., & Ochoa, F. (1989). An investigation of adherence to diagnostic criteria: Clinical diagnosis of the DSM-III personality disorders. *Journal of Personality Disorders, 3*, 180-192.

Perkins, R., & Repper, J. (1998). *Dilemmas in community mental health practice*. Abingdon, England: Radcliffe Medical Press.

Pincus, H.A., Frances, A., Davis, W.W., First, M.B., & Widiger, T.A. (1992). DSM-IV and new diagnostic categories: Holding the line on proliferation. *The American Journal of Psychiatry, 149*, 112-117.

Rogers, D. A. (2000). When, oh when, will psychology lay its own behavioral tracks without relying on psychiatry? *The National Psychologist*. Retrieved July 10, 2002, from http://nationalpsychologist.com/articles/art_v10n2_3.htm.

Schacht, T.E. (1993). How do I diagnose thee? Let me count the dimensions. *Psychological Inquiry, 4*, 115-118.

Schatzberg, A.F., & Rothschild, A.J. (1992). Psychotic (delusional) major depression: Should it be included as a distinct syndrome in DSM-IV? *The American Journal of Psychiatry, 149*, 733-745.

Skodol, A.E. (1991). Axis IV: A reliable and valid measure of psychosocial stressors? *Comprehensive Psychiatry, 32*, 503-515.

Skodol, A.E., & Perry, J.C. (1993). Should an axis for defense mechanisms be included in DSM-IV? *Comprehensive Psychiatry, 34*, 108-119.

Smith, D., & Kraft, W. (1989). Attitudes of psychiatrists toward diagnostic options and issues. *Psychiatry, 52*, 66-77.

Spitzer, R.L. (1991). An outsider-insider's views about revising the DSMs. *Journal of Abnormal Psychology, 100*, 294-296.

Spitzer, R.L., & Wakefield, J.C. (1999). DSM-IV diagnostic criterion for clinical significance: Does it help solve the false positives problem? *The American Journal of Psychiatry, 156*, 1856-1864.

Spitzer, R.L., Endicott, J., & Robins, R.C. (1975). Research diagnostic criteria (RDC). *Psychopharmacology Bulletin, 11*, 22-24.

Spitzer, R.L., Forman, J.B.W., & Nee, J. (1979). DSM-III field trials I: Initial interrater diagnostic reliability. *The American Journal of Psychiatry, 136*, 818-820.

Spitzer, R.L., Skodol, A.E., Gibbon, M., & Williams, J.B.W. (1983). *Psychopathology: A case book*. New York, NY: McGraw-Hill.

Spitzer, R.L., Williams, J.B.W., First, M., & Kendler, K. (1989). A proposal for DSM-IV: Solving the "organic/nonorganic" problem. *Journal of Neuropsychiatry, 1*, 126-127.

Szasz, T. (1974). *The myth of mental illness* (2nd ed.). New York, NY: Harper & Row.

Taylor, R.R., & Jason, L.A. (1998). Comparing the DIS with the SCID: Chronic fatigue syndrome and psychiatric comorbidity. *Psychology and Health, 13*, 1087-1104.

Tsuang, M.T., Stone, W.S., & Faraone, S.V. (2000). Toward reformulating the diagnosis if schizophrenia. *The American Journal of Psychiatry, 157*, 1041-1050.

Wakefield, J.C. (1992). The concept of mental disorder: On the boundary between biological facts and social values. *The American Psychologist, 47*, 373-388.

Wakefield, J.C., & Spitzer, R.L. (2002). Why requiring clinical significance does not solve epidemiology's and DSM's validity problem: Response to Regier and Narrow. In J.E. Helzer & J.J. Hudak (Eds.), *Defining psychopathology in the 21st century: DSM-V and beyond* (pp. 31-40). Washington, DC: American Psychiatric Association.

Widiger, T.A., Frances, A.J., Pincus, H.A., & Davis, W.W. (1990). DSM-IV literature reviews: Rationale, process, and limitations. *Journal of Psychopathology and Behavioral Assessment, 12*, 189-202.

Widiger, T.A., & Shea, T. (1991). Differentiation of Axis I and Axis II disorders. *Journal of Abnormal Psychology, 100*, 399-406.

Williams, J.B.W. (1985). The multiaxial system of DSM-III: Where did it come from and where should it go? *Archives of General Psychiatry, 42*, 181-186.

Williams, J.B.W. (1988) Psychiatric classification. In J.A. Talbott, R.E. Hales, & S.C. Yudofsky (Eds.), *The American psychiatric press textbook of psychiatry* (pp. 201-223). Washington, DC: American Psychiatric Press.

World Health Organization. (1992). *International classification of diseases* (10th ed.). Geneva, Switzerland: Author.

World Health Organization. (2001). *International classification of functioning, disability, and health (ICF)*. Geneva, Switzerland: Author.

Zimmerman, M., Jampala, C., Sierles, F.S., & Taylor, M.A. (1991). DSM-IV: A nosology sold before its time? *The American Journal of Psychiatry, 148*, 463-467.

Chapter 2

DSM-IV and
Occupational Therapy

Occupational therapy "diagnosis" differs substantially from medical and psychological diagnosis. The domain of occupational therapy is occupation (American Occupational Therapy Association [AOTA] Commission on Practice, 2002), meaning that the focus of assessment, goal setting, and intervention is on the daily activities that clients need and want to do. This chapter examines the theoretical bases of psychological and occupational therapy conceptualizations of disorder, the impact of those conceptualizations on diagnosis and beliefs about treatment, and the possibilities for interaction between the two systems. The chapter provides only a general overview, and readers are encouraged to refer to texts that deal with psychosocial considerations in occupational therapy (e.g., Bruce & Borg, 2002; Christiansen & Baum, 1997a; Cottrell, 2000; Scaffa, 2001). To understand how occupational therapy fits in the mental health system, as well as how psychiatric disorders can affect care more generally, some discussion of the differing views of dysfunction is necessary.

PSYCHIATRIC THEORIES OF DYSFUNCTION

What constitutes psychiatric disturbance is not fixed or absolute. Porter (1987) noted that "what is mental and what is physical, what is mad and what is bad, are not fixed points but culture relative" (p. 10). Ideas have changed through the centuries about what mental illness is and what interventions are appropriate. At some points in history, deviant or unusual behavior was accepted in the community; at other points in time, individuals with these behaviors were institutionalized and kept out of sight. Treatment philosophies have shifted from so-called rational to moral to medical and expectations about outcomes from optimistic to pessimistic and back again. All these views have been influenced by and have influenced ideas about the origins and treatments of mental disorder.

Some theorists have speculated that deviance emerges from early childhood experiences (i.e., the analytic view), while others suspect that the problem is faulty learning (i.e., behaviorists), or a skewed set of interpretations about events (cognitive therapies). Other theories emphasize neurobiological explanations for behavior or interactional models (Frager & Fadiman, 1998). As noted in the previous chapter, Szasz (1974) felt that psychiatric disorder did not exist but was, instead, a reflection of lack of acceptance of behavior that was outside the norm, a view that has been reiterated by others over the years (Small & Barnhill, 1998). Some theories (e.g., analytic) focus almost exclusively on internal processes and feelings, while others (e.g., cognitive) focus on thought processes. Still others (e.g., behavioral) focus only on observable behaviors.

DSM-IV purports to be atheoretical (i.e., to apply regardless of one's view of the origins of psychiatric disturbance). However, the diagnostic process itself reflects the medical model (DeAngelis, 1991) and, as discussed in Chapter 1, is becoming increasingly biologically-based. It implies that there are specific syndromes or disorders that constitute discrete and distinguishable entities identified on the basis of a constellation of symptoms, including psychological characteristics, behaviors, and physical findings. This disease model emphasizes cure of illness as the primary focus of intervention.

The disease model has long presented certain dilemmas in mental health care (Antonosky, 1972). Not all psychological theories fit neatly into the medical model. For example, behaviorists attempt to remediate problem behaviors, and cognitive therapists attempt to alter the ways in which clients view the world and their own situations. Neither of these approaches focuses on curing disease. The disease model has also been criticized as being driven by particular segments of the research endeavor, particularly psychopharmacological research (Healy, 2002). Another concern is that diagnosis and symptoms are not good predictors of functional skills, such as work performance and social skills (Tsang, Lam, Ng, & Leung, 2000). Even so, the importance of the medical model to psychiatry continues to be evident in the centrality of the DSM diagnostic process.

It is important to remember that DSM-IV is not only biologically based, but it is culturally based as well. While it includes an appendix listing various mental disorders described by other cultures, the diagnostic system itself is strongly focused on Western beliefs and values about the causes and manifestations of psychological distress. Other explanatory models, including possession by spirits or imbalance of various elements of the self or of the self with nature, are not considered in the Western-based structure of diagnoses. However, large populations both outside and within the United States hold beliefs that are inconsistent with the DSM diagnostic system.

There are a number of reasons why diagnosis is important. Several of these have been noted in the previous chapter. Communication among professionals is facilitated by the common language provided by diagnosis (Spitzer, Skodal, Gibbon, & Williams, 1988). Decisions of third-party payers are simplified by the process of attaching a label to a set of symptoms, and outcomes can be better evaluated based on change in that set of symptoms. For these reasons, it is unlikely that the diagnostic system will disappear any time in the near future.

Psychiatrists have acknowledged that diagnosis is only loosely related to function. It was for this reason that Axis V was developed. It is clear that Axis V correlates with severity of disorder, rather than with specific diagnosis (Klerman, 1988). Individuals who are diagnosed as schizophrenic may present with widely-varying functional abilities; some may be able to hold jobs, for instance, while others may require the constant attention of an in-patient psychiatric facility. (It is also true that individuals diagnosed with a particular disorder may vary. Not all individuals with schizophrenia are alike [APA, 2000]). First and his colleagues (1992) suggest that behaviors may be more helpful than abstract constructs in making diagnoses. Further, there is acknowledgment that once the "disease" has been ameliorated, residual dysfunction in daily life may remain to be addressed (Jaeger & Douglas, 1992). For example, individuals with schizophrenia often develop the disorder in mid to late adolescence. While these individuals learn to deal with the positive symptoms of the disorder (e.g., hallucinations and delusions), they may fail to develop many of the important life skills that are essential elements of normal adolescent development. Once their positive symptoms have been adequately treated, what remains is a set of functional deficits with regard to basic life tasks, such as work and leisure.

The medical community has recognized the limitations of the traditional diagnostic structure. One attempt to deal with these limitations has been the development of the

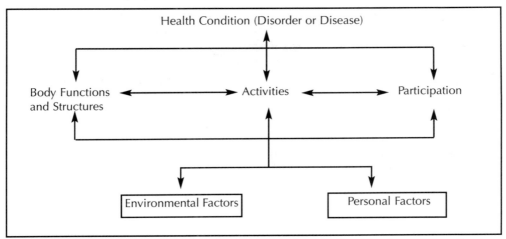

Figure 2-1. Conceptualized interaction of International Classification of Functioning, Disability, and Health factors (reprinted with permission from World Health Organization. (2001). *International classification of function*. Geneva: Author).

International Classification of Functioning, Disability, and Health (ICF) (WHO, 2001). This classification system is based on factors of the individual, including body functions and structures; the interface between the individual and the environment, activities; participation; and the factors in the environment that support or restrict function and context. Figure 2-1 shows how these factors are conceptualized as interacting. This system, like the DSM and the ICD, allows for alphanumeric categorization. Dysfunction related to body function (e.g., a physiological disorder) would be denoted with the letter "b," body structure (e.g., a broken bone or an amputation) is denoted with the letter "s." There are also codes for severity of the problem, ranging from 0 (i.e., no problem) to 4 (i.e., complete problem). Appendix B provides a summary of this system.

The ICF provides a description of function and disability that is separate from, but may be related to, biological disorder. Its creators indicate that it has four major purposes:

1. "To provide a scientific basis for understanding and studying health and health-related states, outcomes, and determinates

2. To establish a common language for describing health and health-related states in order to improve communication between different users, such as health care workers, researchers, policy-makers, and the public, including people with disabilities

3. To permit comparison of data across countries, health care disciplines, services, and time

4. To provide a systematic coding scheme for health information systems" (WHO, 2001, p. 5).

This classification system is much closer to the view promoted by occupational therapy and recognizes that disease and dysfunction are not synonymous. From the perspective of occupational therapy, the emphasis on performance of activity reflects the importance of occupation in constructing meaningful lives both in physical rehabilitation and in mental health, an understanding that is gaining wider recognition (Duncan, 1999).

The ICF was developed through a lengthy process that included research; consensus meetings of researchers, care providers, consumers, and policy makers; and public comment in locations around the world. It was an attempt to be truly international and, therefore, cross-cultural in scope. This effort at cross-cultural awareness is an important attribute of the classification system as it relates to mental health and psychosocial dysfunction. As discussed in Chapter 1, culture clearly influences perceptions of mental health. While DSM-IV-TR (APA, 2000) has incorporated some of this information, the primary categories largely reflect Western, possibly even U.S., beliefs. For example, premenstrual dysphoric disorder, described almost exclusively in industrialized countries and particularly in the United States, is included as a formal diagnosis, while *pribloqtoa*, *susto*, *nervios*, and *amok* are listed only in the appendix. Given the increasingly diverse character of the United States, the existing classification system works poorly across cultures (Bonder, Martin, & Miracle, 2002).

The emphasis in the ICF (WHO, 2001), however, is a helpful step forward for occupational therapists, for whom function is the primary concern. It has brought occupational therapy into the mainstream in international health circles, as others increasingly recognize function as being vital to definitions of health and to quality of life.

OCCUPATIONAL THERAPY VIEW OF MENTAL DISORDER

While physicians focus on disease, occupational therapists focus on function (i.e., the ability of individuals to accomplish their daily occupations) (Christiansen & Baum, 1997a) and performance. It is quite possible to have a disease that results in no functional deficit, or at least one that does not require intervention. An individual who has a head cold has a disease, but he or she may carry on with normal activities (Rogers, 1982).

On the other hand, some individuals who have no diagnosable disease, either physical or psychological, have deficits in performance. Children from socioeconomically deprived backgrounds may have difficulty adapting to the expectations in a school setting; adults from isolated rural settings might show performance deficits when they move to the city to take factory jobs. These do not constitute diseases in the medical sense, but occupational therapists would be concerned about remediating performance deficits. Failure to remediate those deficits could certainly contribute to depression or anxiety.

This view of the individual is a consistent tenet of occupational therapy regardless of the theoretical orientation of the individual. Thus, individuals who adhere to Kielhofner's Model of Human Occupation (MOHO) (Kielhofner, 2002), a general systems model; Allen's cognitive approach (Allen, 1985), a neurobiological model; or the Person-Environment-Occupational Performance (PEO) model (Christiansen & Baum, 1997b) would all focus on function as the central concern of assessment and intervention. The specific problems identified on the basis of these theories would differ. In the case of the MOHO, a deficit might be identified in personal volition (i.e., interests and motivation to accomplish activities). The cognitive approach might lead the individual to identify the cognitive level (i.e., problem solving, the ability to acquire new information) as a source of difficulty in accomplishing activities. The PEO model might lead to identification of a poor fit between environmental demand and individual skills. Likewise, the interventions suggested by the models would vary because the problems identified differed. The long-term goal of each, however, is to enhance performance of everyday occupations.

This perspective is reflected in the *Occupational Therapy Practice Framework: Domain and Process* (AOTA Commission on Practice, 2002), the guiding document for practice developed by the AOTA Commission on Practice. According to this document, the appropriate concern of occupational therapy is engagement in occupation to support participation in context or contexts. To address this concern, therapists may focus on performance areas of

---

Table 2-1

Domain of Occupational Therapy: Engagement in
Occupation to Support Participation in Context or Contexts

Performance in Areas of Occupation

ADLs*
Instrumental activities of daily living (IADLs)
Education
Work
Play
Leisure
Social participation

Performance Skills	Performance Patterns
Motor skills	Habits
Process skills	Routine
Communication/interaction skills	Roles

Context	Activity Demands	Client Factors
Cultural	Objects used and their properties	Body functions
Physical	Space demands	Body structures
Social (For definitions, refer to Table 6)	Social demands	
Personal	Social demands	
Spiritual		Required actions
Temporal	Required body functions	
Virtual	Require body structures	

*Also referred to as basic activities of daily living (BADLs) and personal activities of daily living (PADLs)

Copyright © 2002. American Occupational Therapy Association, Inc. Reprinted with permission.

---

occupation, such as activities of daily living (ADLs), leisure, or social participation; performance skills, such as motor or process skills; or performance pattern, including habits and routines. In doing so, therapists take into account the demands of the activity, client factors, and the context in which occupation is to occur. Like the DSM and the ICF, the *Practice Framework* is a work in progress. It is derived from an earlier document, the Uniform Terminology Checklist (AOTA, 1994), and has been developed through a lengthy process of literature review and discussion. As with these other documents, it can be assumed that new versions of the *Practice Framework* will emerge as it is used in practice and as new developments emerge in occupational therapy. Table 2-1 summarizes the areas included in this conceptualization of the domain of occupational therapy.

Occupational therapy assumes that "people are shaped by what they have done, by their daily patterns of occupation" (Zemke & Clark, 1996, p.vii). The relevant questions for therapy relate to the kinds of choices individuals make about their daily occupations, how those choices contribute to their sense of well-being, and "how occupational therapists are most apt to ignite our patients' intense engagement in a world of productivity and activity" (p. xiv).

Unlike physicians, occupational therapists focus on what it is that the clients need and want to do. Within these broad parameters, therapists develop interventions based on a set of theoretical beliefs about human performance and its enhancement. A number of models assist in understanding behavior. Among these are several noted above, the cognitive disabilities model (Allen, 1985), MOHO (Kielhofner, 2002), and the PEO model (Christiansen & Baum, 1997b). Others include the rehabilitation model (Anthony, 1979) and the Occupational Adaptation model (Schkade & Schultz, 1992; Schultz & Schkade, 1992). Each model suggests a way of conceptualizing occupational function and dysfunction, including the sources of problems and the strategies for intervening. Effective therapists study these models closely, identify the model or combination of models best validated by research, and design their assessment and intervention based on the premises of that model or combination of models. Table 2-2 provides a brief summary of the beliefs of these models. While not an exhaustive list, these are some of the theories in common use that hold promise for enhancement of therapeutic outcomes.

It is important to note that almost all of these models include consideration of the client's cultural background. What it is that the client needs and wants to do varies depending not only on personal and environmental considerations, but also on the cultural values and beliefs that are part of the individual's experience. These beliefs and values are vital when considering therapeutic interactions and can affect both major concerns (e.g., identification of treatment goals) and smaller concerns (e.g., choice of a specific activity to address those goals). Therapists must ensure that in all parts of the therapeutic process they gather and incorporate cultural considerations.

The occupational therapy process in mental health is similar to that in other kinds of intervention. The first step is evaluation to develop an occupational profile and explore the client's current occupational performance profile (AOTA, 2002). Discussion of existing mechanisms for assessment in psychosocial occupational therapy can be found in Bonder (1997) and Kielhofner (2002). It is imperative that occupational therapists focus their assessment on appropriate concerns for their discipline (i.e., on performance) (Bonder, 1993). Therapists, using the *Practice Framework* as a guide, would focus their attention on performance areas such as self-care, leisure, work, and social participation. One effective instrument for accomplishing this level of assessment is the Canadian Occupational Performance Measure (Cresswell, 1998). The Assessment of Motor and Process Skills is an instrument with the potential to measure performance at the skill level in community mental health situations (McNulty & Fisher, 2001). Therapists also need to obtain information about performance patterns, a process that can be accomplished through interview.

Treatment goals are based on the individual's strengths and deficits; the activities the individual needs and wants to perform; and the social, economic, and environmental resources available to the individual. In psychiatry, intervention approaches fall into the following five primary categories (AOTA, 2002):

1. Create and promote (health prevention)
2. Establish and restore (remediation, restoration)
3. Maintain
4. Modify (compensation, adaptation)
5. Prevent (disability prevention).

Table 2-2

Some Theories of Occupational Therapy Practice in Mental Heal~

Theory	Beliefs About Dysfunction	Intervention	Outcomes
Model of Human Occupation (Kielhofner, 2002)	Maladaptive cycles of input, output, and feedback; does not meet need for exploration and mastery; poorly developed or disordered volitional, habituation subsystems	Assessment Evaluation of subsystems, environment, and feedback Intervention Facilitate age appropriate occupation	Adaptive cycles; Age appropriate subsystems
Rehabilitation model (Anthony, 1979)	Psychiatric disability: deficits in skilled performance	Assessment Present and needed skills Intervention Step organized program includes physical fitness and vocational activities	Increased repertoire of skilled behavior: physical, emotional, and intellectual
Person-Environment-Occupation Performance model (Christiansen & Baum, 1997b)	Deficits in person abilities Poor match between person, environment, and occupation Excessive occupational/environmental demands	Assessment Individual skills and wishes Environmental and occupational demands Intervention Enhancement of individual skills, clarification of personal goals, and modification of environment or occupation	Increased personal satisfaction and/or abilities Improved match between environment, occupation, and person
Occupational Adaptation (Schultz & Schkade, 1992; Schkade & Schultz, 1992)	Ineffective adaptive response Ineffective occupational response	Assessment Information about occupational role expectations, person systems, and occupational adaptation Intervention Focuses on enhanced occupational adaptation	Effective occupational performance Effective occupational adaptation

Creating and promoting occupation has a preventive perspective and is intended as a set of strategies to enhance performance. Establishing and restoring occupation focuses on interventions to change the client by enhancing or restoring skills. Maintaining emphasizes efforts to prevent deterioration in function, while modifying emphasizes interventions focused on altering the environment to support performance. Preventing focuses on interventions designed for individuals who are at risk of deficits, with an emphasis on avoiding potential performance problems.

Within each category, the focus of intervention might be on factors such as performance skills and patterns, performance contexts, or client factors (i.e., body functions and structures) (AOTA, 2002). The system suggests that the category of "establish" is most likely to focus on the person (performance skills and patterns, client factors including body functions and structures). The category of "modify," on the other hand, emphasizes context or activity demands. Thus, depending on category, the focus might be on helping the individual to change or on changing the environment or demands of the task.

Four major intervention strategies are incorporated into the system (AOTA, 2002): therapeutic use of self; therapeutic use of occupations, including occupation-based activity, purposeful activity, and preparatory methods; consultation process; and education process.

Therapeutic use of self reflects the reality that interaction with the therapist is, in itself, therapeutic. It has the potential to provide support and encouragement, reinforcement of positive attributes, information, and a role model for behavior and coping. Many occupational therapy interventions expect therapeutic use of self as an essential element. Eklund (1999) describes the importance of the therapeutic relationship in a psychiatric day care unit for individuals with chronic psychiatric disorders. Community-based services for deinstitutionalized or homeless individuals demand thoughtful intervention focused on relationship building (Scaffa, Brownson, & Shordike, 2001).

Activities like cooking skills practice or supported employment (Lloyd & Samra, 2000) are examples of the therapeutic use of occupations. Practical experience, such as assigning a job in the clinic, is another example of use of occupation. This category also includes interventions that remediate underlying skills. These are interventions preparatory to activity (i.e., they are not in and of themselves meaningful occupations, but are skills necessary for participation in those occupations). A child who is retarded might be provided with intense kinesthetic and proprioceptive input through swinging and spinning (Humphries, Snider, & McDougall, 1993). According to sensory integration theory, this might better organize the central nervous system (CNS), thus enhancing higher-level skills in play or school activities (Ayres, 1972). Another example, based on developmental theory, would be providing the same child with practice on lower-level skills (Bruce & Borg, 2002). Having the child balance on a balance beam, for instance, assists the child in gradually achieving higher-order skills, such as running in a step-by-step fashion.

Feelings and attitudes can also be addressed through occupation. For example, inaccurate self-concept and lowered self-esteem are common among individuals with psychiatric disorders regardless of specific diagnosis, and may lead to ineffective performance. Such individuals may not know that they can do particular activities, or they may feel a chronic sense of failure. Providing opportunities for success may bolster sagging self-esteem, and review of performance of a variety of activities may allow for more accurate self-assessment. The MOHO (Kielhofner, 2002) suggests that clients need to have and be aware of their own valued goals in order to perform effectively. They may need practice simply expressing themselves (Gibson & Richert, 1993).

All of these interventions can be accomplished either in individual interaction with clients or in group settings. For some problems, groups have particular advantages. As an example, for a client concerned about self-concept, interaction in a group may provide valuable feedback about self-presentation and the impressions of others. Hearing about the experiences of others can be useful in learning to cope with an array of psychosocial deficits, as well. Because groups can also be a cost-effective way to provide care, it is important for occupational therapists to consider this mechanism.

Modification of occupational demand or context is another strategy for therapeutic use of occupation. It has been theorized that some individuals do not have great capacity to modify their own performance, but that they may benefit from modifications in the activity, which will reduce demand (Allen, 1985). While this somewhat pessimistic view of individual capacity for change is widely challenged in occupational therapy, there is general agreement that environmental modification (i.e., alteration of context) can be an effective strategy for enhancing performance (Christiansen & Baum, 1997a). Another way of viewing this kind of intervention is that many individuals do not know how to construct the most supportive environments for themselves and that they can benefit from learning how to do so. Because setting can influence the performance of the individual, modification of the setting—whether by the therapist or the individual—will maximize function (Kielhofner, 2002).

Educational approaches emphasize teaching of skills that then might be practiced through therapeutic use of occupation. Example of educational approaches are lifestyle training (Lambert, 1998; Salo-Chydenius, 1996), anxiety management (Meeson, 1998), and job exploration (Lloyd & Samra, 2000). This approach is often found in partial hospitalization or day treatment settings (Tomlinson, 1994).

Consultation is a growing arena for occupational therapy practice (Wittman, 1996). Federal legislation, including the Americans with Disabilities Act (ADA) (Crist & Stoffel, 1992) and the Individuals with Disabilities Education Act (IDEA) (Office of Special Education and Rehabilitative Services [OSERS], 1997), has increased the importance of this form of intervention. The ADA specifies that employers must make reasonable accommodations in the workplace for individuals with disabilities, including those with mental disorders. The occupational therapist has valuable expertise to lend to this effort. Specifically, the therapist can help the individual identify the components or characteristics of the job that cause difficulty, then work with the individual and the employer to identify accommodations that are realistic for the situation. More frequent breaks, a less stimulating environment, more specific instructions, and frequent feedback are all examples of modifications that may help an individual with a mental disorder cope with a job. Rather than provide direct care to the individual, the therapist might function to provide advice to the employer (Scott, 1996).

Similarly, there are consultation roles for occupational therapists in substance abuse prevention programs, self-help programs (Moyers & Stoffel, 2001), employment training programs (Scheinholz, 2001), and in schools (Griswold, 1999). In all of these settings, consultation might focus on management of a particular case, understanding the difficulty that led to the case, new program development, or organizational issues.

Using any of these intervention strategies, therapists focus on enhancement of client abilities in performance areas, skills, and patterns. The ultimate goal of occupational therapy, unlike medicine or psychology, is effective function in meaningful occupation. The belief of occupational therapists is that a balance of occupation in all performance areas promotes the best possible quality of life for the individual (Meyer, 1922/1977).

A psychiatrist might look at a client who presents with depressed mood and lethargy and say, "Here is someone who has a dysthymic disorder. Let us treat the client with antidepressant medication and with verbal therapy to allow him to express his feelings." The occupational therapist might look at the same client and say, "Here is someone who has a pervasive sense of failure and no clear goals in life. Let us provide him with activities that will affirm his strengths and help him identify some goals that will give his life meaning." The two approaches are clearly different. In the best possible situation, they are complementary, each providing the client with something that will enhance his or her satisfaction with life, as well as his or her ability to contribute to society.

TRENDS AFFECTING MENTAL HEALTH CARE IN OCCUPATIONAL THERAPY

Occupational therapy, like mental health care in general, must respond to an array of societal and political pressures and changes. Among those that have had the most impact on delivery of occupational therapy services are the following:

1. A trend to provide care in community settings
2. A growing awareness of the interaction of physical and mental conditions
3. Increasing population diversity coupled with growing appreciation of cultural difference in health and disease conceptualizations
4. A trend toward increased interdisciplinary intervention
5. Increasing demands for accountability.

There has been a movement away from in-patient treatment in recent years that has altered occupational therapy practice in mental health in significant ways (Griswold, 1999). Therapists now identify a role for themselves in a wide array of community settings (Scaffa, 2001). Among the emerging forms of mental health treatment are such programs in home health-based (Wooster, Gray, & Gifford, 2001) and community-based social skills and job training programs, such as the Program for Assertive Community Treatment (Allness & Knoedler, 1998) and various versions of the clubhouse approach (Samuel, 1998; Urbaniak, 1995). The clubhouse approach focuses on helping groups of clients organize themselves in much the same way as clubs might, with officers, specific goals, and sometimes, dues. A club might focus on structuring leisure activities for a group of clients or on helping individuals develop work skills. At the same time, the individuals learn organizational, leadership, and communication skills as members of the group.

Work is an area of increasing focus for individuals being treated in the community because psychopharmacological interventions improve the psychological status of the client, but leave residual functional deficits (Diamond, 1998; Eklund, 1996). Because of the push for deinstitutionalization, a significant number of individuals with psychiatric disorders are now homeless, and this is an area in which occupational therapy services are vitally important (Finlayson, Baker, Rodman, & Herzberg, 2002). Leisure continues to be an important focus of intervention in the community (Pegg & Moxham, 2000). Evidence of the effectiveness of community-based occupational therapy interventions is beginning to appear in the literature (Clark et al., 2001; Holm, Santangelo, Fromuth, Brown, & Walter, 2000), providing important support for their value. It is also important to recognize that integration of services is a significant challenge in providing effective community-based care (Burson & Simpatico, 2002). Therapists must inform themselves about available services and mechanisms for ensuring that their clients receive appropriate referral.

Perhaps even more central to practice is the understanding that distinctions between physical and psychological disorder are always arbitrary to some extent. Therapists increasingly recognize that their clients in other settings may have psychiatric disorders (Mayou, Hawton, Feldman, & Ardern, 1991; Stoudemire, 1991). For example, it is well-established that depression is common in individuals who have had cerebrovascular accidents (Allman, 1991). Individuals with arthritis may experience depression resulting from the pain and activity limitations that are consequences of the disease (Penninx et al., 1997). Thus, therapists in rehabilitation settings must be sensitive to the issues of motivation, self-esteem, guilt, and sadness that may accompany this disorder.

Therapists must also be aware of cultural considerations related to mental disorders (Flaskerud, 2000; Lutz & Warren, 2001). As is explicit in DSM-IV (APA, 2000), culture influences diagnosis and treatment, including not only labels for the problem and conceptualizations about etiology and prognosis, but also treatment expectations, cooperation with recommended intervention, family involvement, perceptions of side effects (Bonder et al., 2002; Flaskerud, 2000), and identify as helpful interventions that may not be part of Western psychological tradition. Such treatments include acupuncture (Tukmachi, 2001) and spiritual healing (Meisenhelder & Chandler, 2000). Incorporation of these kinds of beliefs into treatment can have a positive impact on outcomes. For occupational therapists, this means working with clients to identify culturally-relevant activities that are meaningful and motivating to the individual client in the context of his or her environment. Therapists may find that incorporating activities like Tai Chi and meditation into their interventions can be valuable in some situations, and there are many similar examples of non-Western activities that may be the focus of treatment with some clients.

As therapists increasingly work in quarter or half-way houses, community centers, sheltered living facilities, schools, and in client homes, there is much "role blurring" among disciplines (Shackleton & Gage, 1995). In addition to occupational therapists, the client may be treated by the psychiatric nurse; social worker; psychologist; art, music, dance, or recreation therapist; vocational counselor; and psychiatrist, and it can be difficult to maintain effective interaction among these various team members (Hughes, 2001).

The nurse is responsible primarily for nursing care, medical management, and, in inpatient settings, promoting the therapeutic milieu (Gibson & Richert, 1993). Social workers deal with family issues and with discharge planning. Psychologists typically complete psychological assessments and, in some settings, provide individual and group psychotherapy. Art, music, and dance therapists offer opportunities for expression through non-verbal means using the expressive arts as their media. Vocational counselors and job coaches focus on work-related skills and abilities, while recreation therapists focus on leisure abilities and interests. The psychiatrist provides medical care and prescribes medications, including psychotropic medications.

Occupational therapists focus on assessment and remediation of performance of work, leisure, and self-care and the underlying skills required to accomplish those activities. Their holistic view of activity helps them integrate the perspectives of art, music, dance, and recreation therapists and vocational counselors. They emphasize body functions and structures, motor skills, process skills, communication/interaction skills, as well as the habits, routines, and roles required for optimal engagement in occupation (AOTA, 2002).

Ideally, the various mental health professionals work together to provide the best care for the client (Peck & Norman, 1999). However, roles sometimes overlap and as cost containment has become an issue, efforts have been made to reduce the number of different therapists involved with each client. Occupational therapists have a broad perspective and can focus on issues vital to the client; they also have an obligation to recognize their limitations and call on others as appropriate.

Other trends, mentioned in the previous chapter, directly affect the practice of occupational therapy. There is a growing demand for accountability, the demonstration that care is effective, and worth reimbursement (Lloyd, Kanowski, & Samra, 1998). The need for evidence-based practice is particularly vital in a system of care that is attempting to control costs. If occupational therapists expect to continue to be included in this system, they must document their value (Law, 2002). Therapists have an obligation to review current literature and practice standards, a challenge in this era of information overload. One strategy for staying current is to regularly check search engines such as PsychInfo, available through most university libraries. A number of excellent Web sites also provide current and regularly updated information about mental health care. Several of these are listed at the end of this chapter. Therapists should visit these or similar sites on a regular basis to ensure that they are aware of emerging scientific progress and practice trends.

Unfortunately, in the occupational therapy literature, there is a relative scarcity of research about mental health (Craik, 1998; Rebeiro, 1998). This presents significant challenges for the profession as practitioners attempt to implement best practices. Another challenge for therapists is the need to ensure that use of evidence-based practice does not overshadow the views and values of the individual receiving treatment (Feder, 1998). Therapists must be cautious about ignoring individual needs that are not described in the literature or that deviate from the norm.

All these trends make for a complex situation in which occupational therapy services are provided. Therapists must understand the system, the beliefs and values of their clients, and the beliefs and values of other professionals.

The following chapters describe the diagnostic categories in DSM-IV-TR (APA, 2000), including diagnostic criteria, etiology, symptoms, and prognosis. They then describe the functional consequences of each disorder and typical treatment. Those most likely to require occupational therapy services are emphasized, while others are described briefly. In reading these chapters, you will see that individuals with a variety of disorders may benefit from similar occupational therapy interventions because performance-related factors cut across medical diagnoses. It is important to keep in mind the limitations of the diagnostic system, as well as the central goal of occupational therapy: improved occupational performance.

SUGGESTED WEBSITES

ALLPSYCH ONLINE
http://allpsych.com/disorders
Summarizes an array of psychiatric disorders categorized based on DSM groupings. Includes an overview of DSM-IV.

American Occupational Therapy Association
www.aota.org
The professional association for occupational therapists. A variety of publications about mental health can be found at this site. Press releases, special interest group reports, advocacy initiatives, and other information are also included here.

American Psychiatric Association
www.psych.org
This organization is primarily for physicians. Medical research, including new information about diagnosis, lab testing, medication, and other treatments can be found at this site.

American Psychological Association
www.apa.org
Primarily for psychologists, this is a good source of information about nonmedical interventions.

Diversity@work-Disability
www.work.asn.au/disability
Provides information about managing psychiatric disorders in work settings.

Information on Psychiatric Illness
www.nimh.nih.gov/publicat/index.cfm
Posted by the National Institute of Mental Health, this is an excellent site for current information about progress in psychopharmacology.

Mental Health Association in New Jersey
www.mhanj.org
Provides an array of links to sources of information. Most are national or international, not necessarily specific to New Jersey.

National Alliance for the Mentally Ill
www.nami.org
This is the best known consumer organization on mental health and includes excellent information from the perspective of those individuals with mental health problems. Includes educational, research, and advocacy information and is appropriate for both professionals and consumers.

National Library of Medicine
www.nlm.nih.gov
The National Library of Medicine houses both search engines and original documents. It is a comprehensive source for research literature and information about on-going research and policy initiatives.

National Institute of Mental Health
www.nimh.nih.gov
The main body funding research in mental health, this organization provides links to other sources, information about current research, and information about funding opportunities.

Psychiatry, MedMark
www.medmark.org/psy/psychi2.htm
An excellent search engine for a wide array of topics, including various diagnoses, diagnostic testing, medication, and other intervention strategies. Includes a comprehensive list of other sources, including many appropriate for consumers.

PsycPORT.com
www.psycport.com
Produced by the American Psychological Association, this website includes current news reports and press releases.

REFERENCES

Allen, C. (1985). *Occupational therapy for psychiatric diseases: Measurement and management of cognitive disabilities.* Boston: Little, Brown & Co.

Allman, P. (1991). Depressive disorders and emotionalism following stroke. *International Journal of Geriatric Psychiatry, 6,* 377-383.

Allness, D.J., & Knoedler, W.H. (1998). *The PACT model of community-based treatment for persons with severe and persistent mental illness: A manual for PACT start-up.* Arlington, VA: National Alliance for the Mentally Ill.

American Occupational Therapy Association. (1994). *Uniform terminology checklist* (3rd ed.). Rockville, MD: Author.

American Occupational Therapy Association Commission on Practice. (2002). Occupational therapy practice framework: Domain and process. *The American Journal of Occupational Therapy, 56,* 609-639.

American Psychiatric Association. (2000). *Diagnostic and statistical manual of mental disorders* (4th ed., text revision). Washington, DC: Author.

Anthony, W.A. (1979). *The principles of psychiatric rehabilitation.* Amherst, MA: Human Resource Development Press.

Antonosky, A. (1972). Breakdown: A needed fourth step in the conceptual armamentarium of modern medicine. *Social Science & Medicine, 6,* 537-544.

Ayres, A.J. (1972). *Sensory integration and learning disorders.* Los Angeles: Western Psychiatric Services.

Bonder, B.R. (1993). Issues in assessment of psychosocial components of function. *The American Journal of Occupational Therapy, 47,* 211-216.

Bonder, B.R. (1997). Coping with psychological and emotional challenges. In C. Christiansen & C. Baum (Eds.), *Occupational therapy: Enabling function and well-being* (2nd ed., pp. 312-335). Thorofare, NJ: SLACK Incorporated.

Bonder, B.R., Martin, L., & Miracle, A.W. (2002). *Culture in clinical care.* Thorofare, NJ: SLACK Incorporated.

Bruce, M.A., & Borg, B. (2002) *Psychosocial frames of reference: Core for occupation-based practice* (3rd ed.). Thorofare, NJ: SLACK Incorporated.

Burson, K., & Simpatico, T. (2002). Integrating service systems for people with psychiatric disabilities. *OT Practice,* 22-29.

Christiansen, C., & Baum, C. (Eds.). (1997a). *Occupational therapy: Enabling function and well-being* (2nd ed.). Thorofare, NJ: SLACK Incorporated.

Christiansen, C., & Baum, C. (1997b). Person-environment occupational performance: A conceptual model for practice. In C. Christiansen & C. Baum (Eds.), *Occupational therapy: Enabling function and well-being* (2nd ed., pp. 46-70). Thorofare, NJ: SLACK Incorporated.

Clark, F., Azen, S.P., Carlson, M., Mandel, D., LaBree, L., Hay, J., et al. (2001). Embedding health-promoting changes into the daily lives of independent-living older adults: Long-term follow-up of occupational therapy intervention. *Journal of Gerontology: Psychological Sciences, 56B,* P60-P63.

Cottrell, R.J.F. (Ed.). (2000). *Proactive approaches in psychosocial occupational therapy.* Thorofare, NJ: SLACK Incorporated.

Craik, C. (1998). Occupational therapy in mental health: A review of the literature. *British Journal of Occupational Therapy, 61,* 186-192.

Cresswell, M.K.M. (1998). Focus on research... A study to investigate the utility of the Canadian Occupational Performance Measure as an outcome measure in community mental health occupational therapy. *British Journal of Occupational Therapy, 61,* 213.

Crist, P.A.H., & Stoffel, V.C. (1992). The Americans with Disabilities Act of 1990 and employees with mental impairments: Personal efficacy and the environment. *The American Journal of Occupational Therapy, 46,* 434-443.

DeAngelis, T. (1991). DSM being revised, but problems remain. *American Psychological Association Monitor*, 12-13.

Diamond, H. (1998). Vocational decision making in a psychiatric out-patient program. *Occupational Therapy in Mental Health, 14*(3), 67-80.

Duncan, E.A.S. (1999). Occupational therapy in mental health: It is time to recognize that it has come of age. *British Journal of Occupational Therapy, 62,* 521-522.

Eklund, M. (1996). Working relationship, participation and outcome in a psychiatric day care unit based on occupational therapy. *Scandinavian Journal of Occupational Therapy, 3,* 106-113.

Eklund, M. (1999). Outcomes of occupational therapy in a psychiatric day care unit for long-term mentally ill patients. *Occupational Therapy in Mental Health, 14*(4), 21-45.

Feder, J. (1998). Bridging the gap: Integration of consumer needs into a psychiatric rehabilitation program. *Occupational Therapy in Mental Health, 14*(1/2), 89-95.

Finlayson, M., Baker, M., Rodman, L., & Herzberg, G. (2002). The process and outcomes of a multimethod needs assessment at a homeless shelter. *The American Journal of Occupational Therapy, 56,* 313-321.

First, M.B., Frances, A., Widiger, T.A., Pincus, H.A., & Davis, W.W. (1992). *Behavioral Assessment, 14,* 297-306.

Flaskerud, J.H. (2000). Ethnicity, culture, and neuropsychiatry. *Issues in Mental Health Nursing, 21,* 5-29.

Frager, R., & Fadiman, J. (1998). *Personality and personal growth* (4th ed.). New York: Longman.

Gibson, D., & Richert, G.Z. (1993). The therapeutic process. In H.L. Hopkins & H.D. Smith (Eds.), *Occupational therapy* (8th ed., pp. 557-566). Philadelphia, PA: Lippincott.

Griswold, L.A.S. (1999). Community-based practice arenas. In M.E. Neistadt & E.B. Crepeau (Eds.), *Willard and Spackman's Occupational Therapy* (9th ed., pp. 810-815). Philadelphia: Lippincott, Williams, Wilkins.

Healy, D. (2002). *The creation of psychopharmacology.* Cambridge, MA: Harvard University Press.

Holm, M.B., Santangelo, M.A., Fromuth, D.J., Brown, S.O., & Walter, H. (2000). Effectiveness of everyday occupations for changing client behaviors in a community living arrangement. *The American Journal of Occupational Therapy, 54,* 361-371.

Hughes, J. (2001). Occupational therapy in community mental health teams: A continuing dilemma? Role theory offers an explanation. *British Journal of Occupational Therapy, 64*(1), 34-40.

Humphries, T.W., Snider, L., & McDougall, B. (1993). Clinical evaluation of the effectiveness of sensory integrative and perceptual motor therapy in improving sensory integrative function in children with learning disabilities. *Occupational Therapy Journal of Research, 13,* 163-182.

Jaeger, J., & Douglas, E. (1992). Neuropsychiatric rehabilitation for persistent mental illness. *The Psychiatric Quarterly, 63,* 71-94.

Kielhofner, G. (Ed.). (2002). *Model of human occupation* (3rd ed.). Baltimore, MD: Lippincott, Williams & Wilkins.

Klerman, G.L. (1988). Classification and DSM-III-R. In A.M. Nicholi (Ed.), *The new Harvard guide to psychiatry* (pp. 70-87). Cambridge, MA: Belknap Press.

Lambert, R. (1998). Occupation and lifestyle: Implications for mental health practice. *British Journal of Occupational Therapy, 61,* 193-197.

Law, M. (2002). *Evidence-based rehabilitation: A guide to practice.* Thorofare, NJ: SLACK Incorporated.

Lloyd, C., Kanowski, H., & Samra, P. (1998). Developing occupational therapy services within an integrated mental health service. *British Journal of Occupational Therapy, 61,* 214-218.

Lloyd, C., & Samra, P. (2000). OT and work-related programmes for people with a mental illness. *British Journal of Therapy and Rehabilitation, 7,* 254-261.

Lutz, W.J., & Warren, B.J. (2001). Symptomatology and medication for monitoring public mental health consumers: A cultural perspective. *Journal of The American Psychiatric Nurses Association, 7,* 115-124.

Mayou, R., Hawton, K., Feldman, E., & Ardern, M. (1991). Psychiatric problems among medical admissions. *International Journal of Psychiatry in Medicine, 21,* 71-84.

McNulty, M.C., & Fisher, A.G. (2001). Validity of using the Assessment of Motor and Process Skills to estimate overall home safety in persons with psychiatric conditions. *The American Journal of Occupational Therapy, 55,* 649-655.

Meeson, B. (1998). Occupational therapy in community mental health, part 1: Intervention choice. *British Journal of Occupational Therapy, 61,* 7-12.

Meisenhelder, J.B., & Chandler, E.N. (2000). Faith, prayer, and health outcomes in elderly Native Americans. *Clinical Nursing Research, 9,* 191-203.

Meyer, A. (1922/1977). The philosophy of occupational therapy. *The American Journal of Occupational Therapy, 31,* 639-642.

Moyers, P.A., & Stoffel, V.C. (2001). Community-based approaches for substance use disorders. In M. Scaffa (Ed.), *Occupational therapy in community-based practice settings*. Philadelphia: F.A. Davis.

Office of Special Education and Rehabilitative Services. (1997). *IDEA '97: The law*. Retrieved October 29, 2001, from http://www.ed.gov/offices/OSERS/Policy/IDEA/the_law.html.

Peck, E., & Norman, I.J. (1999). Working together in adult community mental health services: Exploring inter-professional role relations. *Journal of Mental Health, 8*, 231-242.

Pegg, S., & Moxham, L. (2000). Getting it right: Appropriate therapeutic recreation programs for community based consumers of mental health services. *Contemporary Nurse, 9*, 295-302.

Penninx, B.W.J.H., Van Tilburg, T., Deeg, D.J.H., Kriegsman, D.M.W., Boeke, A.J., & Van Eijk, J.T.M. (1997). Direct and buffer effects of social support and personal coping resources in individuals with arthritis. *Social Science & Medicine, 44*, 393-402.

Porter, R. (1987). *A social history of madness*. New York: Weidenfeld & Nicolson.

Rebeiro, K.L. (1998). Occupation-as-means to mental health: A review of the literature, and a call for research. *Canadian Journal of Occupational Therapy, 65*, 12-19.

Rogers, J.C. (1982). Order and disorder in medicine and occupational therapy. *The American Journal of Occupational Therapy, 36*, 29-35.

Salo-Chydenius, S. (1996). Changing helplessness to coping: An exploratory study of social skills training with individuals with long-term mental illness. *Occupational Therapy in Mental Health, 8*(2), 21-30.

Samuel, L. (1998). Responsive changes in mental health practice in Wisconsin. *Occupational Therapy in Mental Health, 14*(1/2), 29-34.

Scaffa, M. (Ed.). (2001). *Occupational therapy in community-based practice settings*. Philadelphia: F.A. Davis.

Scaffa, M., Brownson, C.A., & Shordike, A. (2001). Implications for professional education and research. In M. Scaffa (Ed.), *Occupational therapy in community-based practice settings* (pp. 367-390). Philadelphia: F.A. Davis.

Scheinholz, M.K. (2001). Community-based mental health services. In M. Scaffa (Ed.), *Occupational therapy in community-based practice settings*. Philadelphia: F.A. Davis.

Schkade, J.K., & Schultz, S. (1992). Occupational adaptation: Toward a holistic approach for contemporary practice, part 1. *The American Journal of Occupational Therapy, 46*, 829-838.

Schultz, S., & Schkade, J.K. (1992). Occupational adaptation: Toward a holistic approach for contemporary practice, part 2. *The American Journal of Occupational Therapy, 46*, 917-926.

Scott, P. (1996). Employment for individuals with mental disabilities: ADA unlocked the door but who has the handle? *Occupational Therapy in Health Care, 10*(2), 49-64.

Shackleton, T.L., & Gage, M. (1995). Strategic planning: Positioning occupational therapy to be proactive in the new health care paradigm. *Canadian Journal of Occupational Therapy, 62*(4), 188-196.

Small, R.F., & Barnhill, L.R. (Eds.). (1998). *Practicing in the new mental health marketplace: Ethical, legal, and moral issues*. Washington, DC: American Psychological Association.

Spitzer, R.L., Skodal, A.E., Gibbon, M., & Williams, J.B.W. (1988). *Psychopathology: A casebook*. New York: McGraw-Hill.

Stoudemire, A. (1991). Psychological factors affecting physical condition and DSM-IV. *Psychosomatics, 34*, 8-11.

Szasz, T. (1974). *The myth of mental illness* (2nd ed.). New York: Harper & Row.

Tomlinson, J. (1994). The dimensions of occupational therapy in day programs. *Mental Health Special Interest Newsletter, 17*(1), 5-6.

Tsang, H., Lam, P., Ng, B., & Leung, O. (2000). Predictors of employment outcome for people with psychiatric disabilities: A review of the literature since the mid '80's. *Journal of Rehabilitation, 66*(2), 19-31.

Tukmachi, E. (2001). Acupuncture therapy in diseases failing to respond to Western medicine: 6 case reports. *Journal of Chinese Medicine, 67*, 5-10.

Urbaniak, M.A. (1995). Yahara House: A community-based program using the Fountain House model. *Mental Health Special Interest Newsletter, 18*(1), 1-3.

Wittman, P. (1996). Consultation: A vital skill for occupational therapists. *Occupational Therapy in Health Care, 10*(2), 65-71.

Wooster, D.A., Gray, L., & Gifford, K.E. (2001). Specialized practice in home health. In M. Scaffa (Ed.), *Occupational therapy in community-based practice settings* (pp. 223-252). Philadelphia: F.A. Davis.

World Health Organization. (2001). *International classification of functioning, disability and health* (ICF). Geneva, Switzerland: Author.

Zemke, R., & Clark, R. (Eds.). (1996). *Occupational science: The evolving discipline.* Philadelphia: F.A. Davis.

RECOMMENDED READING

Bruce, M.A., & Borg, B. (2002). *Psychosocial frames of reference: Core for occupation-based practice* (3rd ed.). Thorofare, NJ: SLACK Incorporated.

Christiansen, C., & Baum, C. (Eds.). (1997a). *Occupational therapy: Enabling function and well-being* (2nd ed.). Thorofare, NJ: SLACK Incorporated.

Cottrell, R.J.F. (Ed.). (2000). *Proactive approaches in psychosocial occupational therapy.* Thorofare, NJ: SLACK Incorporated.

Scaffa, M. (Ed.). (2001). *Occupational therapy in community-based practice settings.* Philadelphia: F.A. Davis.

Chapter 3

Disorders of Infancy, Childhood, and Adolescence

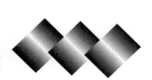
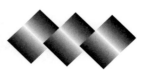

Disorders of infancy, childhood, and adolescence begin in the early years of life and tend to be lifelong conditions with significant impact on functional performance. The disorders may be present at birth, as in the case of some types of mental retardation, or may appear in adolescence, as in the case of some anxiety disorders.

Many of the diagnoses found in other categories of the DSM and covered in later chapters (e.g., mood disorders) may also occur in children or adolescents, with symptoms similar to those seen in adults. The differences in manifestation that are sometimes apparent in children will be discussed in the chapters dealing with adult-onset disorders.

Childhood and adolescence are characterized by numerous stresses, some of which may contribute to diagnosable psychiatric disorders (Newman & Newman, 2003). Sexual, emotional, and/or physical abuse are surprisingly common experiences for children. Peer pressure toward substance use, pressure around school performance, and a wide array of other problems affect the experience of childhood. Depression, suicidal ideation or action, substance abuse, adjustment disorders, and sexual acting-out may result. Some theorists suggest that these difficulties may be part of normal development, particularly during adolescence (Freud, 1958). This view is supported by those who feel that modern society presents more difficult dilemmas than existed in earlier times (Newman & Newman, 2003), among these parental divorce, early placement in day care, and availability of and peer pressure to use drugs and alcohol.

This view has been disputed, however (Newman & Newman, 2003). Some researchers have found adolescents to be largely well-adjusted. The evidence is unclear, and debates rage about the effects of divorce and other societal trends on the well-being of adolescents. These disputes await resolution through further research. There is no question, however, that children and adolescents can experience an array of psychological difficulties.

The process of diagnosing children and adolescents must take into account what reflects normal behavior and what represents dysfunction severe enough to warrant labeling. The DSM-IV-TR (APA, 2000) has attempted to provide very specific criteria about the symptoms required for diagnosis, but there remains an element of subjectivity. Some practitioners suggest that diagnosing the young is particularly challenging because psychiatric disorders still carry a social stigma that may affect the future development of the child.

As with all psychiatric diagnoses, those of childhood and adolescence may occur independently or in conjunction with other problems. The concept of dual diagnosis is a frequent theme in the literature, referring to someone who has two concurrent diagnoses (e.g., retardation and depression) (Dykens & Hodapp, 2001) or any of a number of other psychiatric disorders. By one estimate, 25% of individuals with mental retardation also have some

Table 3-1

Disorders of Infancy, Childhood, and Adolescence

- Mental retardation
- Learning disorders
- Pervasive developmental disorders:
  Autistic disorder
  Asperger's syndrome
- Attention-deficit and disruptive behavior disorders
  Attention deficit hyperactivity disorder
  Conduct disorder
  Oppositional defiant disorder
- Separation anxiety disorder

other psychiatric condition (Dykens & Hodapp, 2001), while other researchers place the figure at anywhere from 20% to 74% (Dosen & Day, 2001). Dual diagnosis complicates both the diagnostic process and treatment, requiring integration of treatment approaches. The issue of dual diagnosis is discussed in greater detail in Chapter 5.

This chapter reviews the diagnoses of infancy, childhood, and adolescence most likely to be seen by occupational therapists. The major diagnoses in this category are listed in Table 3-1.

MENTAL RETARDATION

Three characteristics must be present for this diagnosis: subaverage intelligence, deficits in adaptive functioning in at least two areas, and the fact that subaverage intelligence and deficits in adaptive functioning appear prior to age 18. Intelligence (IQ) is usually measured on any of the standard intelligence tests, such as the Stanford-Binet or Weschler Intelligence Scale for Children III (WISC III) (Frazier, 1999), with 70 being the score used to define retardation. This cut off is arbitrary, as IQ is a continuum and IQ tests typically have standard errors of roughly ±4 points. Further, the tests on which the diagnosis is based have been criticized as being biased toward the majority culture in the United States (Hatton, 2002), complicating diagnosis in minority groups. Cultural factors must be considered in making a diagnosis because abilities common in some groups (e.g., reading) might be less common in a cultural group lacking easy access to educational opportunities. The key issue is the pervasiveness of the developmental delay. Thus, the diagnosis must be made cautiously.

Etiology and Incidence

The etiology of retardation is well established in some cases, but not in others. Some genetic disorders (e.g., trisomy 21 [Down's syndrome] or fragile X syndrome) (Dykens & Hodapp, 2001) cause retardation, as will some prenatal problems such as fetal alcohol syndrome or maternal malnutrition (Chapman & Scott, 2001). A variety of physical problems during early childhood may also lead to retardation (Reber, 1992), including exposure to toxic substances like lead and mercury; diseases, such as meningitis; and injury, especially head trauma. There is a strong association between epilepsy and mental retardation, although whether this is a causative relationship is unclear (Besag, 2002).

Environmental factors may also contribute to retardation (Ramey & Ramey, 1999). Absence of adequate stimulation or parental deprivation may lead to slowed development and low IQ. Early malnutrition is also a factor. Bijou (1992) identifies a number of categories of causes, including biomedical pathology, cultural-familial conditions, and restricted development. At least 30% of cases have no identifiable cause (Reber, 1992).

It is estimated that 5% to 10% of children have developmental disabilities (Shevell, Majnemer, Rosenbaum, & Abrahamowicz, 2001), although not all are severe enough to be diagnosed as mental retardation. The epidemiological studies that have established these incidence figures have been criticized for failing to adequately represent ethnic and cultural minority groups, leading to lack of clarity about incidence in these groups (Hatton, 2002).

Prognosis

To some extent, prognosis is dependent on cause. In some instances, retardation may be reversed when the cause of the retardation is removed (Ramey & Ramey, 1999). Absence of environmental stimulation, for example, may result in developmental lag. If parents can be taught to make the environment more stimulating, the retardation may be remediated and the child may achieve normal function. Some early intervention programs, such as Project Head Start, appear to have positive effects on IQ for many children who are somewhat delayed developmentally. These programs were not designed for children who are mentally retarded, however, and research examining the long-term outcomes of these programs has been equivocal (Bailey, Aytch, Odom, Symons, & Wolery, 1999).

Similarly, where a biological cause can be established, medical treatment of the underlying problem may prevent retardation from worsening, although generally speaking the existing damage will be permanent. For example, if retardation is the result of lead toxicity, agents that remove lead from the system may be introduced. This treatment prevents further damage, but will not generally reverse damage that has already occurred (Galler, Ramsey, Solimano, & Lowell, 1983). Studies suggest that the effects of even minimal lead exposure can be prolonged and persistent (Bellinger, Stiles, & Needleman, 1992). Prompt treatment of diseases such as meningitis, when such treatment exists, may also minimize the probability of retardation or limit damage.

In most cases, however, individuals with mental retardation remain developmentally delayed through life (Dosen & Day, 2001). Functional ability can be enhanced, and most interventions with individuals who are mentally retarded focus on some form of education or training. This may include behavior modification or any of a variety of educational approaches. Depending on the degree of retardation, the individual may learn to cook simple meals, to dress and maintain personal hygiene, and to perform simple vocational tasks, making some individuals relatively independent and self-sufficient. While function may be remediated, individuals who are retarded, by definition, do not achieve the same level as their peers who are not retarded.

Education may extend to the family, both for purposes of prevention (e.g., educating pregnant women about the need for good nutrition), and for management of the retarded child. This may reduce some of the stress that has been noted in families with children who have mental retardation (Hodapp, Ly, Fidler, & Ricci, 2001).

Institutionalization may be necessary, depending on the degree of impairment. Individuals who are profoundly retarded may be unable to learn the skills that would enable them to live even in sheltered environments in the community. For many less severely impaired individuals, however, many types of sheltered environments, special schools, and, later, independent living may provide alternatives to institutionalization. Increasingly, these less restrictive environments are being sought, as children with all types of disabilities are being brought into the mainstream (Blair, 1999). As these children increasingly survive into adulthood, their parents and other family care-takers seek out these kinds of living arrangements to serve their children when they are no longer able to do so.

Implications for Function and Treatment

Retardation is classified as mild (IQ 55 to 70), moderate (IQ 40 to 55), severe (IQ 25 to 40), or profound (IQ below 25). These ranges provide a rough guide to expected function. While IQ and functional ability are correlated, a variety of factors may impact on the functional picture presented by individuals with similar IQ scores. There has been much discussion, for example, about the possibility of cultural bias of IQ tests (Zimmerman & Woo-Sam, 1984), which might cause a low score in someone who otherwise has a reasonable level of function. In fact, there has been much controversy around this point, with some researchers feeling that IQ tests should not be used to identify retardation. As an example, some children from deprived backgrounds may know a great deal of street jargon but have limited vocabularies of words used in the larger society. Furthermore, the concept of environmental press (Lawton, 1980) suggests that the environment can be structured to minimize demands on the individual, thus supporting existing abilities.

Generally speaking, individuals who have low IQs show performance deficits in most areas of function. These may present as delays in the development of specific abilities, the absence of some abilities, or deficits in the skill with which activities are performed. For example, a child who is mentally retarded might learn to sit relatively late, might not sit at all, or might sit with poor control and posture. A individual with profound retardation may never acquire speech or learn to feed him- or herself, while an individual who is only mildly retarded may learn to read and do simple arithmetic problems. In general, individuals with mild to moderate mental retardation tend to be concrete in their thinking and require simple, repeated instructions in order to learn tasks.

Except where there are obvious physical signs of retardation at birth (e.g., in the case of trisomy 21), functional delays observed by parents are most likely to result in the identification of individuals with mental retardation. Parents typically become concerned when a child does not sit, walk, or talk at the expected time.

Functional deficits tend to be pervasive, though as with all children, some areas may be more delayed than others (Dosen & Day, 2001). Functional decrements also are related to the type of retardation (Dykens & Hodapp, 2001). For example, children with Prader-Willi syndrome show a high degree of food-seeking behavior, high rates of tantrums and impulsivity, and increased risk for psychosis in adolescence. ADLs are a relative strength for individuals with fragile X syndrome as compared with individuals with trisomy 21 (Zigler & Hodapp, 1991), while children with trisomy 21 may have better social skills (Dykens & Hodapp, 2001). A child with mental retardation is likely to have motor, social, cognitive, sensory, and psychological deficits, though he or she may have relatively less motor delay than cognitive delay or less social delay than motor delay. For example, some children who are retarded may be quite sociable, but have difficulty with academic skills. Deficits are also roughly correlated with IQ, so that a profoundly retarded child is likely to have severely impaired function in all areas (Dykens & Hodapp, 2001).

Deficits occur in all performance areas: play, social interaction, ADLs, and education. These translate into later deficits in work, play, leisure, and ADLs/IADLs. Hellendoorn and Hoekman (1992) found that play was mental age appropriate rather than chronological age appropriate. From the perspective of occupational therapy, deficits can be anticipated not only in performance areas but also in skills and patterns.

Individuals with mental retardation may have some particular behavioral or situational problems, as well. Self-injurious behavior is noted in a subset of these individuals, particularly those with severe developmental delay (Symons & MacLean, 2000; Thompson & Caruso, 2002). Aggression has also been noted as a problem for some individuals with severe or profound mental retardation (Matson & Mayville, 2001). However, not only are individuals who have mental retardation possible perpetrators of aggression, they are also more likely than others to be victimized (Nettelbeck & Wilson, 2001). Each of these problems calls for particular attention in the assessment and intervention process.

An area of increasing focus is the situation of the adult who has mental retardation. As life expectancy increases for these individuals, and as the trend toward mainstreaming moves them out of institutional care, an array of issues has emerged (Thorpe, Davidson, & Janicki, 2000). Some individuals, particularly those with mild and moderate cognitive limitation, may choose to become parents (Holburn, Perkins, & Vietze, 2001) and will require either training or assistance to successfully manage this role. In addition, new problems may develop. For example, individuals with Down syndrome who survive into their 40s almost universally demonstrate signs of dementia similar to the symptoms of Alzheimer's disease (Thorpe et al., 2000).

A wide array of interventions have a role in the treatment of individuals with mental retardation (Dosen & Day, 2001). Medical treatment focuses on reversing treatable conditions and maximizing health to preserve intact function. Provision of adequate nutrition and exercise and monitoring of health in individuals unable to report symptoms are vital to optimal functioning.

Psychotropic medications can address specific behavioral or emotional correlates of mental retardation (Tyrer & Hill, 2001). Medication may be used by individuals who have accompanying behavioral problems or are self-injurious (Luiselli, Blew, & Thibadeau, 2001). Antidepressants, in particular, have shown promise in reducing these behaviors.

For children, educational approaches are most often employed. For those with mild impairment, "mainstreaming" (i.e., inclusion to the greatest degree possible in the regular school system) is the intervention of choice (Blair, 1999). They may have special classes during the course of the day and attend regular classes when possible. Those more severely impaired will attend special schools.

Behavioral interventions can be valuable both for children and adults (Gardner, Graeber-Whalen, & Ford, 2001). Enhanced social and vocational function can be obtained by carefully outlining the steps involved in each task, and then providing reinforcement as the individual accomplishes each step. Social learning interventions have shown considerable benefit for these individuals (Benson & Valenti-Hein, 2001). Less attention has been paid to leisure and play performance, but there is every reason to believe that this too can be enhanced through behavioral and educational approaches (Lifter, 2000). Community-based instruction (McDonnell, Hardman, Hightower, Keifer-O'Donnell, & Drew, 1993) and job training (Simmons & Flexer, 1992) with emphasis on repeated practice are successful in enhancing adaptive skills. Similarly, functional communication training (Durand & Carr, 1992) can yield long-term improvements in ability.

Residential intervention may be necessary for some individuals (Fleisher, Faulkner, Schalock, & Folk, 2001). In these settings, interaction with staff can lead to more independent functioning (Fleming & Reile, 1993). Fleming and Reile (1993) found that 80% of studies of such programs reported positive or mixed results.

It is important to note, however, that while many types of treatments appear to promote optimal function, none completely reverses retardation, except cases where it is medically possible to do so. On the other hand, recent evidence suggests that some types of retardation (e.g., trisomy 21) have better prognoses than assumed in the past. Some of these individuals achieve quite good function and report very positive levels of life satisfaction.

Implications for Occupational Therapy

For individuals who are retarded, the goal of treatment is most often habilitation (enabling) rather than rehabilitation, since they must acquire skills they never had rather than regain those lost. Since function varies from individual to individual, based both on sociocultural and biological factors (Dosen & Day, 2001), it is important to understand the cause of retardation for the individual, as well as his or her own particular strengths.

In general, goals of occupational therapy focus on facilitating maximal performance. This requires careful assessment of both deficits and strengths in all areas of potential occupational performance deficit (Baloueff, 1999). Individuals with mental retardation often wish to do the same activities as their peers and are able to accomplish many developmental milestones, albeit more slowly than others. Although recognition of strengths is important in working with any client, it is particularly vital with these individuals, as their strengths are often overlooked.

At the same time, realistic appraisal is necessary. It is essential to understand what constitutes the starting point for a particular individual and that the duration of the learning process for a particular skill may place limits on eventual achievement.

Performance areas that are of initial concern include self-care and play. Play is developmentally important for all children, and no less so for those with mental retardation (Lifter, 2000). Limitations in play may restrict later academic ability, social interaction, and language. Play training and play intervention, emphasizing provision of opportunities for play, prompting, and encouraging these behaviors can have an impact beyond that performance area. Educating parents regarding environmental enrichment can be of help in minimizing contextual reasons for limitation (Ramey & Ramey, 1999) and can also reduce family stress (Hodapp et al., 2001).

Skills may also require specific intervention. Motor, language, cognitive, and sensory processing skills can all be delayed. Accomplishment of performance in play, self-care, and academic work may be limited in the absence of adequate skill level. Some therapists have suggested that sensory-integration may be of value in remediating these problems (Gorman, 1997). Individuals who are profoundly retarded are unlikely to acquire more than minimal skills. Early intervention may need to focus on swallowing, in preparation for eating, and on movement to facilitate performance in self-care activities like dressing.

With children who are less severely retarded, training and education may prove quite valuable, particularly when practice is built in. For example, body awareness may facilitate dressing skills. In one school, children aged 6 to 10 years old spent several weeks playing "Simon Says," pointing to body parts on dolls, doing the "Hokey-Pokey" ("you put your left foot in...") and so on. Two months later, they were ready to begin putting legs into pant legs and arms into sleeves. It should be noted that sensory stimulation is a component of these activities and may also have a therapeutic benefit.

It is also important for these children to identify play activities at which they can succeed. Many have siblings they would like to emulate, but Little League may be beyond them unless leagues are specially organized. Not only must the individual identify leisure interests, but he or she must also have the mobility skills to get to those activities (McInerney & McInerney, 1992). Training and practice in use of public transportation is an essential factor in addressing all performance areas.

As these children age, vocational training and training in independent living skills, including training in social skills and sex education (Rhodes, 1993), become increasingly important. Although individuals who are retarded may desire the same activities as their peers who are not retarded, they tend to conceptualize at a concrete level. Because many will live independently or in semi-sheltered environments, they need to understand the accompanying responsibilities. One young woman, for example, expressed a wish for a child until she sat through an independent living group while a baby-doll cried in the background. Another young man planned to go to the movies every day until the therapist had him put his pay from the sheltered workshop in piles to represent rent, food, transportation, etc. This kind of parenting and independent living education is increasingly important as more individuals with mental retardation acquire these roles (Holburn et al., 2001).

Technological devices can provide some assistance (Sandknop, Schuster, Wolery, & Cross, 1992) as a means of structuring the environment to reduce demand. Devices must be carefully evaluated, and training should be provided until the individual is comfortable with their use. It is important to choose wisely because some devices add to rather than reduce complexity of tasks.

Presenting tasks in small steps allows for practice in sequence (Martin, 1989). An additional focus must be on self-esteem because these individuals often compare themselves negatively to others and must deal with pejorative comments by others. Mainstreamed children, for example, must contend with schoolmates who call them "moron" or "dummy."

As can be inferred from this discussion, treatment may occur in a variety of sites, including the home, a special school, a regular school, an institution, a sheltered workshop, or a supervised living facility. Increasingly, as a result of legislative emphasis on allowing every child access to the least restrictive environment, service is being provided in regular schools (Baloueff, 1999). Each setting requires sensitivity on the part of the therapist to the needs of the client, the possibility of movement from setting to setting (e.g., into a supervised apartment when custodial parents die), and the specific requirements for service provision in the setting. Children nearing the end of the educational process may need intensive work on vocational skills.

LEARNING DISORDERS (ACADEMIC SKILLS DISORDERS)

The learning disorders section of the DSM-IV (APA, 1994) was greatly clarified in 2000. In the form of DSM-IV-TR (APA, 2000), it now identifies a number of different conditions, including reading disorder, mathematics disorder, and disorder of written expression. The expansion of this section is particularly important to occupational therapists because of the frequency with which they treat children with academic skills disorders. For each of these diagnoses, characteristics that must be present include achievement substantially below age appropriate expectations and difficulties in daily life and/or academic performance because of the deficit. This category includes three specific disorders that may occur in isolation or in combination: reading disorder, mathematics disorder, and disorder of written expression.

Etiology and Incidence

Taken together, the learning disorders are found in somewhere between 2% and 10% of schoolchildren (APA, 2000). Data for individual disorders are very rough estimates at best because most studies group them together. However, it seems likely that reading disorder may occur in approximately 4% of the school-aged population.

Etiology is not well-established. Most literature supports a biological/neurological component (Gilger & Kaplan, 2001; Grigorenko, 2001; Keogh, 2002), while family studies indicate a genetic factor (Plomin, 2001). Family studies also suggest that prevalence of learning disorders is higher in children whose parents have a history of substance abuse (Martin, Romig, & Kirisci, 2000). It is unclear whether this finding is related to prenatal exposure to drugs or environmental factors during development.

Treatment and Prognosis

Some children grow out of their learning difficulties over time. For these children, the disorder may represent a developmental lag rather than a chronic disorder. It has been suggested by some researchers that learning disorders are developmental variants rather than true psychiatric disorders (Gilger & Kaplan, 2001; Keogh, 2002). If this is true, it might be expected that some of these children would catch up developmentally. For other children, learning disorders have long-term negative consequences. Approximately 5% of people with learning disorders are unresponsive to treatment; these individuals may represent those with true disorder as opposed to developmental variants (Keogh, 2002). Behavior problems are common (McGrath & Grant, 1993), possibly because children with these disorders may have trouble keeping up in class and become frustrated. Similarly, self-esteem may suffer as the child recognizes he or she is not able to do what others can. It appears that good outcomes can be predicted by good phonological processing early in life (Keogh, 2002) and when families provide adequate support (McGrath & Grant, 1993). When teachers and parents work together in planning and implementing treatment, outcomes seem better than when only the school or parent provides intervention (Bowers & Bailey, 2001).

Implications for Function and Treatment

Children with specific learning disorders, by definition, have deficits in the performance area of vocation, which for them is learning. Each of these disorders affects specific skills required to perform effectively in academic settings. Other skill areas may be affected as a consequence. For example, a child who has difficulty learning to read may develop secondary psychosocial difficulties. Patterns are affected in several ways. The child may adopt patterns that allow him or her to mask or manage the deficit. He or she may also develop an array of maladaptive patterns, including school avoidance, "trouble-making" behavior in the classroom, or other kinds of acting-out behavior. Ultimately, the establishment of effective patterns that facilitate compensation or accommodation can be very helpful in managing these disorders.

Identification of the difficulty is a particular concern. Often, these disorders are not noted until the child is in school, sometimes many years down the road (Keogh, 2002). Because many of these children have normal or above average intelligence, they may be able to compensate for their difficulties until schoolwork becomes complex. Late identification causes problems because the child may have already developed a sense of low self-esteem or behavioral deficits.

Treatment must begin with careful assessment to determine the exact nature of the difficulty (Bowers & Bailey, 2001; Gibbs & Priest, 1999). Following assessment, plans can be made to remediate deficits, often through occupational therapy. In addition, teachers can develop instructional plans that make use of alternate pathways available to the child. For example, a child with auditory learning difficulties may be able to make use of visual substitutes, and vice versa. These adaptive mechanisms can be extremely helpful but must be individualized. For example, one child with a disorder of written expression had great difficulty writing, but was able to use a computer with ease.

Implications for Occupational Therapy

There is a vast body of literature about occupational therapy for children with learning disabilities. Treatment of such children is a primary role for therapists in school systems. Screening is a particularly important role because parents and teachers may not know what to look for. Informing parents and teachers about signs of learning disorders can be quite valuable.

Further, occupational therapists assist teachers and parents in managing the difficulties and in providing direct treatment to the child. Sensory-integration is among the interventions that appear to be of value (Bundy, Lane, Fisher, & Murray, 2002). Students also benefit from neuropsychological interventions, cognitive training, accommodation, and compensation (Bowers & Bailey, 2001). One particularly important issue is the transferability of skill from academic to vocational settings as individuals reach adolescence. It is clear that demands of the work place differ from those of academic settings and that skills and accommodations learned in school may not be adequate to the new challenges (Bowers & Bailey, 2001).

MOTOR SKILLS DISORDER

This disorder, also labeled developmental coordination disorder, is characterized by incoordination; clumsiness; or delays in meeting developmental motor milestones for sitting, walking, etc. For a diagnosis to be made, these symptoms must impact on performance and must not be the result of a physical disorder, such as cerebral palsy.

Etiology and Incidence

In children aged 5 to 11, incidence is estimated at about 6% (APA, 2000). Etiology is not clear, although a biological component is suspected (Plomin, 2001).

Prognosis and Treatment

As with learning disorders, some children simply grow out of their difficulties. However, in about half of these children, difficulties persist beyond age 12 (Geuze & Borger, 1993). In those in whom the disorder is more chronic, teachers report behavioral and learning problems. Treatment is similar to that for learning disorders, involving a great deal of motor practice, as well as accommodation and compensation.

Implications for Occupational Therapy

Occupational therapists are very directly involved in treatment of this disorder. In addition to screening, assessment, and consultation with teachers and parents, therapists provide direct treatment (Kinnealey & Miller, 1993). Play that encourages gross motor activity has the potential to strengthen muscles and provide sensory input that may enhance skill.

COMMUNICATION DISORDERS

Included in this category are expressive language disorder, mixed expressive-receptive language disorder, phonological disorder, and stuttering. Expressive language disorder is characterized by difficulty producing sounds in an age-appropriate fashion, as well as difficulty with vocabulary, sentence structure, and grammar. It is very common among young children. By age 17, incidence drops to about 0.5% (APA, 2000). Expressive-receptive language disorder has the above characteristics plus receptive difficulties, such as problems understanding others' language. Phonological disorder is typified by pronunciation difficulties without the accompanying problems with language usage.

Stuttering is an impairment of speech fluency. It may be an inability to produce specific sounds or an inability to control repetitions of sounds or words (Wingate, 2002). As the disorder becomes established, anxiety about speaking appears, exacerbating the problem (Boscolo, Ratner, & Rescorla, 2002). Delay in language development and articulation problems are common among children who stutter. Stuttering almost certainly has a biological substrate (DeNili & Kroll, 2001).

In these disorders, functional impairment depends on the severity of the disorder, the individual's determination, and the understanding of others. Leisure and academic pursuits may be more difficult because of these communication difficulties. Treatment is most often provided by speech therapists, who use such strategies as operant conditioning (Onslow, Ratner, & Packman, 2001) and practice. Occupational therapists may be involved if there is any accompanying learning disability or damage to self-esteem that might be remedied through success with activities.

Co-Occurrence of Learning, Motor, and Expressive Disorders

Several researchers have noted that these disorders frequently occur in combination in children (Gibbs & Priest, 1999; Nippold, 2001). Further, children with these disorders may develop other psychological problems, including anxiety and depression. These findings have obvious implications for screening, requiring therapists, teachers, and others to be alert to signs of difficulties beyond single learning disabilities. They also have implications for treatment, which must take into account the multiple problems that some of these children have. At the same time, therapists are well-advised to keep in mind that, for some children, learning disabilities may represent developmental variants that, with appropriate intervention, can be remediated very successfully. For such children, a major task for occupational therapists is support in maintaining self-esteem and self-concept until development can catch up to task demands.

PERVASIVE DEVELOPMENTAL DISORDERS

Five disorders are included under this heading: autism, Rett syndrome, childhood disintegrative disorder, Asperger's syndrome, and pervasive developmental disorder not otherwise specified. The two most common of these disorders, autism and Asperger's syndrome, will be described in detail here.

Autism

Although this is a relatively rare condition, it has received considerable notice possibly because of the extreme nature of the deficits with which it is associated. A number of popular books (Grandin, 1996; Greenfield, 1986) have brought it to the attention of the general public. In order for the diagnosis to be made, social interaction, communication, and activity must be impaired. Children with autism lack speech or have peculiar speech patterns and have severe social deficits, decreased imitation, and stereotypic gesturing and motor behaviors (Rogers, 2001). Children with autism may sit without making eye contact or speaking while engaging in some self-stimulating behavior, possibly spinning their bodies or twirling their hair for hours on end. They show poor cognitive flexibility, verbal reasoning, complex memory, complex language association, and, in particular, poor social communication (Tanguay, 2000).

Autism often occurs in the presence of other disorders, particularly mental retardation. It must be distinguished from schizophrenia and other psychotic disorders. Differential diagnosis is based on the severe language and social deficits that occur in autism, as well as the probable low IQ. Autism is distinct from pure mental retardation because of the variability of IQ in different areas (performance and verbal), which is a hallmark of autism.

Etiology and Incidence

The etiology of autism is increasingly well-understood. At one point it was considered a problem of inadequate parenting, believed to be associated with maternal coldness, absence, or rejection (Weininger, 1993). This idea has been largely discredited, and current hypotheses center on the possibility of some sort of neurological dysfunction, possibly of genetic origin (Mackowiak, 2000). Brain abnormalities have been found in the cerebellum, limbic system, and cortex, and there is evidence of defective lateralization (Townsend et al., 2001). In addition, neurochemical abnormalities have been found, with suspicion focused on the role of dopamine agonists. A great deal of research interest has focused on genetic causes for these brain and biochemical disorders (Andres, 2002; Cook, 2001). Family studies reveal a risk of 60% for monozygotic twins with a 90% risk for some sort of social/behavioral problems in the second twin. Interest has also focused on the possible role of measles-mumps-rubella (MMR) vaccination, in part because of the epidemiological observation that rates of autism went up at about the time the MMR vaccination became common. However, that theory has been discredited by repeated research study of the issue (DeStefano & Chen, 2001).

According to the APA (2000), incidence is approximately 5 cases per 10,000 individuals, although reports range from 2 to 20 cases per 10,000 individuals. This compares with reports a decade ago of approximately 2 cases per 10,000 individuals (Verheij & van Loon, 1992). More recent reports from the National Institutes of Child Health and Development (2001) suggest rates as high as 1 in 500. The reasons for these disparate estimates are not clear, nor is it clear which is accurate. However, there are concerns about an apparent dramatic increase in reported cases of autism in recent years. The disorder is much more common in males.

It is noteworthy that in about 20% of cases, parents report that the child seems to develop normally for the first year or two of life (Hatton, 2002). It is not clear whether this is a feature of the disorder's onset or whether the symptoms may not be noticed because the skills in which deficits occur do not develop until age 18 months or later. It is also possible that there are two different types of autism: one primary (i.e., present at birth) and one regressive (i.e., emerging after the first 2 years or so of life). Because diagnosis is based on symptoms, not on lab tests, this remains an open question.

Prognosis

In general, prognosis is poor for individuals with autism (Larsen & Mouridsen, 1997). By one estimate only about 20% of individuals with autism are able to lead moderately independent lives as adults (Howlin & Goode, 1998), although it appears that those who have better speech, higher IQ, effective educational interventions, and special skills or interests tend to do better than others. Another estimate is that approximately 25% will experience good quality of life as adults, while another 50% will experience acceptable quality of life (Hameury et al., 1995). While some individuals may show unpredictable improvements, the majority continue to be relatively impaired throughout life and some may deteriorate in adolescence. Long-term consequences include increased stress for families of adolescents and adults with autism because of the additional responsibilities for care of these individuals (Seltzer, Krauss, Orsmond, & Vestal, 2001). These negative reports regarding outcome must be balanced against the occasional reports, like that of Grandin (1996), from individuals with autism who live productive and fulfilling lives, albeit with persistent deficits. Grandin reports having little patience with or understanding of social banter, for example, and her social life is quite circumscribed. On the other hand, she is credited with major advances in animal handling, derived from her sense of empathy for nonhuman beings, and her self-described quality of life is good.

Implications for Function and Treatment

Autistic individuals show extreme impairments in the skill areas of social functioning, ability to communicate, as well as in performance of most activities (Rogers, 2001). These impairments may be characterized by peculiarities in performance or by absence of performance. For example, an autistic individual may be able to speak but may put words together in ways that are not meaningful to others. Similarly, he or she may be able to perform specific fine motor tasks but is unable to put them together into a meaningful sequence of activities to accomplish a specific task.

The deficits in function are quite severe, usually precluding most forms of normal goal-oriented occupation. Autistic individuals are often unable to perform ADLs and IADLs, have disturbed patterns of play, and may be unable to study and, later, to work. Communication skills are particularly poor (Pelios & Lund, 2001). Half of individuals with autism never develop speech, and most fail to use speech in a functional way. Social interaction is severely impaired (Ghuman, Ghuman, & Ford, 1998), with decreased imitation and social response (Rogers, 2001).

Individuals with autism may have areas of unusually good function, such as excellent rote memory, visual/spatial skills, or attention to detail (Pelios & Lund, 2001). These abilities may be associated with selective attention to particular features of the surroundings that other children might not notice. This selective attention may be accompanied by stereotypic interactions with objects, such as spinning them or placing them in particular patterns. Individuals with autism typically display excessively routinized and unproductive patterns of behavior. Their stereotypic movements and verbalizations are quite entrenched but do not contribute to functional outcomes.

Because the etiology is as yet unclear, treatment is not well-established. A wide array of treatments have been attempted, including both psychosocial and biological strategies.

Behavioral interventions are widely recommended (Eikeseth, Smith, Jahr, & Eldevik, 2002), with a focus on developing speech, increasing behaviors such as ADL skills, or decreasing undesirable behaviors such as peculiar movements (Boyd & Corley, 2001). More and more autistic children are in community settings, such as public schools, often in special classes. However, many programs are still provided at special schools or in-patient settings, as they are usually designed to provide high levels of input throughout the day.

Behavior modification has been employed for specific deficits. Early intensive behavioral intervention (EIBI) is advocated by a number of therapists (Boyd & Corley, 2001; Pelios & Lund, 2001). Applied behavior analysis is considered a "best practice" in some areas and involves careful assessment of specific behaviors accompanied by detailed plans for intervention based on behavior modification principles. Because of the severity of dysfunction, behavioral programs usually focus on small components of performance, making global improvement an extremely long-term goal. In an effort to provide more general intervention, environmental enrichment with sensory stimulation has been employed with some success.

Early intervention is increasingly viewed as important (Rogers, 2001). Early intervention can provide families with a sense of relief that their concerns are being taken seriously and can help insure that appropriate treatment strategies are identified. Because of their unique sets of strengths and weaknesses, tailored early intervention can help children with autism learn most effectively. It is possible that early intervention may be associated with better outcomes, although the research on this issue is equivocal.

Biological intervention focuses on drug treatment to ameliorate symptoms such as anxiety and hyperactivity. Clomipramine and pimozide are among the drugs used with some evidence of positive outcome (Ernst et al., 1992; Gordon, State, Nelson, Hamburger, & Rapoport, 1993). Clozapine (Gobbi & Pulvirenti, 2001) and fluoxetine (Peral, Alcami, & Gilaberte, 1999) have also been used. Vitamins (Ferraro, 2001) and special diets (Whiteley, Rodgers, Savery, & Shattock, 1999) are other biological interventions that have been attempted.

It should be noted that over the years, a wide array of interventions of questionable value have been advocated (Ferraro, 2001). One that experiences periodic resurgence of popularity is the Doman-Delcato theory. This theory suggests that children with developmental difficulties have somehow skipped or failed to master earlier developmental stages. By "patterning" these earlier steps (e.g., repeatedly moving the child in a normal creeping pattern), the earlier stages can be mastered, allowing for enhanced function. Research does not support this method, and it has been criticized for creating unrealistic expectations in family members, increasing the already substantial level of stress they are likely to experience (Seltzer et al., 2001).

Implications for Occupational Therapy

Because autistic children are so severely impaired, observation must often substitute for formal assessment, and treatment goals must be sensitive to the probability that change will occur in very small steps. Behavioral and sensory-integration interventions seem to be the treatments of choice for most occupational therapists (Case-Smith & Miller, 1999; Watling et al., 1999).

In general, focus is on basic self-care and communication. Motivation and attention are key issues. Behavioral techniques may be helpful both in enhancing attention and in training autistic children to perform sequences of activities related to self-care.

There is some evidence that play behavior can be enhanced using self-management intervention (Stahmer & Schreibman, 1992). This involves demonstration of appropriate toy use followed by reinforcement of appropriate play. Likewise, sensory integration intervention seems to have the potential to increase goal-directed play (Case-Smith & Bryan, 1999).

Sensory integration interventions are widely used by occupational therapists working with children with autism. These interventions appear to decrease disruptive behavior and increase functional behaviors, including conversation and functional play (Linderman & Stewart, 1999). It is likely that occupational therapy interventions are best provided in the context of multidisciplinary intervention (Aldred et al., 2001; Jordan, 2001; Raffin, 2001), particularly since it is not clear which of the many educational, behavioral, environmental, and biological treatments are most effective (Gabriels et al., 2001).

Asperger's Syndrome

There are those who view autism as a spectrum disorder (i.e., a disorder that can range from mild to severe) (Tanguay, 2000). These individuals hold that Asperger's syndrome is essentially mild autism (Ozonoff, South, & Miller, 2000). However, while Asperger's syndrome does have elements in common with autism and is, indeed, less severe, other researchers believe that there are unique characteristics that distinguish it from so-called mild autism (Gillberg, 1998; Safran, 2001). These researchers suggest that Asperger's syndrome is characterized by higher IQ and absence of language deficits as compared with autism, including mild autism.

To some extent, the debate is irrelevant to occupational therapy. It is clear that there are some children who have autistic-like symptoms, but who are able to function reasonably well. They show some of the stereotypic and obsessive features of autism and lack empathy, but are able to communicate, to learn, and to live independently as adults (Safran, 2001). Parents report that the diagnostic process can be frustrating, as health care providers debate degrees of dysfunction (Schuntermann, 2002). The diagnosis of Asperger's syndrome has become much more common. It is estimated to affect approximately 2 individuals per 1,000 (Tanguay, 2000). From a pragmatic perspective, whether or not it is identical to high functioning autism, the recommendations for intervention are almost identical.

Those recommendations include educational interventions focused on teaching specific social skills (Tanguay, 2000), behavior therapy to improve communication skills and decrease bizarre behaviors, and sensory-integrative approaches to reduce deficits in modulation of sensory input (Dunn, Myles, & Orr, 2002). Structured teaching in the classroom involving careful organization of the physical environment; provision of routines, schedules, and clear expectations; and an emphasis on student interests and skills can also be helpful (Safran, 2001). Medication may be helpful for some of these children in managing anxiety, depression, or hyperactivity. SSRIs and Ritalin are among the medications that may be of help.

The prognosis for individuals with Asperger's syndrome is significantly better than for individuals with autism (Howlin & Goode, 1998; Larsen & Mouridsen, 1997; Nordin &

Gillberg, 1998). While behavioral deficits persist into adulthood, they can often be managed as "quirks" of personality, and the individual can work, manage ADLs and IADLs independently, and sometimes even maintain close relationships. As an example, one child with Asperger's syndrome attended public school and participated in regular classroom activities. He was described by his peers as "odd," but socialized with several classmates nonetheless. He had excellent computer and music skills, and these skills were likely to contribute to later vocational choices.

Other Pervasive Developmental Disorders

DSM-IV-TR (APA, 2000) includes several other pervasive developmental disorders (PDD) distinct from autistic disorder. These other diagnoses are arrived at based on differences in symptoms (Tanguay, 2000). For example, a child with Rett syndrome is more likely to show extreme social aloofness than are those with fragile X syndrome. Subtle differences in symptoms have implications for choice of therapy (Verheij & van Loon, 1992). Verheij and van Loon recommend careful assessment of sensory, sensorimotor, attention, cognitive, emotional, and speech development, and the impact of these on play. Their recommendation is that treatment focus on reducing anxiety, eliminating impeding behavior, and stimulating growth and development, largely through education and behavior modification.

DISRUPTIVE BEHAVIOR DISORDERS

These disorders are reflected in behavior that may initially be more disturbing to others than to the individual. However, the presence of these disorders may have long-term effects on self-esteem and social participation, as the individual is likely to receive considerable social censure and rejection as a result of his or her behavior. In addition, manifested behaviors may interfere with learning, causing long-term academic problems.

Attention-Deficit and Disruptive Behavior Disorders

Included in this category are attention-deficit/hyperactivity disorder (ADHD), both with and without hyperactivity, conduct disorder (CD), oppositional defiant disorder (ODD), and disruptive behavior disorder. These disorders have a very high rate of comorbidity (Lahey, McBurnett, & Loeber, 2000; Loeber, Green, Lahey, Frick, & McBurnett, 2000; Waschbusch, 2002), leading some to speculate that they are spectrum disorders. However, they do also occur as separate disorders, and there is not an absolute or automatic progression from one to another. DSM-IV-TR (APA, 2000) treats them as separate. Occupational therapists are frequently called upon to treat children with ADHD, and often see children with ODD or CD as well.

Attention-Deficit Hyperactivity Disorder

This disorder is characterized by excessive inattention, impulsiveness, and hyperactivity. Typically, the child has difficulty attending to others and is extremely active physically. Problematic behaviors, including at least six specific symptoms of inattention, impulsiveness, or hyperactivity must be present for at least 6 months for the diagnosis to be made. The behaviors must be judged to be more severe than in normal children, a criterion that presents significant diagnostic difficulties, as noted below. In addition, the behaviors must interfere with social, academic, or vocational performance. The problem behaviors must appear prior to age 7 to be diagnosed as ADHD.

Overall, this disorder is reported to be readily diagnosable based on DSM-IV-TR (APA, 2000) criteria (Casat, Pearson, & Casat, 2001). However, in some instances, the diagnosis is difficult, as individual adult perceptions of and tolerance for activity in children varies (Hudziak, 2001). What is labeled "youthful exuberance" in some families may be intolerable to other parents. In some children, the diagnosis is not made until the school years, when ADHD may interfere with the ability to complete school work. In other instances, the diagnosis may be made on the basis of the adult's difficulty accepting the behavior, rather than on clearly disturbed behavior on the part of the child. In addition, there is some evidence that the hyperactivity may be situation specific (Anastopoulos, Klinger & Temple, 2001), so that the child may be impulsive and excessively active in some circumstances but not others. For the most part, however, these children are easily recognizable. They respond to the slightest distraction, running to chase dust, sunlight, and every small sound, rather than focusing on tasks for periods of time. Their level of activity is often exhausting just to watch.

The diagnosis of attention-deficit disorder (ADD) without hyperactivity is even more difficult because inattention may be misunderstood as disinterest, daydreaming, or lack of ability to accomplish required tasks. Persistent inability to focus, inattention to instructions, and, on occasion, stereotypic actions (e.g., doodling rather than doing homework) may suggest ADD without hyperactivity. It is important to distinguish this disorder from boredom or depression.

ADD is an excellent example of a culturally-mediated disorder. In more agricultural societies, ADD is relatively unknown, perhaps because physical activity is more expected and desirable in those circumstances, and the kind of concentration required for school work is less vital. Similarly, some cultures allow more latitude for variation in activity level and educational attainment.

Etiology and Incidence

Etiology of ADHD is not clearly established, although it is suspected that it may occur in the presence of neurological damage or a disordered CNS. First described by Hoffman in 1926, it was originally called minimal brain damage (MBD). Later, it was known as hyperkinetic impulse disorder, then hyperactivity (Casat et al., 2001). ADHD is believed to be a frontal lobe brain dysfunction (Reeve & Schandler, 2001) that affects both executive function (Sergeant, Geurts, & Oosterlaan, 2002) and sensory processing (Dunn & Bennett, 2002).

There is a clear genetic component to the disorder (Bradley & Golden, 2001; Faraone, 2000; Quist & Kennedy, 2001), although there is also speculation that genes alone do not explain the emergence of the disorder. Among the other contributing factors that have been hypothesized, the idea of some sort of dietary influence has been largely discredited (Bradley & Golden, 2001). Hypoxia during birth, maternal smoking, low birth weight, and other environmental factors do seem associated with ADHD (Bradley & Golden, 2001).

This is the most common disorder treated in children (Wilens, Biederman & Spencer, 2002), occurring in 3% to 5% of the population. It is more common in males, although there is some speculation that this is the result of underdiagnosis in girls (Wilens et al., 2002).

Prognosis

Prognosis is good for some children who seem to "outgrow" the disorder as they get older (Lie, 1991). Most children in this group do well, and there is no evidence of higher rates of alcoholism or criminal behavior for these children. Learning disabilities and motor and perceptual problems disappear over time or are compensated for. There is increasing evidence, however, that the disorder persists into adolescence and adulthood for some individuals and that adults can demonstrate symptoms identical to those in children with ADHD (Barkley, Fischer, Smallish, & Fletcher, 2002; Wilens et al., 2002).

A potential negative consequence of ADHD is the possibility that the child will become depressed or develop low self-esteem as a result of the social disapproval or academic difficulties that often accompany the disorder (Faraone & Doyle, 2001). Understandably, the prognosis is less favorable if ADHD is accompanied by retardation or some other behavioral disorder, such as CD or substance abuse (Lynskey & Hall, 2001; Waschbusch, 2002). Comorbidity of these disorders occurs at a relatively high rate among a subset of individuals with ADHD and may account for some of the differences in prognosis reported in various research studies.

Implications for Function and Treatment

Children with ADHD are able to function in many areas. They are usually able to perform age-appropriate ADLs and IADLs, to play, and to interact with peers. Generally speaking, social and academic performance are most impaired (Forness & Kavale, 2001). Peers and adults may find the excessive activity and difficulty concentrating annoying, and avoid or chastise the child. In some instances, poor impulse control leads the child to behave in socially inappropriate or antisocial fashion, again leading to disapproval or legal difficulties. These children may have difficulty in peer relationships persisting into adolescence (Bagwell, Molina, Pelham, & Hoza, 2001).

Developmental stages may alter the ways in which ADHD is expressed (Anastopoulos et al., 2001). In toddlers, it can manifest as impatience to gain desired objects. In preschool children, inattentiveness may be noted, as these children move rapidly from one activity to another. Often, it is entry into kindergarten that brings first recognition of the problem, as the requirement of the situation is that children sit still and attend for increasing time periods. However, the fact that the inattentiveness and hyperactivity may vary with the situation can be challenging, as parents may perceive nothing wrong while teachers are reporting problem behavior in school. In other instances, hyperactivity is clear in the home environment as well. One parent reported that her son routinely ran out into the street while playing, with total disregard for traffic. She indicated that he could sit still for only a few minutes while watching TV or listening to her read. This example may not be typical of all children with ADHD, as some can focus well on particular kinds of activities (e.g., watching TV), while other activities promote significant hyperactivity (particularly in school).

Poor concentration and impulse control present significant problems in the academic sphere (Forness & Kavale, 2001). Not only is learning impaired, but teachers find these children difficult to manage, compounding the students' learning problems. They often do poorly in school and then become anxious about their performance, exacerbating their learning difficulties. Other activities that require concentration or attention may be difficult or impossible for these children, limiting the play and leisure activities in which they are able to participate.

Medication is used frequently to control ADHD (Anastopoulos et al., 2001). Amphetamines, Ritalin in particular, are often used. The exact mechanism by which they work is not known, but they seem helpful in focusing attention. They are reported to be effective in as many as 80% to 90% of children, although somewhat less effective with younger children. There is controversy about the use of these drugs, as their long-term effects are not thought to be adequately understood. Some researchers believe that they are used too freely, particularly in cases where the diagnosis may be marginal. Recently, however, some researchers have begun to suggest that the drugs are actually underutilized (Forness & Kavale, 2001).

Other interventions are both behavioral and environmental (Anastopoulos et al., 2001). Behavioral approaches attempt to reinforce efforts to concentrate and control hyperactivity. Environmental approaches are used to design low stimulus environments in which distractions are kept to a minimum. Parent education can be helpful. Cognitive-behavioral therapy is of value with older children.

Implications for Occupational Therapy

As the name of the disorder implies, attention is an important factor when working with these children. Several approaches may be useful (Florey, 1998). Environmental structuring to minimize distraction may help the child focus on the task at hand. Occupational therapy may also provide patterned, sequenced sensory input to attempt to help the child better organize his or her reactions to the environment. Ideally, this input is provided through play or other meaningful occupations.

Self-esteem is an important issue for these children. Identification of activities they can do well can be enormously helpful in convincing them that they do have strengths, despite repeated scoldings from exasperated adults.

Often, the occupational therapist teaches parents and teachers to manage difficult behaviors. Assisting them in structuring the learning or home environment optimally, breaking tasks into chunks, or providing deep touch to help the child gain control may help the adult cope better and the child function better.

Conduct Disorder

A diagnosis of CD is made when the individual has engaged in at least three episodes of behavior within the past 12 months in which societal norms are violated, such as aggression, destruction of property, lying or theft, or violation of rules. The diagnosis may be made for children, adolescents, or occasionally for adults who do not meet the criteria for antisocial personality disorder.

Etiology and Incidence

Etiology of this disorder is not clearly established. The two main schools of thought are that it is either an environmental or a biological/genetic disorder (Lynam & Henry, 2001; Simonoff, 2001). As the disorder is better understood, it is increasingly clear that the proximal cause of the disorder is misinterpretation of social situations with concomitant inappropriate choice of response (Dodge, 2000). What this means is that when individuals with CD are presented with situations, they may encode cues incorrectly because of attention to the wrong stimuli or an inability to receive sensory input adequately. They may misinterpret the encoded cues or may access ineffective or inappropriate behavioral responses. Finally, they may act inappropriately from the array of responses available to them.

However, this proximal sequence of events in specific situations seems to be caused by a set of complex developmental factors. These include genetic characteristics and *in utero* exposures or experiences (Dodge, 2000; Simonoff, 2001). For example, maternal smoking is associated with CD (Loeber et al., 2000). Autonomic nervous system alterations, such as low heart rate, have been associated with CD, as have deficits in information processing (Dodge, 2000). In addition to biological factors, environmental factors, particularly associated with the family, appear to contribute to the development of CD (Dodge, 2000). Homelessness (Torrance, 1998) and low maternal age (Wakschlag et al., 2000) are among these environmental factors. Parenting style has been strongly implicated, with inconsistent, over-permissive, or excessively harsh parenting all cited as factors (Dodge, 2000). One challenge is in understanding the complex interplay of these many biological and environmental factors (Webster-Stratton, 2000).

CD occurs in roughly 3.6% to 6.6% of children and adolescents (Simonoff, 2001).

Prognosis

With appropriate treatment, approximately one-half (Loeber et al., 2000) to two-thirds (Webster-Stratton, 2000) of children with CD will improve. However, the remainder may well develop antisocial personality disorder, substance abuse, or other disorders of adulthood (Robins, 1999).

Implications for Function and Treatment

Many of these individuals have difficulty with school/work performance, possibly as the result of cognitive or attention deficits, or as a result of attitudinal problems (Webster-Stratton, 2000). For example, reading disabilities have been identified in many of these children. ADL and IADL functions typically are not impaired. Leisure and play tend to focus on socially unacceptable activities, as acting-out may take the place of more normal endeavors. In fact, aggressive behavior and stealing are almost universal among children with CD (Robins, 1999).

These children are more likely to have social difficulties, which may stem from poor ability to detect and understand social cues from others (Dodge, 2000). This finding has led to speculation that training in these skills might improve function and reduce symptoms.

A whole range of treatment options is available, including psychotherapy, behavior therapy, social learning, cognitive therapy, academic intervention, parent training, and recreational programming (Frick, 2000). Pharmacotherapy may also be attempted, including anticonvulsants, antidepressants, and beta blockers. Risperidone is among the medications that have been reported to be of value (Findling et al., 2000).

Implications for Occupational Therapy

Occupational therapists work with children with CD in several ways. First, energy may be channeled to more appropriate activities, with copious reinforcement for acceptable behavior. Expectations for behavior during such activities must be carefully identified and reasonable positive or negative outcomes systematically provided. Engagement in recreation can be of value (Webster-Stratton, 2000) as a way to provide experiences of success in acceptable activities.

Opportunities for appropriate expression of emotion appear to be helpful (Mpofu & Crystal, 2001), as children with CD are often unable to express feelings adequately and are inclined to act out their anger. Providing alternative strategies for emotional expression through play, art, music, or movement may be effective. Experiences of success in positive activities can be of great value in building a more positive self-concept.

Parent training can be effective in situations in which parents lack adequate skills to manage their children (Maughan & Rutter, 2001). Parents can be taught to provide appro-

priate reinforcement of positive behaviors and to provide intervention and negative consequences in the most effective fashion to minimize behavioral problems.

At the same time, the possibility of coexisting deficits must be considered. ADHD should
be addressed, as described above. Specific learning disabilities should also be remediated.

Oppositional Defiant Disorder

A less severe variant of CD is ODD. According to DSM-IV-TR (APA, 2000), this disorder is diagnosed based on a pattern of hostile or defiant behavior of at least 6 months duration that causes noticeable impairment of function. It is reported to be related to CD
(Hoffenaar & Hoeksma, 2002), but diagnostically different enough to be listed separately.
Risk of problems with the legal system is much lower, and school problems tend to be less
severe. Similarly, prognosis is better over the long term. Interventions are similar to those
used with individuals with CD.

Separation Anxiety Disorder

This disorder is typified by anxiety or panic related to threatened separation from familiar caretakers or presence of unfamiliar adults. Onset is prior to age 18, duration is at least 4
weeks, and the disorder causes functional decline. The decline relates to reluctance to go to
school or engage in other activities away from the immediate family (Chandler, 2002).

Other anxiety disorders, including obsessive-compulsive disorder (Swedo, Leonard, &
Rapoport, 1992; Thomsen, 1992), can occur in children and adolescents. Other anxiety disorders in children are discussed in Chapter 8.

Etiology and Incidence

The etiology of this disorder is not well understood, although it may have a biological
basis, as is suspected of some of the adult anxiety disorders. There has also been speculation
about premature separation from a primary caregiver (Bowlby, 1969). More recent theories
focus on the role of learning and of neurobiology (Chandler, 2002).

This disorder occurs in 4% of the population and is more common in females (APA, 2000).

Prognosis

In some instances, the disorder disappears spontaneously, sometimes after only one
episode. In other cases, it may become severe and disabling, as the individual may develop
a social phobia or school phobia and refuse to leave the home. The child may have a stom-
ach-ache every morning or cry and scream when the school bus comes (Chandler, 2002).
Remediation is easiest in those situations in which there are clear environmental factors,
such as excessive pressure to perform well in school, contributing to the problem. Altering
the environment may be quite effective in those situations. One child got sick at school
every morning before computer class. She improved when she received individual tutoring
that convinced her she could handle the work.

Implications for Function and Treatment

As noted, in severe cases, school, social, and leisure activities may be severely compromised. Individuals may become so anxious at the thought of having to perform in one of

these spheres that they become physically ill. ADLs are usually not affected, nor are IADLs, which may be performed in the home. However, activities that require interacting with strangers or leaving familiar environments may be all but impossible. It appears to be performance (i.e., school and leisure activity) rather than motor, social, or other skill that is impaired.

Treatment is not well understood, although some theorists suspect that altering home circumstances to provide a more stable, less pressuring environment may be helpful. Some behavioral techniques are also valuable, as are relaxation techniques (Chandler, 2002). Cognitive therapy, often useful for adults with anxiety disorders, works best for older children and adolescents (Chandler, 2002). Antianxiety and antidepressant medications are also useful in some situations.

Implications for Occupational Therapy

Relaxation techniques may be helpful to children with anxiety disorders. Using mental imagery to picture success, enjoyment, and relaxation can provide a useful prelude to anxiety-provoking activities.

In addition, activities in and of themselves can be relaxing, particularly if those that are enjoyable to the child can be identified. Sometimes pairing a pleasant activity with one that evokes anxiety can relieve feelings of distress. The student who felt sick before computer class did well when the task was playing computer games rather than doing schoolwork. The positive association later generalized to other computer activities.

Expressive arts may be beneficial as a way to uncover and explore fears. A child who was afraid to leave his room drew pictures of enormous snakes and spiders. It turned out that he had encountered a snake in his basement that had greatly frightened him. It was then possible to address his fear.

OTHER DISORDERS OF INFANCY, CHILDHOOD, AND ADOLESCENCE

There are numerous other disorders that may occur in younger individuals. Some are the same as those that occur in adults, including schizophrenia (Kumra, Nicolson, & Rapoport, 2002), obsessive-compulsive disorder (Wever & Rey, 1997), and mood disorders (Akin, 2001). Suicidal behavior has been noted in children as young as preschool, although the reasons for the behavior differ from those of adults (Fasko & Fasko, 1991). The most common cause was expected punishment; other reasons were escape from an unpleasant situation and a desire for reunion with a significant other who had died.

Table 3-2 provides a brief summary of the symptoms and functional implications of the most common disorders of childhood. There are a number of other childhood disorders (APA, 2000), including eating, tic, and elimination disorders; elective mutism; stereotypic movement disorder; and reactive attachment disorder, that are discussed briefly in Chapter 10.

Table 3-2
Developmental Disorders

Disorder	Symptoms	Functional Deficits
Mental retardation	I. Subaverage	Potential deficit in intelligence and all performance areas Roles may not be affected, but habit and routine may be difficult to establish
	2. Deficits in adaptive function cognitive	Deficits in process and communication likely Motor skills may or may not be affected
	3. Appears before age 18	Range from mild to severe
Autistic disorder	1. Impaired social interaction	All performance areas show substantial deficits May exhibit excessively patterned behavior
	2. Impaired communication process	Deficits in process skills pronounced, motor skills may be impaired Motor performance may not be goal-directed
	3. Restricted activity	Severe
	4. Onset during infancy or childhood	
ADHD	1. Restlessness, distractability	Affects education, work, social participation particularly; may also affect play, leisure, and ADLs/IADLs Habits and routines impaired Roles are not typically affected
	2. Excessive activity	Motor skills not impaired, process skills affected, manifested by impulsivity, poor control Communication minimally affected
	3. Impulsivity	May improve during adolescence
	4. Onset before age 7	

(continued)

Table 3-2 (Continued)		
Disorder	**Symptoms**	**Functional Deficits**
CD	1. Has engaged in at least three antisocial acts within the past 12 months	Self-care may be impaired Work and education typically the most seriously affected Patterns focus on anti-social roles and activities
Separation anxiety disorder	1. Excessive anxiety	School, social, and leisure patterns affected

REFERENCES

Akin, L.K. (2001). Pediatric and adolescent bipolar disorder: Medical resources. *Medical Reference Services Quarterly, 20*(3), 31-44.

Aldred, C., Pollard, C., Phillips, R., & Adams, C. (2001). Multidisciplinary social communication intervention for children with autism and pervasive developmental disorder: The Child's Talk project. *Educational and Child Psychology, 18*(2), 76-87.

American Psychiatric Association. (1994). *Diagnostic and statistical manual of mental disorders* (4th ed.). Washington, DC: Author.

American Psychiatric Association. (2000). *Diagnostic and statistical manual of mental disorders* (4th ed., text revision). Washington, DC: Author.

Anastopoulos, A.D., Klinger, E.E., & Temple, E.P. (2001). Treating children and adolescents with attention-deficit/hyperactivity disorder. In J.N. Hughes, A.M. LaGreca, & J.C. Close (Eds.), *Handbook of psychological services for children and adolescents* (pp. 245-266). Oxford: Oxford University Press.

Andres, C. (2002). Molecular genetics and animal models in autistic disorder. *Brain Research Bulletin, 57*, 109-119.

Bagwell, C.L., Molina, B.S.G., Pelham, W.E., & Hoza, B. (2001). Attention-deficit hyperactivity disorder and problems in peer relations: Predictions from childhood to adolescence. *Journal of the American Academy of Child and Adolescent Psychiatry, 40*, 1285-1292.

Bailey, D.B., Aytch, L.S., Odom, S.L., Symons, F., & Wolery, M. (1999). Early intervention as we know it. *Mental Retardation and Developmental Disabilities Research Reviews, 5*, 11-20

Baloueff, O. (1999). Developmental delay and mental retardation. In M.E. Neistadt & E.B. Crepeau (Eds.), *Willard & Spackman's occupational therapy* (9th ed., pp. 576-581). Baltimore, MD: Lippincott, Williams & Wilkins.

Barkley, R.A., Fischer, M., Smallish, L., & Fletcher, K. (2002). The persistence of attention-deficit/hyperactivity disorder into young adulthood as a function of reporting source and definition of disorder. *Journal of Abnormal Psychiatry, 111*, 279-289.

Bellinger, D.C., Stiles, K.M., & Needleman, H.L. (1992). Low-level lead exposure, intelligence and academic achievement: A long-term follow-up study. *Pediatrics, 90*, 855-861.

Benson, B.A., & Valenti-Hein, D.C. (2001). Cognitive and social learning treatment. In A. Dosen & K. Day (Eds.), *Treating mental illness and behavior disorders in children and adults with mental retardation* (pp. 101-118). Washington, DC: American Psychiatric Press.

Besag, F.M. (2002). Childhood epilepsy in relation to mental handicap and behavioural disorders. *Journal of Child Psychology and Psychiatry, and Allied Disciplines, 43*, 103-131.

Bijou, S.W. (1992). Concepts of mental retardation. *The Psychological Record, 42*, 305-322.

Blair, C. (1999). Science, policy, and early intervention. *Intelligence, 27*, 93-110.

Boscolo, B., Ratner, N.B., & Rescorla, L. (2002). Fluency of school-aged children with a history of specific expressive language impairment: An exploratory study. *American Journal of Speech-Language Pathology, 11*, 41-49.

Bowers, T.G., & Bailey, M.D. (2001). Specific learning disorders: Neuropsychological aspects of psychoeducational remediation. *Innovations in Clinical Practice: A Source Book, 19,* 49-61.

Bowlby, J. (1969). *Attachment and Loss.* New York: Basic Books.

Boyd, R.D., & Corley, M.J. (2001). Outcome survey of early intensive behavioral intervention for young children with autism in a community setting. *Autism, 5,* 430-441.

Bradley, J.D.D., & Golden, C.J. (2001). Biological contributions to the presentation and understanding of attention-deficit/hyperactivity disorder: A review. *Child Psychology Review, 21,* 907-929.

Bundy, A.C., Lane, S.J., Fisher, A.G., & Murray, E.A. (2002). *Sensory integration theory and practice* (2nd ed.). Philadelphia: F.A. Davis.

Casat, C.D., Pearson, D.A., & Casat, J.P. (2001). Attention-deficit/hyperactivity disorder. *Clinical Assessment of Child and Adolescent Behavior, 16,* 263-306.

Case-Smith, J., & Bryan, T. (1999). The effects of occupational therapy with sensory integration emphasis on preschool-age children with autism. *The American Journal of Occupational Therapy, 53,* 489-497.

Case-Smith, J., & Miller, H. (1999). Occupational therapy with children with pervasive developmental disorders. *The American Journal of Occupational Therapy, 53,* 506-513.

Chandler, J. (2002). *Panic disorder, separation anxiety disorder, and agoraphobia in children and adolescents.* Retrieved October 23, 2002, from http://www.klis.com/chandler/pamphlet/panic/panicpamphlet.htm.

Chapman, D.A., & Scott, K.G. (2001). The impact of maternal intergenerational risk factors on adverse developmental outcomes. *Developmental Review, 21,* 305-325.

Cook, E.H. (2001). Genetics of autism. *Child and Adolescent Psychiatric Clinics of North America, 10,* 333-350.

DeNili, L.F., & Kroll, R.M. (2001). Searching for the neural basis of stuttering treatment outcome: Recent neuroimaging studies. *Clinical Linguistics & Phonetics, 15*(1-2), 163-168.

DeStefano, F., & Chen, R.T. (2001). Autism and measles-mumps-rubella vaccination. Controversy laid to rest? *CNS Drugs, 15,* 831-837.

Dodge, K.A. (2000). Conduct disorder. In A.J. Sameroff, M. Lewis, & S.M. Miller (Eds.), *Handbook of developmental psychopathology* (2nd ed., pp. 447-463). New York: Kluwer Academic/Plenum Publishers.

Dosen, A., & Day, K. (2001). Epidemiology, etiology, and presentation of mental illness and behavior disorders in persons with mental retardation. In A. Dosen & K. Day (Eds.), *Treating mental illness and behavior disorders in children and adults with mental retardation* (pp. 3-24). Washington, DC: American Psychiatric Press.

Dunn, W., & Bennett, D. (2002). Patterns of sensory processing in children with attention deficit hyperactivity disorder. *Occupational Therapy Journal of Research, 22,* 4-15.

Dunn, W., Myles, B.S., & Orr, S. (2002). Sensory processing issues associated with Asperger's syndrome: A preliminary investigation. *The American Journal of Occupational Therapy, 56,* 97-102.

Durand, V.M., & Carr, E.G. (1992). An analysis of maintenance following functional communication training. *Journal of Applied Behavior Analysis, 25,* 777-794.

Dykens, E.M., & Hodapp, R.M. (2001). *Journal of Child Psychology and Psychiatry, and Allied Disciplines, 42,* 49-71.

Eikeseth, S., Smith, T., Jahr, E., & Eldevik, S. (2002). Intensive behavioral treatment at school for 4- to 7- year-old children with autism. *Behavior Modification, 26,* 49-68.

Ernst, M., Magee, H.J., Gonzalez, N.M., Locascio, J.J., Rosenberg, C.R., & Campbell, M. (1992). Pimozide in autistic children. *Psychopharmacology Bulletin, 28,* 187-191.

Faraone, S.V. (2000). Genetics of childhood disorders: XX. ADHD, Part 4: Is ADHD genetically heterogeneous? *Journal of the American Academy Child and Adolescent Psychiatry, 39,* 1455-1457.

Faraone, S.V., & Doyle, A.E. (2001). The nature and heritability of attention-deficit/hyperactivity disorder. *Child and Adolescent Psychiatric Clinics of North America, 10,* 299-316.

Fasko, S.N., & Fasko, D. (1991). Suicidal behavior in children. *Psychology: A Journal of Human Behavior, 27-28,* 10-16.

Ferraro, F.R. (2001). Survey of treatments for childhood autism. *Psychology and Education, 38*(2), 29-41.

Findling, R.L., McNamara, N.K., Branicky, L.A., Schluchter, M.D., Lemon, E., & Blaumer, J.L. (2000). A double-blind pilot study of risperidone in the treatment of conduct disorder. *Journal of the American Academy Child and Adolescent Psychiatry, 39,* 509-516.

Fleisher, M., Faulkner, E.H., Schalock, R.L., & Folk, L. (2001). A model for in-patient services for persons with mental retardation and mental illness. In A. Dosen & K. Day (Eds.), *Treating mental illness and behavior disorders in children and adults with mental retardation* (pp. 503-516). Washington, DC: American Psychiatric Press.

Fleming, R.K., & Reile, P.A. (1993). A descriptive analysis of client outcomes associated with staff interventions in developmental disabilities. *Behavioral Residential Treatment, 8,* 29-43.

Florey, L. (1998). Psychosocial dysfunction in childhood and adolescence. In M.E. Neistadt & E.B. Crepeau (Eds.), *Willard & Spackman's occupational therapy* (9th ed., pp. 622-635). Baltimore, MD: Lippincott, Williams & Wilkins.

Forness, S.R., & Kavale, K.A. (2001). ADHD and a return to the medical model of special education. *Education and Treatment of Children, 24,* 224-247.

Frazier, J.A. (1999). The person with mental retardation. In A.M. Nicholi, Jr. (Ed.). *The Harvard guide to psychiatry* (3rd ed., pp. 660-671). Cambridge, MA: Harvard University Press.

Freud, A. (1958). Adolescence. *Psychoanalytic Study of Children, 13,* 255-278.

Frick, P.J. (2000). A comprehensive and individualized treatment approach for children and adolescents with conduct disorders. *Cognitive and Behavioral Practice, 7,* 30-37.

Gabriels, R.L., Hill, D.E., Pierce, R.A., Rogers, S.J., & Wehner, B. (2001). Predictors of treatment outcome in young children with autism. *Autism, 5,* 407-429.

Galler, J.R., Ramsey, F., Solimano, G., & Lowell, W.E. (1983). The influence of early malnutrition on subsequent behavioral development: II. Classroom behavior. *Journal of the American Academy Child and Adolescent Psychiatry, 22,* 16-22.

Gardner, W.I., Graeber-Whalen, J.L., & Ford, D.R. (2001). Behavioral therapies: Individualizing interventions through treatment formulations. In A. Dosen & K. Day (Eds.), *Treating mental illness and behavior disorders in children and adults with mental retardation* (pp. 69-100). Washington, DC: American Psychiatric Press.

Geuze, R., & Borger, H. (1993). Children who are clumsy: Five years later. *Adapted Physical Activity Quarterly, 10,* 10-21.

Ghuman, H.S., Ghuman, J.K., & Ford, L.W. (1998). Pervasive developmental disorders and learning disorders. In H.S. Ghuman & R.M. Sarles (Eds.), *Handbook of child and adolescent out-patient day treatment and community psychiatry* (pp. 197-212). Philadelphia: Brunner/Mazel.

Gibbs, M., & Priest, H.M. (1999). Designing and implementing a 'dual diagnosis' module: A review of the literature and some preliminary findings. *Nurse Education Today, 19,* 357-363.

Gilger, J.W., & Kaplan, B.J. (2001). Atypical brain development: A conceptual framework for understanding developmental learning disabilities. *Developmental Neuropsychology, 20,* 465-481.

Gillberg, C. (1998). Asperger's syndrome and high-functioning autism. *British Journal of Psychiatry, 172,* 200-209.

Gobbi, G., & Pulvirenti, L. (2001). Long-term treatment with clozapine in an adult with autistic disorder accompanied by aggressive behavior. *Journal of Psychiatry & Neuroscience, 26,* 340-341.

Gordon, C., State, R.C., Nelson, J.E., Hamburger, S.D., & Rapoport, J. (1993). A double-blind comparison of clomipramine, desipramine, and placebo in the treatment of autistic disorder. *Archives of General Psychiatry, 50,* 441-447.

Gorman, P.A. (1997). Sensory dysfunction in dual diagnosis: Mental retardation/mental illness and autism. *Occupational Therapy in Mental Health, 13*(1), 3-22.

Grandin, T. (1996). *Thinking in pictures and other reports from my life with autism.* New York: Vintage Books.

Greenfield, J. (1986). *A client called Noah.* New York: Henry Holt and Co.

Grigorenko, E.L. (2001). Developmental dyslexia: An update on genes, brains, and environments. *Journal of Child Psychology and Psychiatry, and Alllied Disciplines, 42,* 91-125.

Hameury, L., Roux, S., Lenoir, P., Adrien, J.L., Sauvage, D., Barthelemy, C., et al. (1995). Longitudinal study of autism and other pervasive developmental disorders: A review of 125 cases. *Development and Brain Dysfunction, 8,* 51-65.

Hatton, C. (2002). People with intellectual disabilities from ethnic minority communities in the United States and the United Kingdom. In L.M. Glidden (Ed.), *International review of research in mental retardation* (pp. 209-240). San Diego: Academic Press.

Hellendoorn, J., & Hoekman, J. (1992). Imaginative play in children with mental retardation. *Mental Retardation, 30,* 255-263.

Hodapp, R.M., Ly, T.M., Fidler, D.J., & Ricci, L.A. (2001). Less stress, more rewarding: Parenting children with Down syndrome. *Parenting Science and Practice, 1,* 317-337.

Hoffenaar, P.J., & Hoeksma, J.B. (2002). The structure of oppositionality: Response dispositions and situational aspects. *Journal of Child Psychology and Psychiatry, and Allied Disciplines, 43,* 375-385.

Holburn, S., Perkins, T., & Vietze, P. (2001). The parent with mental retardation. *International Review of Research in Mental Retardation, 24,* 171-210.

Howlin, P., & Goode, S. (1998). Outcome in adult life for people with autism and Asperger's syndrome. In F.R. Volkmar (Ed.), *Autism and pervasive developmental disorders* (pp. 209-241). Cambridge, England: Cambridge University Press.

Hudziak, J.J. (2001). The role of phenotypes (diagnoses) in genetic studies of attention-deficit/hyperactivity disorder and related child psychopathology. *Child and Adolescent Psychiatric Clinics of North America, 10,* 279-297.

Jordan, R. (2001). Multidisciplinary work for children with autism. *Educational and Child Psychology, 18*(2), 5-14.

Keogh, B.K. (2002). Research on reading and reading problems: Findings, limitations, and future directions. In K.G. Butler & E.R. Silliman (Eds.), *Speaking, reading, and writing in children with language learning disabilities: New paradigms in research and practice* (pp. 27-44). Mahwah, NJ: Erlbaum Associates.

Kinnealey, M., & Miller, L.J. (1993). Sensory integration/learning disabilities. In H.L. Hopkins & H.D. Smith (Eds.), *Occupational therapy* (8th ed., pp. 489-494). Philadelphia: Lippincott, Williams & Wilkins.

Kumra, S., Nicholson, R., & Rapoport, J.L. (2002). Childhood-onset schizophrenia: Research data. In R.B. Zipursky & S.C. Schulz (Eds.), *The early stages of schizophrenia* (pp. 161-190). Washington, DC: American Psychiatric Publishing.

Lahey, B.B., McBurnett, K., & Loeber, R. (2000). Are attention-deficit/hyperactivity disorder and oppositional defiant disorder developmental precursors to conduct disorder?. In A.J. Sameroff, M. Lewis, & S.M. Miller (Eds.), *Handbook of developmental psychopathology* (2nd ed., pp. 431-446). New York: Kluwer Academic/ Plenum Publishers.

Larsen, F.W., & Mouridsen, S.E. (1997).The outcome in children with childhood autism and Asperger's syndrome originally diagnosed as psychotic. A 30-year follow-up study of subjects hospitalized as children. *Eur Child Adolesc Psychiatry, 6,* 181-190.

Lawton, M.P. (1980). *Environment and aging.* Monterey, CA: Brooks-Cole.

Lie, N. (1991). Follow-ups of children with attention deficit hyperactivity disorder. *Acta Psychiatrica Scandinavica, 85,* 5-40.

Lifter, K. (2000). Linking assessment to intervention for children with developmental disabilities or at-risk for developmental delay: The Developmental Play Assessment (DPA) instrument. In K. Gitlin-Weiner, A. Sandgrund, & C.E. Schaefer (Eds.), *Play diagnosis and assessment* (2nd ed., pp. 228-261). New York: Wiley.

Linderman, T.M., & Stewart, K.B. (1999). Sensory integrative-based occupational therapy and functional outcomes in young children with pervasive developmental disorders: A single-subject study. *The American Journal of Occupational Therapy, 53,* 207-213.

Loeber, R., Green, S.M., Lahey, B.B., Frick, P.J., & McBurnett, K. (2000). Findings on disruptive behavior disorders from the first decade of the developmental trends study. *Clinical Child and Family Psychology Review, 3,* 37-60.

Luiselli, J.K., Blew, P., & Thibadeau, S. (2001). Therapeutic effects and long-term efficacy of antidepressant medication for persons with developmental disabilities. *Behavior Modification, 25,* 62-78.

Lynam, D.R., & Henry, B. (2001). The role of neuropsychological deficits in conduct disorders. In J. Hill & B. Maughan (Eds.), *Conduct disorders in childhood and adolescence* (pp. 235-263). Cambridge, England: Cambridge University Press.

Lynskey, M.T., & Hall, W. (2001). Attention deficit hyperactivity disorder and substance use disorders: Is there a causal link? *Addiction, 96,* 815-822.

Mackowiak, M. (2000). Aetiology of autism: Focus on the biological perspective. *Early Child Development and Care, 160,* 77-84.

Martin, C.S., Romig, C.J., & Kirisci, L. (2000). DSM-IV learning disorders in 10- to 12-year-old boys with and without a parental history of substance use disorders. *Preventive Science, 1,* 107-113.

Martin, M.J. (1989). Children with mental retardation. In P.N. Pratt and A.S. Allen (Eds.), *Occupational Therapy for Children* (2nd ed., pp. 422-441). Los Angeles: Times Mirror Company.

Matson, J.L., & Mayville, E.A. (2001). The relationship of functional variables and psychopathology to aggressive behavior in persons with severe and profound mental retardation. *Journal of Psychopathology and Behavioral Assessment, 23,* 3-9.

Maughan, B., & Rutter, M. (2001). Antisocial children grown up. In J. Hill & B. Maughan (Eds.), *Conduct disorders in childhood and adolescence* (pp. 507-552). Cambridge: Cambridge University Press.

McDonnell, J., Hardman, M.L., Hightower, J., Keifer-O'Donnell, R., & Drew, C. (1993). Impact of community-based instruction on the development of adaptive behavior of secondary-level students with mental retardation. *American Journal of Mental Retardation, 97,* 575-584.

McGrath, M., & Grant, G. (1993). The life cycle and support networks of families with a person with a learning difficulty. *Disability, Handicap & Society, 8,* 25-41.

McInerney, C.A., & McInerney, M. (1992). A mobility skills training program for adults with developmental disabilities. *The American Journal of Occupational Therapy, 46,* 233-239.

Mpofu, E., & Crystal, R. (2001). Conduct disorder in children: Challenges, and prospective cognitive behavioural treatments. *Counseling Psychology Quarterly, 14,* 21-32.

National Institute of Child Health and Development. (2001). Facts about autism. Retrieved October 21, 2003, from http://www.nichd.nih.gov/publications/pubs/autism1.htm.

Nettelbeck, T., & Wilson, C. (2001). Criminal victimization of persons with mental retardation: The influence of interpersonal competence on risk. *International Review of Research in Mental Retardation, 24,* 137-169.

Newman, B.M., & Newman, P.R. (2003). *Development through life: A psychosocial approach* (8th ed.). Belmont, CA: Wadsworth/Thomson Learning.

Nippold, M.A. (2001). Phonological disorders and stuttering in children: What is the frequency of co-occurrence? *Clinical Linguistics & Phonetics, 15,* 219-228.

Nordin, V., & Gillberg, C. (1998). The long-term course of autistic disorders: Update on follow-up studies. *Acta Psychiatrica Scandinavica, 97,* 99-108.

Onslow, M., Ratner, N.B., & Packman, A. (2001). Changes in linguistic variables during operant, laboratory control of stuttering in children. *Clinical Linguistics & Phonetics, 15,* 651-662.

Ozonoff, S., South, M., & Miller, J.N. (2000). DSM-IV-defined Asperger's syndrome: Cognitive, behavioral and early history differentiation from high-functioning autism. *Autism, 4,* 29-46.

Pelios, L.V., & Lund, S.K. (2001). A selective overview of issues on classification, causation, and early intensive behavioral intervention for autism. *Behavior Modification, 25,* 678-697.

Peral, M., Alcami, M., & Gilaberte, I. (1999). Fluoxetine in children with autism. *Journal of the American Academy of Child and Adolescent Psychiatry, 38,* 1472-1473.

Plomin, R. (2001). Genetic factors contributing to learning and language delays and disabilities. *Child and Adolescent Psychiatric Clinics of North America, 10,* 259-277.

Quist, J.F., & Kennedy, J.L. (2001). Genetics of childhood disorders: XXIII. ADHD, Part 7: The serotonin system. *Journal of the American Academy of Child and Adolescent Psychiatry, 40,* 253-256.

Raffin, C. (2001). A multidisciplinary approach to working with autistic children. *Educational and Child Psychology, 18*(2), 15-27.

Ramey, S.L., & Ramey, C.T. (1999). Early experience and early intervention for children "at risk" for developmental delay and mental retardation. *Mental Retardation and Developmental Disabilities Research Reviews, 5,* 1-10.

Reber, M. (1992). Mental retardation. *The Interface of Psychiatry and Neurology, 15,* 511-522.

Reeve, W.V., & Schandler, S.L. (2001). Frontal lobe functioning in adolescents with attention deficit hyperactivity disorder. *Adolescence, 36,* 749-765.

Rhodes, R. (1993). Mental retardation and sexual expression: A historical perspective. *Sexuality and Disabilities, 8,* 1-27.

Robins, L.N. (1999). A 70 year history of conduct disorder: Variations in definition, prevalence, and correlates. In P. Cohen, S. Slomkowski, & L.N. Robins (Eds.), *Historical and geographical influences on psychopathology* (pp. 37-56). Mahwah, NJ: L. Erlbaum Associates.

Rogers, S. (2001). Diagnosis of autism before the age of 3. *International Review of Research in Mental Retardation, 23,* 1-31.

Safran, S.P. (2001). Asperger's syndrome: The emerging challenge to special education. *Exceptional Children, 67,* 151-160.

Sandknop P., Schuster, J., Wolery, M., and Cross, D., (1992). The use of an adaptive device to teach students with moderate mental retardation to select lower priced grocery items, *Education and Training in Mental Retardation, 27,* 219-229.

Schuntermann, P. (2002). Pervasive developmental disorder and parental adaptation: Previewing and reviewing atypical development with parents in child psychiatric consultation. *Harvard Review of Psychiatry, 10*(1), 16-27.

Seltzer, M.M., Krauss, M.W., Orsmond, G.I., & Vestal, C. (2001). Families of adolescents and adults with autism: Uncharted territory. *International Review of Research in Mental Retardation, 23,* 267-294.

Sergeant, J.A., Geurts. H., & Oosterlaan, J. (2002). How specific is a deficit of executive functioning for attention-deficit/hyperactivity disorder? *Behavioural Brain Research, 130,* 3-28.

Shevell, M. I., Majnemer, A., Rosenbaum, P., & Abrahamowicz, M. (2001). Provide of referrals for early childhood developmental delay to ambulatory subspecialty clinics. *Journal of Child Neurology, 16,* 645-650.

Simmons, T.J., & Flexer, R.W. (1992). Community-based job training for persons with mental retardation: an acquisition and performance replication. *Community-Based Job Training,* 261-272.

Simonoff, E. (2001). Gene-environment interplay in oppositional defiant and conduct disorder. *Child and Adolescent Psychiatric Clinics of North America, 10,* 351-374.

Stahmer, A.C., and Schreibman, L. (1992). Teaching children with autism appropriate play in unsupervised environments using a self-management treatment package. *Journal of Applied Behavior Analysis, 25,* 447-459.

Swedo, S.E., Leonard, H.L., & Rapoport, J.L. (1992). Childhood-onset obsessive compulsive disorder. *Obsessional Disorders, 15,* 767-775.

Symons, F.J., & MacLean, W.E. (2000). Analyzing and treating severe behavior problems in people with developmental disabilities. Observational methods using computer-assisted technology. In T. Thompson, D. Felce, & F.J. Symons (Eds.), *Behavioral observation: Technology and applications in developmental disabilities* (pp. 143-157). Baltimore, MD: Paul H. Brookes.

Tanguay, P.E. (2000). Pervasive developmental disorders: A 10-year review. *Journal of the American Academy of Child and Adolescent Psychiatry, 39,* 1079-1095.

Thompson, T., & Caruso, M. (2002). Self-injury: Knowing what we're looking for. In S.R. Schroeder, M.L. Oster-Granite, & T. Thompson (Eds.), *Self-injurious behavior* (pp. 3-21). Washington, DC: American Psychological Association.

Thomsen, P.H. (1992). Obsessive-compulsive disorder in adolescence. *Psychopathology, 25,* 301-310.

Thorpe, L., Davidson, P., & Janicki, M. (2000). Healthy aging: Adults with intellectual disabilities: Biobehavioural issues. *Journal of Applied Research in Intellectual Disabilities, 14,* 218-228.

Torrance, A.F.M. (1998). Does homelessness predict conduct disorder? A causal model of risk factors among low socioeconomic status children. *Dissertation Abstracts International: Section B: The Sciences & Engineering, 58,* 5659.

Townsend, J., Westerfield, M., Leaver, E., Makeig, S., Jung, T. Pierce, K., et al. (2001). Event-related brain response abnormalities in autism: Evidence for impaired cerebello-frontal spatial attention networks. *Cognitive Brain Research, 11,* 127-145.

Tyrer, S., & Hill, S. (2001). Psychopharmacological approaches. In A. Dosen & K. Day (Eds.), *Treating mental illness and behavior disorders in children and adults with mental retardation* (pp. 45-68). Washington, DC: American Psychiatric Press.

Verheij, F., and van Loon, H. (1992). Pervasive developmental disorders not otherwise specified: A developmental-psychopathological approach for the development of made-to-measure treatment planning. *Acta Paedopsychiatrica, 55,* 235-242.

Wakschlag, L.S., Gordon, R.A., Lahey, B.B., Loeber, R., Green, S.M., & Leventhal, B.L. (2000). Maternal age at first birth and boys' risk for conduct disorder. *Journal of Research on Adolescence, 10,* 417-441.

Waschbusch, D.A. (2002). A meta-analytic examination of comorbid hyperactive-impulsive-attention problems and conduct problems. *Psychological Bulletin, 128,* 118-150.

Watling, R., Deitz, J., Kanny, E.M., & McLaughlin, J.F. (1999). Current practice of occupational therapy for children with autism. *The American Journal of Occupational Therapy, 53,* 498-505.

Webster-Stratton, C. (2000). Oppositional-defiant and conduct-disordered children. In M. Hersen & R.T. Ammerman (Eds.), *Advanced abnormal child psychology* (pp. 387-412). Mahwah, NJ: Lawrence Erlbaum Associates.

Weininger, O. (1993). Attachment, affective contact, and autism. *Psychoanalytic Inquiry, 13,* 49-62.

Wever, C., & Rey, J.M. (1997). Juvenile obsessive-compulsive disorder. *The Australian and New Zealand Journal of Psychiatry, 31,* 105-113.

Whitely, P., Rodgers, J., Savery, D., & Shattock, P. (1999). A gluten-free diet as an intervention for autism and associated spectrum disorders: Preliminary findings. *Autism, 3,* 45-65.

Wilens, T.E., Biederman, J., & Spencer, T.J. (2002). Attention deficit/hyperactivity disorder across the lifespan. *Annual Review of Medicine, 53,* 113-131.

Wingate, M.E. (2002). *Foundations of stuttering.* San Diego, CA: Academic Press.

Zigler, E., & Hodapp, R.M. (1991). Behavioral functioning in individuals with mental retardation. *Ann Rev Psychol, 42,* 29-50.

Zimmerman, I.L., & Woo-Sam, J.M. (1984). Intellectual assessment of children. In G. Goldstein and M. Hersen (Eds.), *Handbook of psychological assessment* (pp. 57-76). New York: Pergamon Press.

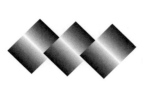
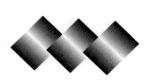

Chapter 4

Delirium, Dementia, Amnestic, and Other Cognitive Disorders

This section of the DSM-IV-TR (APA, 2000) includes diagnoses characterized by cognitive dysfunction. The majority also have etiologies that have been demonstrated to be biological. There are three major categories: delirium (i.e., a disturbance of consciousness and cognition developed over a short time), dementia (i.e., multiple cognitive deficits without change in consciousness), and amnestic disorder (i.e., disturbance in memory without other cognitive impairments). Table 4-1 shows the distinctions between delirium and dementia.

DELIRIUM

Delirium is characterized by global changes in cognition, with accompanying alteration of consciousness. The individual has diminished awareness of the environment and is disoriented to time, place, and, sometimes, to person as well. In addition to altered consciousness, delirium presents with inability to maintain attention, disorganized thinking, changes in psychomotor activity or sleep, perceptual disturbances, and memory impairment. Onset is generally rapid, and a precipitating event can frequently be identified.

Etiology and Incidence

Delirium may accompany a high fever, head trauma, encephalitis, substance abuse, tumors, and many other physical conditions. Differential diagnosis on Axis III is critical, as the cause of delirium defines its treatment. Delirium is extremely common, occurring in 10% to 15% of individuals in medical and surgical wards (Lipowski, 1992). It is typically transient, resolving in days or weeks, either through cure of the underlying biological disorder, or through death, which occurs in about 14% of cases (Lipowski, 1992).

Implications for Function

Individuals with delirium show marked functional decrements in all spheres as a result of altered consciousness and diminished cognition. They are unable to accomplish normal daily activities, and cognitive, motor, and sensory abilities are likewise impaired. Occupational therapists are only occasionally involved in treatment of individuals with delirium, most often when the delirium persists accompanying a prolonged state of coma. In

Table 4-1
Distinguishing Delirium From Dementia

Delirium (i.e., cognitive change and altered consciousness)

Substance intoxication delirium
Substance withdrawal delirium

Dementia (i.e., cognitive change and full consciousness)

Dementia of the Alzheimer's type
Vascular dementia

these instances, the therapist may be asked to provide patterned sensory stimulation to encourage resolution of the coma and to provide range of motion to minimize contractures that might occur as a result of prolonged bed rest and inactivity.

DEMENTIA

Dementia is characterized by memory loss in the presence of full consciousness. Abstract thinking and judgment are impaired. Aphasia, apraxia, and other cognitive and motor dysfunction may be noted, along with personality changes, such as newly-developing paranoia. The diagnosis requires symptoms sufficiently severe to interfere with vocational or social functioning. Changes in consciousness are not noted.

Cognitive loss in dementia is far beyond age-associated memory impairment (AAMI) (Larabee & Crook, 1994), the sort of minor memory change that is characteristic of normal aging but is not disabling. One longitudinal study suggested that about one-third of individuals who show signs of AAMI later develop dementia (Helkala et al., 1997). Given the relatively high incidence of dementia in older populations, this finding may not have particular predictive or etiological significance, however.

Etiology and Incidence

There are a large number of possible causes of dementia. They include Alzheimer's disease (AD), vascular disease (multi-infarct dementia), Huntington's chorea, Pick's disease, Jakob-Creutzfeldt disease, and multiple sclerosis (Corcoran, 2001), all of which cause irreversible cognitive damage. Among the reversible causes of dementia are depression and metabolic and nutritional problems (Corcoran, 2001). There is a group of dementias labeled pseudodementia (e.g., Ganser syndrome) that are thought to be psychogenic rather than biological in origin (Jeste, Gierz, & Harris, 1990). Recent research suggests that even some cases of Ganser syndrome may have a biological origin, specifically, traumatic brain injury (TBI) (Dalfen & Feinstein, 2000). Differential diagnosis is difficult at present but vital to effective treatment. By far the most common dementing illness is dementia of the Alzheimer's type (DAT) or AD (Guttman, Altman, & Nielsen, 1999). It is believed to affect approximately 2.1 million individuals, with a projection of 2.9 million by 2015 (United States General Accounting Office, 1998).

Distinguishing among the dementias is done on the basis of both laboratory findings and the nature of the symptoms. DAT and Pick's are primarily cortical, while Huntington's and Parkinson's diseases are subcortical (Cummings, 1982). Multi-infarct and Jakob-Creutzfeldt are mixed. The subcortical dementias have more extrapyramidal signs, such as ataxia and tremor, while the cortical dementias have more cognitive symptoms, such as memory loss, personality change, and visuospatial impairment. Identification of these symptom differences is an important step in diagnosis.

Multi-infarct dementia, a vascular dementia, can be diagnosed by computerized axial tomography (CT scan), as it is caused by small infarcts in the cerebral vascular system (Alzheimer's Disease Education and Referral Center, 2002a). The main symptom is spotty loss of function that progresses through rather abrupt changes in performance followed by periods of relative stability. This stair-step progression is in contrast to DAT, which shows more global loss and more gradual, continuous progression. The difference may be quite subtle, however.

Pseudodementia (i.e., Ganser syndrome) is characterized by a course that is not deteriorating and by differences between the subjective report of the individual about severity and the objective findings. Typically, objective signs are less severe than those reported by the individual (Jeste et al., 1990). "Approximate answers" to questions (for example, 2 + 2 = 5) (Dalfen & Feinstein, 2000) are also typical. This disorder is not a form of malingering, as there is no conscious attempt to mislead. It may, instead, be a hysterical or psychotic episode or the result of a closed-head injury. Prevalence is uncertain, but probably about 2% of dementias are pseudodementia.

Depressive dementia is characterized by slowing and poverty of response (Corcoran, 2001; Riley, 2001). The individual may not respond to questions at all or may give very brief responses. Psychomotor slowing is also a sign of this type of dementia, which is responsive to psychotropic medication. A caution for caregivers is the possibility that a depressive dementia may be superimposed on another irreversible dementia, causing excess disability (Gitlin & Corcoran, 1996). If the depression is treated, symptoms may be reduced, although the course of the underlying dementia will not be altered. One caregiver reported that his mother, when moved from the isolation of her apartment to an assisted-living facility, regained significant function as a result of diminished depression. Although she still had substantial functional loss as a result of DAT, she was able to play bridge again—an activity that was important to her quality of life.

Diagnosis of DAT must be made by exclusion. It can be confirmed only through brain biopsy or autopsy, although laboratory and cognitive testing has become increasingly effective in identifying the disorder early in its course (Boyd, 2001). If other causes of dementia, including depression, metabolic disorders, and multi-infarct dementia, can be ruled out, a diagnosis of DAT will be made.

The precise etiology of DAT is not known, although autopsy reveals a characteristic pattern of neuritic plaques and tangles (Boyd, 2001) as well as changes in the hippocampus. A variety of etiological factors have been hypothesized. The most prevalent theories at present include a genetic explanation (Boyd, 2001) possibly related to defects of chromosomes 21, 14, or 1. The finding that chromosome 21 is involved was related to the observation that individuals with trisomy 21 who live into their 40s almost all show characteristic symptoms and cortical changes associated with Alzheimer's disease (Devenny, Krinsky-McHale,

Sersen, & Silverman, 2000). A slow virus (as has been demonstrated in Jakob-Creutzfeldt disease) or some unexplained loss of neurotransmitters, particularly cholinesterase (Alzheimer's Disease Education and Referral Center, 2002a), have been suggested as causes. A buildup of a protein known as amyloid has been identified (Boyd, 2001), although the reason for this buildup is not established.

It appears that there may be more than one type of DAT (Fenn, Luby, & Yesavage, 1993). A number of researchers speculate that there is a familial (i.e., genetic) form of DAT that differs symptomatically from other forms, as well as having a different etiology (Boyd, 2001). While this type of Alzheimer's disease has been difficult to document because of diagnostic problems and deaths from unrelated causes, an autosomal dominant familial form has been identified.

A distinction has been made between early and late onset dementia (Alzheimer's Disease Education and Referral Center, 2000a). Early onset dementia is more severe, with worse aphasia (i.e., speech difficulty) and presence of agraphia (i.e., difficulty writing) earlier in the course of the disorder (Brandt et al., 1989). Some researchers theorize that the early onset type is familial, but this contention is still open to debate.

There has been increasing research about DAT, which accounts for approximately 65% to 75% of cases of dementia (Richards & Hendrie, 1999). Since the numbers are likely to increase, considerable attention has been given to the disorder. Rates for other dementias are also increasing. Possibly because of differential life expectancies, the disorders are more common in women.

Prognosis

Prognosis for DAT is always poor. The disease progresses to total incapacity and death. The speed of progress is quite variable, however. Some researchers speculate that early-onset DAT is more likely to progress rapidly, to result in greater dysfunction, and to cause death within a few years. By contrast, later-onset DAT is thought to progress more slowly, with the possibility of functional plateaus that last for long periods of time. Different course as a result of age of onset is not clearly established, but it is known that DAT will progress over time and always ends in death.

Prognosis for multi-infarct dementia is variable. Existing damage is irreversible, but the progress of the disease may be slow. In some cases it may not be progressive. Treatment of coexisting high blood pressure or vascular disease may slow or stop deterioration of function.

The other irreversible dementias also have poor long-term prognoses. The only one with any particularly effective treatment is Parkinson's disease, which can be treated symptomatically with medication, levodopamine (L-dopa) being the most commonly used (Neurosurgery://on-call, 2000). In some instances, surgery may be used, either pallidotomy, in which portions of the global pallidus are destroyed, or thalamotomy, in which a small, specific portion of the thalamus is destroyed (Neurosurgery://on-call, 2000). Otherwise, management rather than treatment is the goal of intervention.

When the dementia is a pseudodementia or is caused by depression, prognosis is relatively good (Riley, 2001). The underlying psychological disorder is often treatable with psychotherapy and with a variety of psychotropic medications. Improvement in the depressive symptoms leads to improved cognitive function. As noted previously, this is true even when the individual has AD.

Implications for Function and Treatment

Dementia has a devastating impact on all areas of function. As it progresses, occupational, social, and ADL/IADL performance areas become increasingly impaired. Ultimately, basic skills, including swallowing and even breathing, may become difficult. In fact, death often occurs as a result of pneumonia that results from inability to clear the lungs (Burns, 1992). As noted above, the progress of the diseases is somewhat variable and rather unpredictable. Some residual function may be retained for long periods of time.

DAT has been described as progressing through three stages (Corcoran, 2001). The first symptom identified is usually memory impairment. The individual may put water on the stove to boil and forget to turn it off or may go out and forget how to get back home. Memory difficulties may lead to work problems and carelessness in personal grooming. For example, the individual may forget how to do work tasks or forget to bathe. During the second stage, aphasia, apraxia, disorientation, and restlessness appear. It is common during this phase to see the individual pacing around the house for hours on end; forgetting who people are, even those closest to him or her; and having difficulty finding words. In some individuals, an attempt to deal with the word-finding problem is made by talking around the word. Thus, the "radio" may be called "the machine with a switch that talks."

Personality changes also occur. Temper outbursts are common as the individual finds his or her limitations extremely frustrating. In addition, as ability to understand the environment worsens, the individual becomes fearful and often paranoid. When personal items are missing, the individual often assumes that they have been stolen. Finally, memory becomes severely impaired, and total loss of sensory, motor, and cognitive abilities occurs. The individual becomes bedridden and incontinent, unable to chew or swallow.

Clearly, patterns are significantly affected by DAT. Routines are affected early on as the individual begins to lose ability in performance areas. Some habits are retained until later in the progression of the disease. In fact, it has been noted that procedural memory is relatively spared and allows for continuation of well-learned skills until late in the course of the disorder (Camp, Foss, Stevens, & O'Hanlon, 1996).

Some specific characteristics of the symptoms are worth noting. First, personality and social behavior may be maintained well into the disease. In fact, some individuals learn to cover their impairment so well that it is not recognized by others until the disease is well along. It is only after listening for awhile that the other person becomes aware that verbalizations, however pleasant, make no sense. The memory and sensory losses also have some specific characteristics. Problems seem to arise in the encoding of information, so the defect is in recent rather than immediate or remote memory (LaRue, 1982). This means that the individual will be able to process what is happening at the moment and what happened 50 years ago, but not what happened that morning or 15 minutes ago. In addition, extraneous memories seem to intrude on function, leading to confabulation and perseveration. An individual who is questioned about family members may present a long, rambling description of sisters and brothers but not remember spouse and children. This is a characteristic that distinguishes DAT from depression, which is more likely to lead to absence of response.

Language, especially word-finding, is almost universally impaired. Articulation, however, remains intact until very late in the disease course (Murdoch, Chenery, Wilks, & Boyle, 1987). The individual can say words but not put them together in a meaningful way. Aphasia is thought to be worse in the familial type, and agraphia is a defining feature of familial DAT. Visuospatial deficits are common, as are visual field losses (Steffes & Thralow, 1987). Therefore, the individual has difficulty with walking and other activities that require spatial discrimination. Temporal distortions are also common, with the person unable to keep track of time, day, or season.

Other dementias are characterized by different functional deficits. Pick's disease, which has an earlier onset than DAT (usually age 40 to 60), manifests itself first with behavioral and affective changes (Alzheimer's Disease Education and Referral Center, 2002a). Cognitive changes, including aphasia, occur later. Unlike DAT, motor and sensory changes are rare, and occur later in the disease course. Visuospatial deficits are also rare.

Multi-infarct dementia has less predictable functional consequences, as changes are dependent on the location and extent of cerebral damage (Alzheimer's Disease Education and Referral Center, 2002b). In addition, progress of the disease is inconsistent. There may be long periods of plateau and sudden decrements in performance.

Depressive dementias are a manifestation of depression most likely to appear in the elderly (Riley, 2001). Instead of symptoms of sadness and hopelessness, this depression presents with confusion and memory impairment. Unlike the dementias described above, however, motor slowing and reduced levels of response to the environment are seen. This type of dementia is reversible through drug therapy. Hysterical dementias are those that have no identifiable biological base and seem to be the result of psychological conflict and stress rather than biology. They are usually identifiable by the course, which is atypical for any of the known dementias, and by the fact that the dementia may come and go, with periods of normal function interspersed with problem behavior. Usual treatment for these dementias is psychotherapy and possibly drug therapy.

There are other causes of dementia, as well, including Korsakoff's, Wernicke's, and syphilitic dementia. Korsakoff's and Wernicke's are attributable to long-term alcoholism, while syphilitic is attributable to tertiary syphilis. All are irreversible, although they may stabilize rather than progress. Each has its own particular course and symptoms. Korsakoff's, for example, presents with amnesia of recent events. The individual remembers quite clearly up to a particular point in time, perhaps 10 years ago, and has no memory of anything that occurred from that time to the present.

A new dementia, emerging in rapidly-growing numbers, is that related to human immunodeficiency virus (HIV)(McArthur, 1998). Approximately 5% to 10% of the HIV-infected population has signs of dementia, even before development of acquired immunodeficiency syndrome (AIDS). The rate of such dementia has been steadily declining as antiretrovirus therapies show effectiveness in preventing symptoms. However, the absolute number of individuals affected has been increasing as more people with HIV infection survive for longer periods.

AIDS dementia complex has many of the features of other dementias but progresses very rapidly. It is separate from some of the opportunistic infections that cause encephalitis or other CNS diseases. Its manifestations are global cognitive impairment, including memory deficits, intellectual impairment, and poor concentration and memory. According to Buckingham and Shernoff (1998), infected individuals have social, leisure, and vocational functioning decrements. They also show emotional lability, disorientation, and occasionally psychotic symptoms. Late-stage individuals are severely dysfunctional in all spheres.

Available treatment of individuals with dementing illnesses is minimal, except in those cases in which a reversible cause can be identified. In the majority of cases, however, treatment is symptomatic and behavioral. If the individual is wandering at night, for example, a low dose of a sleeping medication may be administered (Boyd, 2001). In cases in which severe paranoia appears, antipsychotic medication may also be tried. Medical intervention presents problems, though, as drugs may be sedating, making symptoms such as confusion worse (Jeste, Rockwell, Harris, Lohr, & Lacro, 1999). Some symptoms can be reasonably well-managed for some period of time.

Experimentation with new medications is on-going. One that has received considerable notice is donepezil (i.e., Aricept) (Stahl, 2000). The drug seems to have a modest impact on cognition as measured by neuropsychological tests. However, no improvement on self-care measures has been noted, and only about one-third of individuals show any improvement at all. In addition, Aricept has serious side effects, including the potential of liver damage. Research is also underway for rivistigmine (Corey-Bloom, Anand, & Veach, 1998), and galantamine (Raskind, Peskind, Wessel, Parys, & the Galantamine USA-1 Study Group, 2000) among others. These drugs seem more promising and are now used in practice more frequently than Aricept.

The most common dementias, however, cannot be cured, nor can the progression be stopped or even slowed in many cases. Much intervention focuses on the individual's caregiver, who must learn how to manage the behaviors. The caregiver may be taught how to give simple instructions, how to deal with temper outbursts, and so on (Boyd, 2001; Corcoran, 2001).

Implications for Occupational Therapy

Occupational therapists have a vital role to play in the treatment of dementing illnesses. Because of the incurable and usually progressive nature of the disorders, interventions that focus on management and maximizing quality of life are quite valuable. In the early stages of these disorders, efforts can be made to help the individual maintain function and autonomy (Trace & Howell, 1991). This may be done through environmental adaptation, education, and use of assistive devices, particularly memory aids. Van Deusen (1992) recommends teaching compensatory techniques for visuospatial problems and apraxia during the early stages of the disorder.

There are several major strategies that can be employed for most dementias. The first of these is prevention. There has been some suggestion that individuals who are active cognitively show fewer signs of cognitive deterioration (Azar, 2002). Taking classes, attending lectures, working crossword puzzles, and other cognitively-challenging activities may delay symptoms of DAT, although this is far from certain. However, mental activity cannot possibly harm the individual, so recommendations that people engage in mentally-challenging activities are warranted.

Once signs of dementia appear, strategies include restoration of function where possible, optimization of remaining abilities, compensation for abilities lost, and substitution of remaining skills (Glisky & Glisky, 2002). Restoration is reflected in attempts to restore damaged function through repetitive drills and practice. This strategy does not currently have research evidence to support its value. Optimization of function may include such strategies as use of mnemonic devices; these may be challenging for individuals as dementia progresses and are, therefore, useful only in the early stages. Compensation involves an array of environmental or contextual strategies, such as labeling doors with pictures of the rooms behind them and using technological devices, such as timers, to provide reminders. Substitution uses intact memory processes to enhance function. Camp and his colleagues (1996) have used Montessori methods to capitalize on procedural memory, which appears to remain relatively intact quite late in the process of DAT. These methods involve careful preparation of the environment to cue behaviors, and engaging the individual in activities that are well-entrenched (perhaps a card game of "go fish" or a "proverb completion" game) can enhance both function and quality of life.

As the individual's function declines, focus shifts to helping caregivers cope with emerging deficits (Corcoran, 2001). Again, environmental adaptation can be useful. This includes simplifying the environment; reducing the number of stimuli; and also adding various safety devices, such as automatic turn-off switches for stoves and door alarms to warn of wandering. The caregiver must be educated about the course of the disease and given information on how to deal with problems. It may be helpful to provide information on how to feed the person, how to modify clothing, and so on.

Other suggestions include careful use of community services to reduce caregiver burden (Scaffa, 2001), carefully patterned sensory stimulation to minimize the potential for sensory deprivation, and exercise to reduce potential for motor impairment (Corcoran, 2001).

Many of these interventions are effective when provided in groups. Support groups for both the individual and caregivers are a valuable emotional outlet. Reminiscence or remotivation groups for the individual can support function and improve quality of life by providing pleasant and engaging activities.

For both the individual and the caregiver, quality of life is a major issue. For the individual, activity should be encouraged at whatever level he or she can perform. Day treatment programs provide structured activities and stimulation at a level that the individual can manage. The caregiver is often overwhelmed and exhausted by the needs of the individual and must be encouraged to take time for his or her own leisure. At some point, nursing home placement may be necessary, and the occupational therapist may join with others who are involved in care to help the informal caregiver make this decision.

At all stages of the disorder, psychotherapy and other expressive therapies should be considered (Bonder, 1994). The individual often needs to express emotions and this becomes increasingly possible through verbal therapies, particularly as the disorder is diagnosed earlier. Where verbal expression is not possible, art, music, and dance may be valuable in assisting the individual to cope. A number of first person accounts of the disorder are now available (Davis, 1989; McGowan, 1993) and it is clear that such expression makes a significant difference in quality of life. Table 4-2 summarizes the symptoms and functional deficits found in delirium and dementia.

AMNESTIC DISORDER

Unlike delirium and dementia, amnestic disorders are focal cognitive disorders (Caine, 1993; Reinvang, 1998). This means that only memory is affected, rather than cognition, more globally. Amnestic disorder may be due to substance abuse (Jacobson & Lishman, 1987) or to a variety of medical conditions. These conditions are characterized by inability to learn new material or to recall previously learned material to an extent that impairs function (APA, 2000).

Amnestic disorders can be caused by illness, such as encephalitis (Hokkanen & Launes, 2000); normal aging; anxiety; depression; use of certain drugs, including some over-the-counter medicines; and hypoxia (Erikson, 1990), including carbon monoxide poisoning (Ali-Cherif et al., 1984). A particular kind of amnesia is found in Korsakoff's syndrome (Nickel, 1990), a potential consequence of long-term alcohol abuse. In this form of amnesia, memory is intact to a particular point in the individual's life history. Past that point, the individual is unable recall events (i.e., retrograde amnesia), and he or she will be unable to create new memories (i.e., anterograde amnesia).

Amnesia can also be caused by trauma, with individuals sometimes demonstrating difficulty recalling events surrounding an automobile accident or other traumatic event. The majority of amnestic disorders are characterized by difficulty remembering a particular brief

Table 4-2

Organic Mental Syndromes and Disorders

Disorder	Symptoms	Functional Deficits
A. Syndromes		
Delirium	1. Reduced attention 2. Disorganized thinking 3. Altered consciousness 4. Rapid onset	All areas affected. Patterns disrupted Motor, process, and communication impaired
Dementia	1. Memory impairment 2. Cognitive impairment 3. Symptoms one and two interfere with function 4. No altered consciousness	All performance areas impaired; Work and leisure deteriorate first Roles, habits, and routines deteriorate over time Process skills and communication affected early; motor later May be mild to severe; often progressive
Intoxication	1. Evidence of recent ingestion of a psychoactive substance 2. Substance causes maladaptive behavior	Work, play, social participation, and leisure are all affected Roles, habits, and routines are all disrupted Process skills affected Probable impairment of motor and communication skills
Withdrawal	1. Symptoms of organic disorder as a result of substance withdrawal	May affect any area, and all patterns
B. Disorders		
Dementia of the Alzheimer type	1. Dementia 2. Insidious onset 3. Deteriorating course	Global and progressive
Multi-infarct	1. Dementia 2. Step-wise deteriorating ability 3. Focal neurological signs (e.g., weakness, altered reflexes) 4. Laboratory evidence of cerebrovascular disease	Unpredictable and patchy with stable plateaus

period of time, and most resolve relatively quickly. In spite of the popular portrayals of amnestic disorder in movies and TV shows, occupational therapists are unlikely to encounter individuals with these disorders.

REFERENCES

Ali-Cherif, A., Royere, M.L., Gosset, A., Poncet, M., Salamon, G., & Khalil, R. (1984). Behavior and mental activity disorders after carbon monoxide poisoning. Bilateral pallidal lesions. *Revue d'Neurologie, 140,* 401-405.

Alzheimer's Disease Education and Referral Center. (2002a). Stockholm sessions cover emerging and established therapies. *Advance, 22*(3), 2-3.

Alzheimer Disease Education and Referral Center. (2002b). *Multi-infarct dementia fact sheet.* Retrieved September 19, 2002, from http://www.alzheimers.org/pubs/mid.htm.

American Psychiatric Association. (2000). *Diagnostic and statistical manual of mental disorders* (4th ed., text revision). Washington, DC: Author.

Azar, B. (2002). Use it or lose it? *Monitor on Psychology, May,* 48-50.

Bonder, B.R. (1994). Psychotherapy for individuals with Alzheimer disease. *Alzheimer Disease and Associated Disorders, 8* (suppl.), 75-81.

Boyd, M.A. (2001). Behavioral disturbances associated with dementia: Nursing implications. *Journal of the American Psychiatric Nurses Association, 7*(6), S14-S22.

Brandt, J., Mellits, E.D., Rovner, B., et al. (1989). Relation of age at onset and duration of illness to cognitive functioning in Alzheimer's Disease. *Neuropsychiatry, Neuropsychology, and Behavioural Neurology, 2,* 93-101.

Buckingham, S.L., & Shernoff, M. (1998). Psychosocial interventions in persons with HIV-associated neuropsychiatric compromise. In W. VanGorp & S. Buckingham (Eds.), *A mental health practitioner's guide to the neuropsychiatric complications of HIV/AIDS* (pp. 228-240). New York: Guilford Publications.

Burns, A. (1992). Cause of death in dementia. *International Journal of Geriatric Psychiatry, 7,* 461-464.

Caine, E.D. (1993). Should aging-associated cognitive decline be included in DSM-IV? *Journal of Neuropsychiatry, 5,* 1-5.

Camp, C.J., Foss, J.W., Stevens, A.I., & O'Hanlon, A.M. (1996) Improving prospective memory task performance in persons with Alzheimer's disease. In M. Brandimonte, G.O. Einstein, & M.A. McDaniel (Eds.), *Prospective memory: Theory and applications* (pp. 351-367). Mahwah, NJ: Lawrence Erlbaum Associates.

Corey-Bloom, J., Anand, R., & Veach, J. (1998). A randomized tiral evaluating the efficacy and safety of ENA 713 (rivastigmine tartrate), a new acetylcholinesterase inhibitor, in patients with mild to moderately severe Alzheimer's disease. *International Journal of Geriatric Psychopharmacology, 1,* 55-65.

Corcoran, M. (2001). Dementia. In B.R. Bonder & M. Wagner (Eds.), *Functional performance in older adults* (2nd ed., pp. 287-304). Philadelphia: F.A. Davis.

Cummings, J.I. (1982). Cortical dementias. In D.F. Benson & D. Blume (Eds.), *Psychiatric aspects of neurologic disease*, Vol. 2 (pp. 93-121). New York: Grune and Stratton.

Dalfen, A.K., & Feinstein, A. (2000). Head injury, dissociation, and the Ganser syndrome. *Brain Injury, 14,* 1101-1105.

Davis, R. (1989). *My journey into Alzheimer's disease.* Wheaton, IL: Tyndale House Publishers, Inc.

Devenny, D.A., Krinsky-McHale, S.J., Sersen, G., & Silverman, W.P. (2000). Sequence of cognitive decline in dementia in adults with Down's syndrome. *Journal of Intellectual Disability Research, 44*(Pt. 6), 68-69.

Erikson, K.R. (1990). Amnestic disorders. Pathophysiology and patterns of memory dysfunction. *The Western Journal of Medicine, 152,* 159-166.

Fenn, H., Luby, V., & Yesavage, J.A. (1993). Subtypes in Alzheimer's disease and the impact of excess disability: Recent findings. *International Journal of Geriatric Psychiatry, 8,* 67-73.

Gitlin, L.N., & Corcoran, M.A. (1996). Managing dementia at home: The role of home environmental modifications. *Topics in Geriatric Rehabilitation, 12*(2), 28-39.

Glisky, E.L., & Glisky, M.L. (2002). Learning and memory impairments. In P.J. Eslinger (Ed.), *Neuropsychological interventions: Clinical research and practice* (pp. 137-162). New York: Guilford Press.

Guttman, R., Altman, R.D., & Nielsen, N.H. (1999). Alzheimer disease. Report of the Council on Scientific Affairs. *Archives of Family Medicine, 8,* 347-353.

Helkala, E.L., Koivisto, K., Hanninen, T., Vanhanen, M., Kuusisto, J., Mykkanen, L., et al. (1997). Stability of age-associated memory impairment during a longitudinal population-based study. *Journal of the American Geriatrics Society, 45,* 120-122.

Hokkanen, L., & Launes, J. (2000). Cognitive outcome in acute sporadic encephalitis. *Neuropsychology Review, 10*(3), 151-167.

Jacobson, R.R., & Lishman, W.A. (1987). Selective memory losss and global intellectual deficits in alcoholic Korsakoff's syndrome. *Psychological Medicine, 17,* 649-655.

Jeste, D.V., Gierz, M., & Harris, M.J. (1990). Pseudodementia: Myths and reality. *Psychiatric Annals, 20*(2), 71-79.

Jeste, D.V., Rockwell, E., Harris, M.J., Lohr, J.B., & Lacro, J. (1999). Conventional vs. newer antipsychotics in elderly patients. *The American Journal of Geriatric Psychiatry, 7,* 70-76.

Larabee, G.J., & Crook, T.H. (1994). Estimated prevalence of age-associated memory impairment derived from standardized tests of memory function. *International Psychogeriatrics, 6,* 95-104.

LaRue, A. (1982). Memory loss and aging. *The Psychiatric Clinics of North America, 5,* 89-103.

Lipowski, Z.J. (1992). Update on delirium. *The Interface of Psychiatry and Neurology, 15,* 335-346.

McArthur, J. (1998). *Update on neurology. The GENEVA report.* Retrieved September 15, 2002, from http://www.hopkins-aids.edu/geneva/hilitex_ mcar_dem.html.

McGowan, D.F. (1993). *Living in the labyrinth: A personal journey through the maze of Alzheimer's.* San Francisco, CA: Elder Books.

Murdoch, B.E., Chenery, H.J., Wilks, V., & Boyle, R.S. (1987). Language in Alzheimer dementia. *Brain and Language, 31,* 122-137.

Neurosurgery://on-call. (2000). *Parkinson's disease.* Retrieved September 15, 2002, from http://www.neuro surgery.org/health/patient/detail.asp?DisorderID=46.

Nickel, B. (1990). The Korsakoff concept of Karl Bonhoeffer and its relation to the psychometrics of amnestic disorders. *Psychiatry, Neurology, and Medical Psychology, 42*(1), 42-50.

Raskind, M.A., Peskind, E.R., Wessel, T., Parys, W., & the Galantamine USA-1 Study Group (2000). Galantamine in Alzheimer's disease: A 6-month randomized placebo-controlled trial with a 6-month extension. *Neurology, 54,* 2261-2268.

Reinvang, I. (1998). Amnestic disorders and their role in cognitive theory. *Scandinavian Journal of Psychology, 39,* 141-143.

Richards, S.S., & Hendrie, H.S. (1999). Diagnosis, management, and treatment of Alzheimer disease. *Archives of Internal Medicine, 159,* 789-798.

Riley, K.P. (2001). Depression. In B.R. Bonder & M. Wagner (Eds.), *Functional performance in older adults* (2nd ed., pp. 287-318). Philadelphia: F.A. Davis.

Scaffa, M. (Ed.). (2001). *Occupational therapy in community-based practice settings.* Philadelphia: F.A. Davis.

Stahl, S. (2000). *Essential psychopharmacology: Neuroscientific basis of practical applications.* Cambridge, United Kingdom: Cambridge University Press.

Steffes, R., & Thralow, J. (1987). Visual field limitation in the patient with dementia of the Alzheimer's type. *Journal of the American Geriatrics Society, 35,* 198-204.

Trace, S., & Howell, T. (1991). Occupational therapy in geriatric mental health. *The American Journal of Occupational Therapy, 45,* 833-838.

United States General Accounting Office. (1998). *Alzheimer's disease: Estimates of prevalence in the United States* (GAO/HEHS-98-16). Washington, DC: Author.

Van Deusen, J. (1992). Perceptual dysfunction in persons with dementia of the Alzheimer's type: A literature review. *Physical & Occupational Therapy in Geriatrics, 10*(4), 33-46.

Chapter 5

Substance-Related Disorders

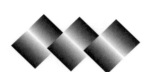
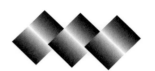

In our society, substance abuse is a pervasive problem. Among the many substances that are abused, some are illicit—among them cannabis, cocaine, PCP, hallucinogens, and some opiates. Others (e.g., sedatives and some of the opioids) are available as prescription medications, useful for specific purposes, but hazardous if misused. Still other substances are intended for other purposes but subject to abuse (e.g., glues, paints, and solvents may be inhaled). One of the most commonly abused substances is alcohol, which is legal, widely available, and socially accepted under many circumstances. Similarly, nicotine is a legal and readily available psychoactive substance with potentially devastating health effects. The illegal substances have been recognized as problematic for years, while disapproval of alcohol and nicotine abuse has ebbed and flowed. Prohibition of alcohol in the 1920s and '30s has been replaced by general acceptance of alcohol use, while there is a strong push currently to reduce smoking. Table 5-1 shows the categories of abused substances found in DSM-IV-TR (APA, 2000).

DSM-IV-TR (APA, 2000) has four general categories to describe the nature of substance use that can be applied regardless of the substance and also in cases in which several are abused simultaneously. These categories are dependence, intoxication, abuse, and withdrawal. Dependence and abuse are considered "use disorders," intoxication and withdrawal, "substance-induced disorders." In DSM, each substance is then described separately. There are also categories for alcohol- or drug-induced mood, anxiety, and psychotic disorders.

Dependence is diagnosed when at least three of the following signs occur within a 12-month period: the substance is taken in larger amounts or over more time than the individual planned, efforts to cut down are unsuccessful, and much of the person's activity revolves around getting the substance, and other activities are reduced as a result, even though the individual may know that this is a harmful pattern. Obligations are not met, and dangerous behavior may result from intoxication. For example, the individual may miss work, spend paychecks on the substance rather than on food, and may drive while intoxicated or begin to steal to have money to pay for the substance. The individual is aware that the problem exists but develops tolerance (i.e., increasing amounts are needed to obtain an effect). In addition, for most substances, withdrawal symptoms can occur and the individual may take the substance to avoid these symptoms. Thus, even though the individual knows that he or she has a problem, withdrawal becomes so unpleasant that the individual expends considerable effort to continue the substance.

Some earlier descriptions of substance abuse sought to distinguish between dependence (i.e., the psychological need for a substance) and addiction (i.e., the physical need for a substance to avoid physical withdrawal symptoms). DSM-IV-TR handles this by allowing a distinction between dependence with and dependence without physiological characteristics.

```
┌─────────────────────────────────────────────────────────────────┐
│                          Table 5-1                                │
│                  Substance-Related Disorders                      │
│                                                                   │
│   • Alcohol and sedatives           • Opioids                     │
│   • Cocaine and amphetamines        • Cannabis                    │
│   • Hallucinogens and phencyclidines • Nicotine                   │
│   • Inhalants                                                     │
└─────────────────────────────────────────────────────────────────┘
```

Abuse is diagnosed when criteria for dependence are not met, but the individual has noticeable behavioral problems related to substance use. The symptoms will not be as global or persistent as those for dependence.

Intoxication describes single episodes of substance use during which behavior is affected. Behavior during intoxication may include belligerence; emotional lability; and cognitive, judgment, social, or vocational impairment, all directly due to recent ingestion of a substance.

Withdrawal describes emotional distress or impairment in functioning directly due to efforts to stop using a substance. This does not include short-term effects (e.g., hangover), that result from single episodes of use and cessation.

The types of substance abuse that are most likely to come to the attention of the occupational therapist are described in detail here; those less commonly seen by occupational therapists are discussed briefly. Substances with similar physiological actions are discussed together. Because occupational therapy interventions for substance abuse are similar regardless of substance, these are presented together later in the chapter.

It is important for therapists to remember that individuals with substance abuse disorders may present in other areas of practice. For example, an individual in a rehabilitation setting may have been injured in an accident while impaired by substance abuse. Callahan (1990), a well-known cartoonist, is a quadriplegic as a result of an auto accident he experienced while driving intoxicated. Even after the accident, he described his main problem as substance abuse, not paralysis. Screening to identify problematic substance use is essential regardless of setting. Treatment for other conditions must take a client's substance use or abuse into consideration.

ALCOHOL AND SEDATIVES

Both alcohol and sedatives are CNS depressants. While alcohol may cause a brief sense of excitement, both have the effect of slowing responses over time. The "high" that accompanies them is actually a slowing of CNS and autonomic function. In cases of overdose, death may occur as a result of respiratory or cardiac slowing.

Alcohol use and abuse are common in the United States, with 5.7% of the population over the age of 12 reporting heavy drinking (Substance Abuse and Mental Health Services Administration [SAMHSA], 2002a). Different cultural and religious groups vary in their patterns of use, some abstaining totally, others using alcohol in specific ceremonial contexts, others using alcohol liberally (Straussner, 2001). As an example, Native-American adolescents are particularly likely to use alcohol (and other substances) with particularly dire consequences (Schinke, Tepavac, & Cole, 2000). Contrary to the common stereotype, African-

Americans are less likely to abuse alcohol than non-Hispanic whites, although those who do abuse alcohol are much more likely to be dysfunctional (Gerstein & Green, 1993). Three main patterns of abuse appear among heavy drinkers (SAMHSA, 2002a). One is characterized by daily intake of large amounts of alcohol. The second by regular binges (e.g., on weekends). This pattern is particularly common among adolescents (SAMHSA, 2002b). The third pattern is characterized by long periods of abstinence interspersed with heavy binges. Other substance abuse, particularly for nicotine, is frequently present in this last group of individuals.

Sedatives are characterized by two common patterns of abuse. In some individuals, the drug may be prescribed for a specific purpose, but tolerance may develop and symptoms of dependence appear. Cases in which these drugs are prescribed for long periods of time in order to allow an individual to function, as in the case of severe anxiety, do not qualify as substance abuse. In other cases, however, obtaining the drug becomes primary, and function changes in negative ways as a result. The second pattern of abuse is seen in individuals who obtain the drug through illicit means, specifically for purposes of abuse (i.e., for the "high"). In both cases, tolerance is marked.

Etiology and Incidence

There are several theories about the emergence of alcoholism. During the early part of the century (i.e., the preprohibition and prohibition years), alcoholism was thought to be a moral failure. Since that time, it has come to be viewed as a disease and that is now the commonly held explanation. One theory holds that a genetic predisposition to alcoholism may be triggered by certain environmental factors (Dantzer & Ollat, 1991). A familial pattern, evident even when children are raised by adoptive parents, suggests some genetic component in at least some cases (Schuckit, 1999). Familial alcoholism seems to have an earlier onset and worse prognosis than the nonfamilial type (Nathan, 1991). Evidence from cognitive studies supports the idea that there is a difference between familial and nonfamilial alcoholism (Ward, Mangold, El Deiry, McCaul, & Hoover, 1998), as opioid activity has been found to differ in the brains of individuals with familial alcohol dependency. While the origins of alcoholism are not entirely clear, individual and racial differences in alcohol tolerance, separate from dependence and abuse, have been noted. For example, individuals of some races are much more likely to have severe reactions to alcohol than Caucasians and, therefore, to drink less. On the other hand, diminished ability to metabolize alcohol, as found in Native American populations, for example, can lead to increased rates of alcoholism (French, 2000).

Women who are alcoholic have later onset and drink less, but progress more rapidly through the stages of the disorder (Lex, 1991). There is strong evidence of a link between trauma (e.g., sexual and physical abuse) and substance abuse among women (Wing & Oertle, 1999). Female alcoholism is of particular concern because of the potential for harm to the fetus during pregnancy. Chronic alcohol abuse during pregnancy causes fetal alcohol syndrome in the infant, manifested by retardation and CNS damage (Roebuck, Mattson, & Riley, 1999).

As will be discussed later in this chapter, alcohol abuse is often seen in combination with other psychiatric disorders. This "dual diagnosis" is a particular problem as the two or more different disorders affecting these individuals may reinforce each other, as in the case of an individual who self-medicates with sedatives to reduce symptoms of an anxiety disorder, thereby complicating treatment (Harrison & Precin, 1996; Hilarski & Wodarski, 2001).

Alcohol abuse is of particular importance in adolescents. After decreasing in the late 1980s, drug use overall has been increasing among adolescents by 1% to 2% per year since 1991 (Johnston, O'Malley, & Bachman, 1997). As with women, there is a link between early experiences of abuse and substance abuse and from substance abuse to juvenile violence. Because their abuse starts early in life, adolescents are at risk for significant additional problems throughout life, including health consequences, disruptions in developmental tasks, and disordered interpersonal relationships (Interdisciplinary Faculty Development Program in Substance Abuse Education [IFDPSAE], 2000). Further, alcohol is one of several so-called "gateway" drugs (i.e., a drug that has the potential to lead to abuse of other substances, such as cocaine, marijuana, and heroin) (Bachman, Wadsworth, O'Malley, & Johnston, 1997).

At the other end of the life span, older adults may also abuse alcohol or become alcoholic (Liberto, Oslin, & Ruskin, 1992). Older men become alcoholic more often than women. Older adults who are long-standing alcohol abusers or become alcoholic late in life are particularly vulnerable to adverse medical consequences of their abuse (Fingerhood, 2000).

Dependence on sedatives is less well-explained. For individuals who are exposed to the drugs as a result of some other condition, dependence probably results from the effects of the drug itself. Among those who experiment with sedatives as illicit drugs, personality disorders that may predispose to drug experimentation (e.g., antisocial personality) may be precursors of the problem. In addition, sedative abuse may result from efforts to self-treat panic disorder (Cox, Norton, Swinson, & Endler, 1990). Physicians often prescribe sedatives to control anxiety.

Approximately 15% of the adult population of the United States has had problems with alcohol dependence at some point during their lives (APA, 2000). According to the National Household Survey (SAMHSA, 2001), 12.4 million individuals in the United States are heavy drinkers. The incidence of sedative dependence is roughly 1.1% of the population (APA, 2000).

Prognosis

Some individuals simply stop abusing alcohol (Klingemann, 1991) or sedatives. The exact percentage of spontaneous remissions is not known. Others benefit from treatment, while some continue abuse throughout their lives, which are often shortened by the dependence. While previous research suggests that some alcoholics go on to drink more moderately (Gottheil, Thornton, Skoloda, & Alterman, 1982), this finding is controversial, as the vast majority of treatment programs hold that alcoholics must be totally abstinent to avoid relapse. Without further evidence on the point, the latter view must be taken as accurate.

The most effective interventions are those that emphasize social support, such as Alcoholics Anonymous (AA) (Vaillant, 1999). Prognosis is good for individuals who identify such interventions and make use of them. Vaillant uses the analogy of diabetes to describe the needed course of treatment (i.e., alcoholism is a chronic disease that requires careful monitoring over the long term). The worst prognosis is for polysubstance users (i.e., those who abuse alcohol along with other substances).

Alcoholism is a serious problem with major physical and lifestyle consequences (IFDP-SAE, 2000). Individuals who continue abuse may suffer liver damage, cognitive impairment, peripheral neuropathy, cardiomyopathy, chronic pancreatitis, and various cancers of the upper respiratory or gastrointestinal tract. In addition, social isolation, unemployment, and possibly homelessness or incarceration may occur for long-term chronic alcohol abusers.

Implications for Function and Treatment

These diagnoses are made only if functional impairment is present. Since these substances are all CNS depressants, recent ingestion leads to drowsiness, reduction in perceptual and motor function, with accompanying problems in an array of skills. Vocational and social performance are the areas most commonly affected, although later stages of dependence, particularly if organic signs appear, may result in decrements in all areas of function. Early in the disease, leisure time is most affected, with the individual's primary leisure activity being substance ingestion. Many alcoholics are quite lonely, though cause and effect are hard to determine. As time goes on, family life suffers as the individual spends more time drinking. Work behavior is impaired as the individual either misses time from work as a result of hangovers or performs poorly because of intoxication on the job.

Auto and industrial accidents may result from impaired motor and perceptual abilities while under the influence. Withdrawal symptoms may lead the individual to spend a great deal of time obtaining the substance or to become irritable or enraged. The skills required to accomplish ADLs and IADLs are rarely severely impaired, but individuals lose interest in performing these activities (Fishman, 2002). Some individuals lose interest in eating as the disorder progresses. Nutritional deficiencies may result from poor diet. Similarly, individuals may become forgetful, resulting in chores undone, checkbooks unbalanced, and so on.

Patterns for individuals actively abusing alcohol tend to revolve around drinking. Routines involve drinking with friends or alone, getting alcohol, and avoiding withdrawal. Other habits deteriorate, so that the individual may begin to fail to attend to basic needs.

Special note should be made of social role performance. Individuals who are dependent on these substances spend much of their leisure time obtaining and using the substance. They prefer the company of others who are dependent. In addition, if their spouses and family members do not desert them, the family members may feel compelled to hide the abuse, thereby supporting it. This pattern has been described as "codependence" and is problematic in efforts to treat dependence.

Performance decrements may well be due to CNS changes. It is clear that intoxication causes such alterations. While the changes diminish to some extent following detoxification, subtle neurological signs may persist and, if abuse continues over time, become more prominent (IFDPSAE, 2000).

A wide variety of treatments have been attempted. Medications used include sertraline (Pettinati et al., 2001), naltrexone (Monterosso et al., 2001), and SSRIs (Pettinati, 2001). Medications are used for a number of other substance abuse problems as well—to blunt the effects of withdrawal, to reduce craving, or to treat underlying depression or anxiety that might contribute to self-medication through abuse. However, most interventions that involve medications also include one or more psychosocial treatments at the same time.

One of the best known, and apparently most successful, psychosocial interventions is AA. This is a self-help group that has a philosophy based in a specific set of religious and moral beliefs. AA or other self-help groups may be linked to formal alcoholism treatment programs. Medical interventions include detoxification/withdrawal assistance and relapse prevention (Gorelick, 1993). In addition, various family interventions seem helpful (O'Farrell, 1992). Typically for both sedative and alcohol abuse, recognition of the problem and a willingness to do something about it are important first steps (Vaillant, 1999).

Increasingly, there has been a focus on prevention and early identification (Toomey et al., 1996). The main goal of such programs has been to delay onset of use and progression from lower to higher use frequency or decrease in consumption (Pentz, 1999). Relapse prevention is equally important, requiring emphasis on strategies to avoid situations in which abuse would be likely and on establishing alternative and satisfying lifestyles (Rawson, Obert, McCann, & Ling, 1991).

COCAINE AND AMPHETAMINES

Unlike alcohol and sedatives, these substances are stimulants that result in a psychological "high" and psychomotor excitement, both of which are brief (Weddington, 1993), encouraging increasing use. Cocaine is most commonly inhaled, though it may also be smoked (in the case of the "freebase" or "crack" form) or injected.

Etiology and Incidence

Cocaine and amphetamines tend to be abused in similar patterns. Two are prominent. The first involves daily use of the substance; the second, binges of varying frequency. Amphetamine abuse can emerge following use of the medications to assist in dieting. Although this use of the drug for this purpose has been largely discredited, some physicians still prescribe it. Cocaine is strictly illicit, although it has been considered trendy by middle and upper class individuals. At the same time, the numbers of lower class individuals abusing cocaine increased dramatically as crack has become more readily available and cheaper. Both can be highly addictive, with only a few exposures leading to both withdrawal symptoms and increasing desire for the effects.

Of these two dependencies, cocaine is by far the greater concern at present in this country. Estimates probably understate incidence. It was estimated in the early 1980s that 0.2% of the population used cocaine, but use increased dramatically until leveling off in the early 1990s (SAMHSA, 2002c).

One reason for concern is the teratogenic effect on fetuses (Gingras, Weese-Mayer, Hume, & O'Donnell, 1992). Given the number of pregnant women who abuse cocaine, and the fact that cocaine crosses the placental barrier, increasing numbers of infants have been born cocaine addicted and have lasting neurological damage as a result.

Another group of drugs in this category are the so-called "club drugs" (Drug Abuse Warning Network [DAWN], 2000), including LSD, GHB, ketamine, amphetamines, rohypnol, and MDMA (i.e., ecstasy). Ecstasy is now a frequent substance of choice among this group, particularly as associated with "raves" (i.e., parties that are based on its use) (National Institute on Drug Abuse [NIDA], 2002a). Use is most common among Caucasian adolescents and young adults (DAWN, 2000). MDMA is a neurotoxin, and it can cause a sharp increase in body temperature. There are reports of mortality either as a result of high body temperature or due to excessive water intake that upsets body chemistry.

Prognosis

Prognosis for abuse of these drugs is variable. They are highly addictive and have a somewhat glamorous image. Reported deaths of movie stars and athletes as a result of cocaine ingestion has changed that image somewhat. Although these individuals have received much attention, the problem is probably worse among individuals in lower socioeconomic groups (Smart, 1991). The increased availability of crack (a smoked form of cocaine) and the reductions in cost have increased the probability that individuals will continue to abuse the drug. While the pleasurable effects of these substances diminish over time, the craving does not. In addition, abuse of sedatives or alcohol frequently accompanies abuse of these substances to reduce some of the undesirable effects of the drugs, such as anxiety and insomnia. Thus, the picture is complicated by addiction to several substances at once.

Implications for Function and Treatment

As with alcohol and sedative dependence, abuse of these substances is most likely to affect vocational and social performance. Irritability is pronounced, and social withdrawal may develop and become severe. Use of the drug becomes the primary avocational interest, thus affecting function in this sphere as well. ADLs and IADLs are affected as organic (i.e., CNS) signs begin to appear or as need for the drug begins to supersede the wish to attend to these activities (Fishman, 2002).

Some individuals who abuse these drugs turn to criminal activity to support the habit. They may steal or become prostitutes to pay for the drug as their ability to hold jobs decreases and their need for the drug increases. Others become drug pushers themselves.

Treatment is problematic and still poorly developed. AA-type interventions may be valuable. Some medical attention may be necessary to prevent complications during withdrawal. The array of treatments includes medications to avoid withdrawal symptoms and reduce anxiety (Tutton & Crayton, 1993), 28-day in-patient stays, 12-step programs modeled after AA, and out-patient group and individual therapy (Rawson et al., 1991).

In general, however, current efforts to treat these types of abuse are not particularly effective. Several problems have been noted in treatment efforts. First, there is no medication to ameliorate withdrawal effects. Second, unlike some other substances, the pleasurable effect, though diminished over time, continues to occur. Third, there is an increasingly well-developed culture around these drugs, particularly in "ghetto" environments. Thus, while some individuals simply stop using, for many there may be little motivation to withdraw and little medical help for those who do wish to do so. Hardcore use is associated with particularly poor outcomes (Silkharev & Bryun, 1998).

HALLUCINOGENS AND PCP

Etiology and Incidence

Initial use usually occurs as a result of experimentation with drugs. Personality disorders or adjustment problems may be considered as predisposing factors because they might encourage such experimentation. Hallucinogens and PCP may be contaminated with or taken with other substances, particularly cannabis and alcohol. After a decline during the 1970s and 1980s, these drugs are becoming more popular, with a threefold increase in new users in the 1990s (SAMHSA, 2002c)

Users find the effects unpredictable (NIDA, 2002a). For some individuals, one exposure to the negative effects, particularly during an early experience with the drug, is sufficient to end its use. Occasionally, a pattern of long-term abuse may emerge. Heavier use has been correlated with flashbacks, possibly resulting from neurological changes caused by the drug or as a result of a hysterical reaction. There is not unanimity about the existence of this phenomenon.

Prognosis

Most individuals abuse these drugs for relatively short periods of time before resuming previous activities or moving on to other substances. For most people, these are drugs that prompt experimentation but not usually long-term addiction. PCP is the more dangerous, as it is easily produced in a laboratory, thus it is readily available. It has particularly damaging consequences, including the potential for brain damage, sometimes after very few uses (NIDA, 2002b); psychotic reactions; and violent rage. PCP users are frequently brought to emergency rooms as a result of either unpleasant psychological effects or because of overdoses. These individuals can become violent or suicidal and must be watched closely.

Implications for Function and Treatment

While the drugs are being abused, performance is severely impaired in all spheres. This is a direct result of the effects of the drugs, which cause hallucinations and cognitive and perceptual dysfunction. It is rare, however, to see such individuals in treatment as a result of dependence or abuse of these two classes of drugs. The exception is when an organic mental disorder appears, as is more likely to be the case with PCP (NIDA, 2002b).

OPIOIDS

Among this group of drugs are some that are clearly illicit, such as heroin, and others that may be prescribed as analgesics, anesthetics, or cough-suppressants. The latter group includes codeine, hydromorphone (e.g., Dilaudid), methadone, hydrocodone (e.g., Vicodin), oxycodone (e.g., Percodan, Percocet), and, most recently, oxycodone (e.g., Oxycontin) (NIDA, 2002c). Used in properly supervised medical settings, none of the latter group should lead to dependence, but many of them are used without supervision, or obtained through illicit sources. Methadone is a special problem. Used as a treatment for opioid addiction, it is itself addicting, leading to abuse in some situations. Newer drugs have the same effect in minimizing withdrawal symptoms from opioids but without producing the high that is associated with methadone.

Etiology and Incidence

In many cases, dependence on these substances is a reflection of other problems in an individual's life. These may be related to a pre-existing or coexisting character disorder, situational problems, or adjustment difficulties (Hilarski & Wodarski, 2001). Since abuse of these substances requires contact with illicit sources, establishment of dependence requires action on the part of the individual. It is common, for example, to find this sort of addiction in individuals with prior histories of delinquency or unstable home situations. Almost all have a history of prior other substance abuse (Dinwiddie, Reich, & Cloninger, 1992). It should be noted, however, that these addictions can be found in individuals from all sorts of life circumstances (SAMHSA, 2002c).

After diminishing in the 1980s, use of opioids increased during the 1990s (SAMHSA, 2002c). In 2000 alone, 2 million new users were identified for the pain relievers in this category alone. There were 146,000 new heroin users in the same year.

Prognosis

Dependence on these drugs is intractable, although apparently less so than cocaine. The drugs cause significant tolerance effects fairly rapidly, and withdrawal symptoms are severe and unpleasant. Thus, after initial experiences with the drugs for the "high" they cause, later experiences are often attempts to avoid withdrawal symptoms. In addition, since these drugs are related to lifestyle and personality characteristics, the environment tends to support the addiction. In order to successfully withdraw, individuals may have to cope not only with withdrawal, but also with making necessary changes in lifestyle to avoid encouragement to continue abusing the substance. Tolerance is a particular problem. As it develops, increasing amounts are required to experience the euphoria it causes. However, these drugs are also CNS depressants. Many individuals die of overdoses, particularly of heroin. As with other substances, there are "nuclear" users (i.e., those who use the substance frequently and at substantial doses) and "marginal" users (i.e., those who use infrequently and at relatively lower doses). Outcomes tend to be better for the marginal users (Silkharev & Bryun, 1998).

While prognosis is generally thought to be poor, there is not absolute agreement on this. Klingemann (1991) reports instances of "auto-remission," although the reasons for this occurrence are not clear. As with other abuse, coexisting psychosis is a predictor of poor prognosis (Harrison & Precin, 1996). Newer medical interventions, including use of naloxone and buprenorphine, have shown great promise (Tai, 2002).

Implications for Function and Treatment

These addictions have a particularly severe impact on function. The drugs are illicit and expensive, and tolerance develops quickly. Thus, individuals who become dependent on these substances are likely to redefine their valued performance areas as they spend much of their time in pursuit of their next "fix." Once ingested, the drugs cause lethargy and withdrawal, making it difficult to maintain a stable employment. The need for money to purchase the drug, accompanied by its effects, means that these individuals often turn to crime as a means to support the habit. Stealing and prostitution are common among opioid addicts.

In addition to impact on ability to maintain vocational function, dependence has a severe impact on social function. Social life also focuses on the drug. Friends tend to be involved with it, and relationships are tenuous, as the drug assumes primary importance in the individual's life. Similarly, leisure activities are replaced by the drug, which becomes the individual's vocation, avocation, and social life.

ADL and IADL function becomes impaired as dependence increases. The lethargy while under the influence of the drug leads to lessened interest in self-maintenance and maintenance of the surroundings. Individuals may have little interest in appearance and hygiene or in the environment. In addition, financial woes tend to be severe, leaving little for food, shelter, or clothing.

Treatment often begins in in-patient settings. "Cold turkey" withdrawal is held by some to be most effective (i.e., the individual must simply stop taking the substance, rather than withdrawing from it gradually). For most individuals, withdrawal is aided by use of medications such as methadone or buprenorphine (Kosten, Schottenfeld, Ziedonis, & Falcioni, 1993), which is discussed below. Medical management may be necessary to deal with complications of withdrawal. At the same time, other interventions must be made. Twelve-step interventions similar to AA have been reported to be successful with some individuals. A dilemma with this sort of treatment is that some individuals use it as a way to lower their tolerance for the drug, so that when they leave the in-patient setting, their dose requirement of the drug will be less.

In some cases, out-patient treatment may be an option. Methadone, which can cause dependence if taken in an unsupervised setting, is often used as a mechanism for withdrawing individuals from opioids. It prevents the withdrawal symptoms, with a less pronounced "high" than other narcotics. However, it must be continued once started, or withdrawal symptoms will occur. Increasingly, naloxone and buprenorphine are being used, and reports of their effectiveness are encouraging (Tai, 2002).

Social circumstances also affect outcomes. Individuals who have supportive and involved families do better than others (Grinspoon, Bakalar, & Weiss, 1999). This is problematic, however, as opioid addiction often involves a whole lifestyle supported and encouraged by the social system.

CANNABIS

This is a commonly used illicit substance, with approximately 2.4 million new initiates per year (SAMHSA, 2002c). It is popularly conceived as one of the less dangerous drugs. Many individuals begin using marijuana and hashish in social settings, believing them to be relatively harmless. Psychoactive symptoms appear to be less than those of other substances, making it unlikely that individuals with dependence will be seen in treatment. Chronic cannabis use seems to interfere with motivation and, therefore, with function (Grinspoon et al., 1999). In addition, a fairly high proportion of individuals with other psychiatric disturbances and alcoholics are also problematic cannabis abusers and these individuals have a much worse course. The best documented negative effects of cannabis are delirium, panic, and acute paranoia or mania. No catastrophic health effects have been found. However, the risk of accident while under the influence is cause for concern, particularly among adolescents who may be likely to try to drive while using marijuana.

Dependence and abuse generally develop over a relatively long period of time (Grinspoon et al., 1999). They are characterized by increasing frequency of use, rather than increased amounts at a given time. Prolonged use may lead to lethargy, anhedonia, and memory and attention deficits. Some changes in perceptual skills have also been noted. However, function is not as severely impaired as in other forms of substance abuse. Prognosis is better in many cases; cannabis seems to be a drug with which many adolescents experiment but then stop using.

INHALANTS

A wide variety of substances may be inhaled, including gasoline, paint thinners, glue, and various cleaners. The active ingredients are aliphatic and aromatic hydrocarbons that cause intoxication, resulting in a "high."

This type of substance abuse most often appears in children and adolescents, particularly those from disadvantaged backgrounds (SAMHSA, 2002d). Young people with a grade average of "D" are three times as likely as those with grades of "A" to use inhalants. These children are often from dysfunctional families and show significant adjustment problems, including truancy, poor grades, delinquency, and so forth. It appears that these adjustment problems predate the substance abuse. It also appears that abuse of inhalants leads to abuse of other substances. Inhalants are extremely dangerous, leading to physical and mental problems, including kidney and liver disease, even when used for only short periods of time.

Tolerance and withdrawal symptoms have been reported, but it is not clear that either phenomenon occurs. It is clear, however, that this type of abuse is intractable, recurring even after treatment. Furthermore, the effects of the drugs exacerbate existing functional difficulties. Performance of vocational, leisure, and self-care are all affected, probably with some coexisting decrements in cognitive and psychological skills due to CNS damage.

NICOTINE

Nicotine is the drug that makes cigarette smoking appealing. It is a highly addictive substance (Fiore, 2000). It is a mild stimulant that is difficult to stop once an addiction has developed, usually over the course of time. Smoking is a leading cause of preventable disease, and over 25% of Americans smoke (Fiore, 2000).

While some individuals are able to withdraw from smoking, the majority have considerable difficulty doing so. Behavioral techniques have been found to be effective in highly motivated individuals, but for many, the effects of nicotine are too reinforcing to be given up (Fiore, 2000).

For most, however, symptoms and interference with function are minimal, at least from a psychological perspective. Some individuals may have increasing problems in work situations as smoking is increasingly prohibited. Most, however, continue to perform in their typical fashion. Major problems with this type of addiction are physical and appear over long periods of time. Development of lung, larynx, and oral cancer, as well as cardiovascular problems, is common, but usually occurs after decades of smoking. Such long-term hazards tend to be disregarded by smokers or do not provide sufficient motivation to stop a severe addiction. Other hazards (e.g., fire from careless smoking) are less well-publicized. It does appear that some CNS function is compromised, possibly leading to such problems as auto accidents.

CAFFEINE

Caffeine was newly included in DSM-IV (APA, 1994) as an abused substance. It is the most widely used psychoactive substance in the United States and elsewhere (Heishman &

Henningfield, 1992). It is a mild stimulant but has the potential for excessive dose, resulting in jitteriness, anxiety, insomnia, and tachycardia. It also has withdrawal symptoms, most notabley fatigue and headache.

However, caffeine is rarely addressed as a drug in treatment settings. As compared with other drugs, its negative consequences are minimal, thus treatment is rare. Pregnant women are encouraged to limit consumption, although even the evidence about potential harm to a fetus is equivocal.

GENERAL TREATMENT CONSIDERATIONS

Many of the reports of addiction note the clustering of substance use (Strain, Brooner, & Bigelow, 1991). Recent and on-going research is focused on both medical interventions and on an array of behavioral interventions (Tai, 2002). Among the behavioral interventions considered effective or promising are cognitive-behavioral therapy, contingency management (a form of behavioral intervention in which reinforcements or outcomes of behavior are carefully managed), family therapy, and couples therapy. Relapse prevention strategies in out-patient care (Obert, Rawson, & Miotto, 1997) include education, identification of strategies for dealing with high-risk situations, development of coping skills, and development of new lifestyle behaviors. Ward (1998) notes that use of leisure time is a problem for individuals who are substance abusers. Substance abuse education, coping skills training, and lifestyle interventions are appropriate goals for occupational therapy.

Prevention of substance abuse is a central focus of many programs (Perry et al., 2002). As in relapse prevention, emphasis on lifestyle is crucial to efforts to prevent substance abuse. Similarly, screening and brief intervention are strategies increasingly viewed as valuable in preventing or minimizing substance abuse problems (IFDPSAE, 2000).

Dual Diagnosis

Substance abuse can coexist with CD, depression, developmental disabilities, schizophrenia, manic depressive disorder, and personality disorders (Harrison & Precin, 1996; Hilarski & Wodarski, 2001).

This so-called "dual diagnosis" is extremely problematic in that treatment efforts are confounded by the combination of problems. In general, such patients have very poor problem-solving ability that complicates intervention. It is also difficult to know if one condition led to the other or if they emerged separately. Substance abuse can lead to mood, anxiety, and psychotic disorders. Among adolescents who are substance abusers, various forms of violence are common, both with the adolescent as a victim of abuse and as a perpetrator of violent acts (Van Dalen, 2001). It is also possible that individuals abuse substances secondary to, or as a result of, another disorder. Alcohol abuse may emerge as a means to self-treat anxiety, for example. Understanding the etiology of the coexisting disorder(s) is essential to satisfactory intervention.

Treatment recommendations vary. Shilony, Lacey, O'Hagen, & Curto (1993) recommend a continuum from 6 months to 1 year of residential treatment to sheltered housing to out-patient aftercare. They note that lack of housing and aftercare presents significant problems. Recommendations for care emphasize the need for careful assessment to ensure that the approach is tailored to the individual (Harrison & Precin, 1996). However, data regarding effectiveness of various forms of treatment are sparse, with preliminary studies showing no increased positive effect when programs are specially planned for individuals with dual diagnosis (Lehman, Herron, Schwartz, & Myers, 1993).

IMPLICATIONS FOR OCCUPATIONAL THERAPY

Substance abuse, regardless of the drug, can interfere with performance of ADLs/IADLs and vocational and leisure activities (Moyers & Stoffel, 2001). In addition, there is reason to believe that CNS processing is impaired by some of the substances discussed in this chapter. Thus, intervention must occur at the level of both performance and skill.

Van Deusen (1989) discusses the impact of alcohol abuse on fine motor skills, tactile and figure-ground perception, and visual spatial function. She notes that there seems to be some spontaneous recovery of these skills in individuals who abstain from drinking but that practice may enhance this recovery. Her recommendation is that occupational therapy focus on remediating motor and sensory-motor deficits by way of sports activities, computer games, and so on. It is reasonable to assume that other substance abusers might respond to similar intervention.

A second area of concern is use of time, particularly leisure time (Harrison & Precin, 1996; Moyers & Stoffel, 2001). Substance abuse often becomes the primary focus of activity, and individuals with abuse disorders need to learn through education and experimentation about alternative uses of time. Identification of new and satisfying leisure activities can have a significant impact on outcomes of treatment. The individual must learn to fill newly free time with meaningful activities that will divert attention from the desire for the abused substance and provide satisfaction (Moyers, 1997). In addition, social skills training may help the individual to acquire new friends to replace those who were fellow alcoholics. Family treatment can also be helpful in resolving feelings of loneliness and enhancing relationships that are almost certainly damaged by substance abuse (Moyers, 1992). It is recommended that spiritual aspects of recovery be emphasized (Moyers, 1997).

The issue of time use is closely related to sociocultural considerations about work and work skills. Many substance abusers lose their jobs because of their addiction and must relearn job skills as well as work-related skills, such as following directions and relating to supervisors. Time management is a particular problem related to work as well as other activities (Moyers & Stoffel, 2001).

More problematic is the issue of individuals who turn to substance abuse specifically because they feel hopeless about future prospects. In inner city areas, substance abusers often have no job experience or skills and no hope of acquiring them. Training in work and work-related skills may mean starting at square one with reading and writing. Although this approach can be very valuable, it is time and cost intensive. Linkage with community services and constant follow-up is vital. All these difficulties contribute to, or are caused by, poor self-esteem. Experiences that can provide both motivation and hope are essential.

Finally, learning new methods for managing stress and experiencing successes that build self-esteem can assist individuals to remain substance-free. Ward (1998) notes that all of these approaches can be used successfully in group treatment, and that the group itself may have positive benefit in terms of providing realistic feedback, as well as an opportunity to practice interpersonal skills. Since loneliness is a problem for individuals who are substance abusers, group therapy can provide important social support.

Screening and Brief Intervention

Recent research suggests that every health care provider should practice screening and brief intervention in every practice setting (Haack & Adger, 2002). Screening can be done informally or with a variety of brief interviews, such as the CAGE (Ewing, 1984). The acronym CAGE reflects the four questions that are included in this assessment, specifically:

- C: Has anyone ever felt you should Cut down on your drinking?

- A: Have people Annoyed you by criticizing your drinking?

- G: Have you ever felt Guilty about your drinking?

- E: Have you ever had a drink first thing in the morning (Eye-opener) to steady your nerves or to get rid of a hangover?

A positive response to one of these questions suggests a problem. Such individuals might benefit either from motivational interviewing that encourages efforts to reduce use or by referral to a substance abuse program (Fleming, Barry, Manwell, Johnson, & London, 1997). Clinicians do not need to be experts at intervening with long-term substance abusers but can be very effective in reducing the impact on individuals in the early stages, or making sure that those who are having serious problems receive help (Bonaguro, Nalette, & Seibert, 2002).

REFERENCES

American Psychiatric Association. (1994). *Diagnostic and statistical manual of mental disorders* (4th ed.). Washington, DC: Author.

American Psychiatric Association. (2000). *Diagnostic and statistical manual of mental disorders* (4th ed., text revision). Washington, DC: Author.

Bachman, J.G., Wadsworth, K.N., O'Malley, P.M., & Johnston, L.D. (1997). *Smoking, drinking, and drug use in young adulthood: The impacts of new freedoms and new responsibilities.* Ann Arbor, MI: University of Michigan Institute for Social Research.

Bonaguro, J.A., Nalette, E., & Seibert, M.L. (2002). The role of allied health professionals in substance abuse education. In M.R. Haack & H. Adger (Eds.), *Strategic plan for interdisciplinary faculty development: Arming the nation's health professional workforce for a new approach to substance use disorders* (pp. 169-184). Providence, RI: Association for Medical Education and Research in Substance Abuse.

Callahan, J. (1990). *Don't worry, he won't get far on foot.* New York: Vintage Books.

Cox, M.J., Norton, G.R., Swinson, R.P., & Endler, N.S. (1990). Substance abuse and panic-related anxiety: A critical review. *Behavioral Research Therapy, 28,* 385-393.

Dantzer, R., & Ollat, H. (1991). Alcoholism: A psychobiological perspective. *European Psychiatry, 6,* 209-215.

Dinwiddie, S.H., Reich, T., & Cloninger, C.R. (1992). Patterns of lifetime drug use among intravenous drug users. *Journal of Substance Abuse, 4,* 1-11.

Drug Abuse Warning Network (DAWN). (2000). *The DAWN report: Club drugs.* SAMHSA Office of Applied Studies. Retrieved October 29, 2002, from http://222.samhsa.gov/oas/DAWN/clubdrug.htm.

Ewing, J.A. (1984). Detecting alcoholism: The CAGE questionnaire. *The Journal of the American Medical Association, 252,* 1095-1097.

Fingerhood, M. (2000). Substance abuse in older people. *Journal of the American Geriatrics Society, 48,* 985-995.

Fiore, M.C. (2000). Treating tobacco use and dependence: An introduction to the US Public Health Service clinical practice guideline. *Respiratory Care, 45,* 1196-1262.

Fishman, M. (2002). Treatment of HIV and addiction: Preserving therapeutic optimism. *Advanced Studies in Medicine, 2,* 189-194.

Fleming, M.F., Barry, K.L., Manwell, L.B., Johnson, K., & London, R. (1997). Brief physician advice for problem alcohol drinkers. A randomized controlled trial in community-based primary care practices. *The Journal of the American Medical Association, 277,* 1039-1045.

French, L.A. (2000). *Addictions and Native Americans.* Westport, CT: Praeger.

Gerstein, R.D., & Green, L.W. (Eds.). (1993). *Preventing drug abuse: What do we know?* Washington, DC: National Academy Press.

Gingras, J.L., Weese-Mayer, D.E., Hume, R.F., & O'Donnell, K.J. (1992). Cocaine and development: Mechanisms of fetal toxicity and neonatal consequences of prenatal cocaine exposure. *Early Human Development, 31,* 1-24.

Gorelick, D.A. (1993). Overview of pharmacologic treatment approaches for alcohol and other drug addiction. *Psychiatric Clinics of North America, 16,* 141-156.

Gottheil, E., Thornton, C.C., Skoloda, T.E., & Alterman, A.I. (1982). Follow-up of abstinent and nonabstinent alcoholics. *The American Journal of Psychiatry, 139,* 560-565.

Grinspoon, L., Bakalar, J., & Weiss, R. (1999). Substance use disorders. In A.M. Nicholi (Ed.), *The Harvard guide to psychiatry* (3rd ed., pp. 390-399). Cambridge, MA: Harvard University Press.

Haack, M.R., & Adger, H. (Eds.). (2002). *Strategic plan for interdisciplinary faculty development: Arming the nation's health professional workforce for a new approach to substance use disorders.* Providence, RI: Association for Medical Education and Research in Substance Abuse (AMERSA).

Harrison, T.S., & Precin, P. (1996). Cognitive impairments in clients with dual diagnosis (chronic psychotic disorders and substance abuse): Considerations for treatment. *Occupational Therapy International, 3,* 122-141.

Heishman, S.J., & Henningfield, J.E. (1992). Stimulus functions of caffeine in humans: Relation to dependence potential. *Neuroscience and Biobehavioral Reviews, 16,* 273-287.

Hilarski, C., & Wodarski, J.S. (2001). Comorbid substance abuse and mental illness: Diagnosis and treatment. *Journal of Social Work Practice in the Addictions, 1,* 105-119.

Interdisciplinary Faculty Development Program in Substance Abuse Prevention. (2000). *Curriculum on substance abuse screening and brief intervention.* Providence, RI: AMERSA.

Johnston, L.D., O'Malley, P.M., & Bachman, J.G. (1997). *National survey results on drug use from the monitoring the future study, 1975-1996, Vol 1: Secondary school students* (NIH Publication No. 94-3809). Rockville, MD: U.S. Department of Health and Human Services.

Klingemann, H.K.H. (1991). The motivation for change from problem alcohol and heroin use. *British Journal of Addiction, 86,* 727-744.

Kosten, T.R., Schottenfeld, R., Ziedonis, D., & Falcioni, J. (1993). Buprenorphine versus methadone maintenance for opioid dependence. *The Journal of Nervous and Mental Disease, 181,* 358-364.

Lehman, A.F., Herron, J.D., Schwartz, R.P., & Myers, C.P. (1993). Rehabilitation for adults with severe mental illness and substance use disorders. *The Journal of Nervous and Mental Disease, 181,* 86-90.

Lex, B.W. (1991). Some gender differences in alcohol and polysubstance users. *Health Psychology: Official Journal of the Decision of Health Psychology, American Psychological Association, 10,* 121-132.

Liberto, J.G., Oslin, D.W., & Ruskin, P.E. (1992). Alcoholism in older persons: A review of the literature. *Hospital and Community Psychiatry, 43,* 975-984.

Monterosso, J.R., Flannery, B.A., Pettinati, H.M., Oslin, D.W., Rukstalis, M., O'Brien, C.P., et al. (2001). Predicting treatment response to naltrexone: The influence of craving and family history. *American Journal of Addictions, 10,* 258-268.

Moyers, P.A. (1992). Occupational therapy intervention with the alcoholic's family. *The American Journal of Occupational Therapy, 46,* 105-111.

Moyers, P.A. (1997). Occupational meanings and spirituality: The quest for sobriety. *The American Journal of Occupational Therapy, 51,* 207-214.

Moyers, P.A., & Stoffel, V.C. (2001). Community-based approaches for substance use disorders. In M.E. Scaffa (Ed.), *Occupational therapy in community-based practice settings* (pp. 319-342). Philadelphia: F.A. Davis.

Nathan, P.E. (1991). Substance use disorders in the DSM-IV. *Journal of Abnormal Psychology, 100,* 356-361.

National Institute on Drug Abuse. (2002a). *NIDA InfoFacts: MDMA (Ecstasy).* Retrieved October 10, 2002, from http://www.nida.nih.gov/infofax/ecstasy.html.

National Institute on Drug Abuse. (2002b). *NIDA InfoFacts: PCP (Phencyclidine).* Retrieved October 14, 2002, from http://www.nida.nih.gov/infofax/pcp/html.

National Institute on Drug Abuse. (2002c). *NIDA InfoFacts: LSD.* Retrieved October 14, 2002, from http://www.nida.nih.gov/infofax/lsd.html.

Obert, J.L., Rawson, R.A., & Miotto, K. (1997). Substance abuse treatment for "hazardous users": An early intervention. *Journal of Psychoactive Drugs, 29,* 291-298.

O'Farrell, T.J. (1992). Families and alcohol problems: An overview of treatment research. *Journal of Family Psychology, 5,* 339-359.

Pentz, M.A. (1999). Prevention. In M. Galanter & H.S. Kleber (Eds.), *Textbook of substance abuse treatment* (2nd ed., pp. 535-544). Washington, DC: American Psychiatric Press.

Perry, C., Williams, C.L., Komro, K.A., Veblen-Mortenson, S., Stigler, M.H., Munson, K.A., et al. (2002). Project Northland: Long-term outcomes of community action to reduce adolescent alcohol use. *Health Education Research, 17,* 117-132.

Perry, C.L. (1999). *Creating behavior change: How to develop community-wide programs for youth.* Thousand Oaks, CA: Sage Publications, Inc.

Pettinati, H.M. (2001). The use of selective serotonin reuptake inhibitors in treating alcoholic subtypes. *Journal of Clinical Psychiatry, 62*(Suppl.20), 26-31.

Pettinati, H.M., Volpicelli, J.R., Luck, G., Kranzler, H.R., Rukstalis, M.R., & Cnaan, A. (2001). Double-blind clinical trial of sertraline treatment for alcohol dependence. *Journal of Clinical Psychopharmacology, 21,* 143-153.

Rawson, R.A., Obert, J.L., McCann, M.J., & Ling, W. (1991). Psychological approaches for the treatment of cocaine dependence: A neurobehavioral approach. *Journal of Addictive Diseases, 11,* 97-119.

Roebuck, T.M., Mattson, S.N., & Riley, E.P. (1999). Behavioral and psychosocial profiles of alcohol-exposed children. *Alcoholism, Clinical and Experimental Research, 23,* 1070-1076.

Schinke, S.P., Tepavac, L., & Cole, K.C. (2000). Preventing substance use among Native American young: Three years results. *Addiction Behavior, 25,* 387-397.

Schuckit, M. (1999). New findings in the genetics of alcoholism. *The Journal of the American Medical Association, 281,* 1875-1876.

Shilony, E., Lacey, D., O'Hagen, P., & Curto, M. (1993). All in one neighborhood: A community-based rehabilitation treatment program for homeless adults with mental illness and alcohol/substance abuse disorders. *Psychosocial Rehabilitation Journal, 16,* 103-116.

Silkharev, A.V., & Bryun, E.A. (1998). Comparative psychological study of the ethnofunctional discoordination in patients with heroin addiction, alcoholism and affective disorders. *Psychological Journal, 19,* 282-296.

Smart, R.G. (1991). Crack cocaine use: A review of prevalence and adverse effects. *The American Journal of Drug and Alcohol Abuse, 17,* 13-26.

Strain, E.C., Brooner, R.K., & Bigelow, G.E. (1991). Clustering of multiple substance use and psychiatric diagnoses in opiate addicts. *Drug and Alcohol Dependence, 27,* 127-134.

Straussner, S.L.A. (2001). *Ethnocultural factors in substance abuse treatment.* New York: Guilford Press.

Substance Abuse and Mental Health Services Administration. (SAMHSA) (2001). *The National household survey on drug abuse.* Retrieved October 29, 2002, from http://www.samhsa.gov/oas/nhsda/2k1nhsda/vol1/highlights.htm

Substance Abuse and Mental Health Services Administration (SAMHSA). (2002a). *Alcohol use.* Retrieved September 10, 2002, from http://www.samhsa.gov/oas/nhsda/2k1nhsda/vol1/Chapter3.htm.

Substance Abuse and Mental Health Services Administration (SAMHSA). (2002b). *The NHSDA report: Alcohol use.* Retrieved September 10, 2002, from http://www.samhsa.gov/oas/2k2/alcNS/alcNS.cfm.

Substance Abuse and Mental Health Services Administration (SAMHSA). (2002c). *Trends in initiation of substance use.* Retrieved September 10, 2002, from http://www.samhsa.gov/oas/nhsda/2k1nhsda/vol1/Chapter5.htm.

Substance Abuse and Mental Health Services Administration (SAMHSA). (2002d) *The NHSDA report: Inhalant use among youths.* Retrieved September 10, 2002, from http://www.samhsa.gov/oas/2k2/inhalNS/inhalNS/cfm.

Tai, B. (2002, November). *US national drug abuse treatment clinical trials network.* Paper presented at the AMERSA Annual Meeting, Washington, DC.

Toomey, T.L., Williams, C.L., Perry, C.L., Murray, D.L., et al. (1996). An alcohol primary prevention program for parents of 7th graders: The amazing alternatives! Home program. *Journal of Child and Adolescent Substance Abuse, 5*(4), 35-53.

Tutton, C.S., & Crayton, J.W. (1993). Current pharmacotherapies for cocaine abuse: A review. *Journal of Addictive Diseases, 12,* 109-126.

Vaillant, G.E. (1999). *The alcohol-dependent and drug-dependent person.* In A.M. Nicholi (Ed.), *The Harvard guide to psychiatry* (3rd ed., pp. 672-683). Cambridge, MA: Harvard University Press.

Van Dalen, A. (2001). Juvenile violence and addiction: Tangled roots in childhood trauma. *Journal of Social Work Practice in the Addictions, 1*(1), 25-40.

Van Deusen, J. (1989). Alcohol abuse and perceptual-motor dysfunction: The occupational therapist's role. *The American Journal of Occupational Therapy, 43,* 384-390.

Ward, J.D. (1998). Psychosocial dysfunction in adults. In M.E. Neistadt & E.B. Crepeau (Eds.), *Willard and Spackman's occupational therapy* (9th ed., pp. 716-740). Philadelphia: Lippincott, Williams & Wilkins.

Ward, G.S., Mangold, D., El Deiry, S.M., McCaul, M.E., & Hoover, D. (1998). Family history of alcoholism and hypothalamic opioidergic activity. *Archives of General Psychiatry, 55,* 1114-1119.

Weddington, W.W. (1993). Cocaine: Diagnosis and treatment. *Psychiatric Clinics of North America, 16,* 87-95.

Wing, D.M., & Oertle, J.R. (1999). Patterns of chemical addiction in women veterans with posttraumatic stress disorder. *Journal of Addictions Nursing, 11,* 107-111.

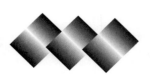

Chapter 6

Schizophrenia and Other Psychotic Disorders

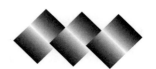

The psychotic disorders, including schizophrenia, are among the most disabling. Perhaps for that reason, they have received a great deal of attention. Of the psychotic disorders, schizophrenia is the best known, although media portrayals of the disorder tend to be somewhat misleading. DSM-IV-TR (APA, 2000) identifies the characteristics that must be present for the diagnosis to be made, including a minimum duration and a specific constellation of symptoms that must include at least some positive symptoms of psychosis: hallucinations, delusions, disorganized thinking, or some combination of these. Note that the term "positive" refers to the fact that a symptom is present and does not imply that it is good. Schizophrenia also includes "negative" symptoms such as flat affect and anhedonia.

As discussed in Chapter 1, the diagnoses in this category are likely to be carefully examined in the development of DSM-V. It has been suggested that the concept of "schizotaxia" may provide helpful explanation of the whole spectrum of schizophrenic-type disorders described here (Tsuang, Stone, & Faraone, 2000). This concept suggests that the range of schizophrenia-like disorders, including schizotypal personality disorder and schizoaffective disorder, is a set of alternative expressions of the same etiologic factors. Table 6-1 shows the main types of schizophrenia listed in DSM-IV-TR (APA, 2000).

SCHIZOPHRENIA

This is one of the mental disorders that is defined relative to function. In order for the diagnosis to be made, functional level must be below the highest level previously achieved in one or more areas. In addition, thought, including both content and form, is disturbed. Delusions (i.e., beliefs that are firmly held but not true) occur frequently in these individuals. The most common types of delusions are delusions of persecution (i.e., fear that one is being followed or will be harmed by others), delusions of reference (i.e., the belief that one is being talked about by others), or delusions of grandeur (i.e., the belief that one possesses special powers, abilities, or gifts). Loosening of associations, incoherence, or excessively concrete or abstract thought are also characteristic. Someone with loose associations might answer a question about the weather by launching into a discussion of weather patterns in outer space. An excessively concrete response might be that there are two rain drops on the window of a red car outside, while an excessively abstract answer might be that weather is in the eye of the beholder and relates to the meaning of life.

> Table 6-1
> ### Common Types of Schizophrenia
>
> - Paranoid type
> - Disorganized type
> - Catatonic type
>
> - Undifferentiated type
> - Residual type

Perception and affect are also disturbed. Hallucinations (i.e., sensory experiences such as seeing visions or feeling ants crawling under the skin) are typical. Auditory hallucinations (i.e., hearing voices) are most common, although any sense may be involved. The individual may smell peculiar smells and think that poison gas is in the room or see strange figures in the mirror. Affect is either flat or inappropriate. Some individuals with schizophrenia are totally expressionless, while others may have bizarre smiles, laugh inappropriately, and so on.

Peculiar psychomotor behavior may be present. Odd mannerisms, grimacing, hyperactivity or, conversely, waxy rigidity may be observed. Sense of self is also impaired. The individual may have difficulty discriminating between self and others or between self and the environment.

Most often, the disorder appears during adolescence or early adulthood, with an average age of onset between 20 and 25 (Grothe et al., 2000). Less often, the schizophrenia develops in childhood (Eggers, Bunk, & Kraus, 2000) or later in life (Citrone, 1998). The childhood form is thought to be most severe and chronic (Levitt et al., 2001). The late onset form is extremely rare and almost always associated with dysfunctional behavior earlier in life and/or previous psychiatric diagnosis (Howard, 1996).

This diagnosis is made only if symptoms have persisted for at least 6 months. Within the most recent month, the individual must experience at least two of the following:

- Delusions
- Hallucinations
- Disorganized speech or behavior
- Catatonic symptoms
- Negative symptoms, such as flat effect or avolition (APA, 2000).

Schizophrenic symptoms occur in three predictable phases (Furlow, 2000). The first is a prodromal phase in which function begins to deteriorate. The individual withdraws from friends and family. Work, self-care, and avocational activities suffer. The individual may stop bathing, begin to have trouble relating to people at work or school, and spend most free time staring in a mirror or just sitting. The active phase is characterized by delusions and hallucinations, thought disorder, and other psychotic symptoms. This phase may occur spontaneously or as a result of stress. The residual phase is often similar to the prodromal phase in terms of symptomatology. During this phase, functional level continues to be below the highest level ever achieved by the individual. Most individuals continue to have flat affect, peculiar behavior, and functional difficulties between active phases. They usually have few friends or interests, ignore self-care, and may have problems concentrating well enough to work.

Several types of schizophrenia are identified in DSM-IV-TR (APA, 2000), with differing constellations of symptoms. Each may occur in an episodic pattern, as a continuous state, or, least common, as a single episode. Catatonic schizophrenia is characterized by immobility or catatonic excitement (motor excitation that is purposeless and not affected by external stim-

Table 6-2

Symptoms and Functional Deficits Associated With Schizophrenia

Disorder	Symptoms (Duration of at least 6 months with two or more symptoms for at least 1 month)	Functional Deficits
Schizophrenia	1. Delusions 2. Hallucinations 3. Disorganized speech 4. Disorganized behavior 5. Negative symptoms 6. Flat or inappropriate affect 7. Episodic deterioration of function	All performance areas Worst with adolescent onset Habits, routines, and roles either not established or impaired during exacerbations Process skills and communication are significantly affected Motor skills may be intact
A. Catatonic	1. Catatonia is most marked symptom	
B. Disorganized	1. Above symptoms plus disorganized speech 2. Incoherence or severely disorganized behavior 3. Flat affect	
C. Paranoid	1. Preoccupation with delusional system and/or auditory hallucinations 2. Absence of loose associations, flat or inappropriate affect, catatonic or disorganized behavior	Usually less impaired ADLs/IADLs Significant impairment in work May establish acceptable roles, but more typically impaired Usually little motor impairment Substantial process deficits

uli), echolalia or echopraxia, absence of response to external stimuli that should encourage movement, peculiar movements, or mutism. Individuals with catatonic schizophrenia may sit rigid for hours without moving, often in positions that appear very uncomfortable. They may not eat, speak, or in any way acknowledge the environment during these periods. This is an uncommon type of schizophrenia, occurring in approximately 10% of all cases (Fink & Taylor, 1991). Table 6-2 shows the symptoms and functional deficits associated with the main forms of schizophrenia.

Disorganized schizophrenia is characterized by flat or inappropriate affect and disorganization of behavior or speech. Individuals who are diagnosed with this type of schizophrenia are usually unkempt and disheveled, walk with a shuffling gait and stooped posture, and may mutter unintelligibly. Conversations with such individuals may be incomprehensible, or they may exclaim with great fear about voices telling them terrible things or figures appearing to them. They tend to be lethargic and difficult to engage in activity, or occasionally, to be excessively active but not engaged in any purposeful activity.

Paranoid schizophrenia is noticeably different from the other schizophrenias. Its predominant feature is a well-developed system of delusions, particularly delusions of persecution. Catatonic behavior, inappropriate affect, disorganized behavior, and loose associations are not present. The presenting features are auditory hallucinations with disorganized, flat, or inappropriate affect. Hallucinations tend to feed into a sense of persecution. These individuals, if willing to discuss their fears at all, may complain of being followed by the FBI, for example. This type of schizophrenia seems markedly different in terms of etiology. Findings demonstrate that, unlike those with other types of schizophrenia, individuals with the paranoid form show few, if any, impairments on neuropsychological testing (Tsuang, Faraone, & Green, 1999). Typically, these individuals have better premorbid social, marital, and instrumental functioning. The diagnosis is more stable than other types (McGlashan & Fenton, 1991), and the long-term outcome is more favorable (Tsuang et al., 1999).

Residual schizophrenia is diagnosed when the individual has psychotic symptoms but does not fit the criteria for other forms of schizophrenia. Catatonic and undifferentiated schizophrenia may develop over time into the residual type (Tsuang et al., 1999), while paranoid type does not.

Etiology and Incidence

There are a variety of theories about the emergence of schizophrenia. There is a family pattern that can be demonstrated even when the individual is not raised by the biological family (Kumra, Nicolson, & Rapoport, 2002). The risk for first-degree relatives of an individual with schizophrenia is 10 times higher than the general population, and a child whose two parents have schizophrenia has a 40% risk of developing the disorder (Keks, Mazumdar, & Shields, 2000)

However, the genetic component does not seem sufficient to cause the emergence of the disease (Harvey, 2001). Not all individuals who are genetically predisposed develop schizophrenia, even if they are identical twins. Some theorists suggest that environmental factors, including a variety of psychosocial stressors, such as maladjusted family relationships, contribute as well. This vulnerability model (Harvey, 2001) suggests that multiple factors, both biological and psychosocial, must be present for the disorder to emerge.

Stress has been examined as an etiologic factor, and while it seems unlikely that it causes schizophrenia, it appears to be a factor in exacerbations (Wuerker, 2000). The stress explanation has replaced earlier theories about the role of poor parenting in the development of schizophrenia, suggesting that family dysfunction may play a role in the emergence of the disorder in individuals with a predisposition, but that poor parenting alone is insufficient to cause the disorder.

There is evidence that the diagnosis is more common in lower socioeconomic groups, but this may be an outcome of the disease rather than a predisposing factor. Since the disease is marked by functional decline, the individual may have difficulty holding a job and, therefore, move downward in terms of socioeconomic factors. There is clear evidence that poor premorbid functioning characterizes individuals who ultimately develop schizophrenia (Furlow, 2000; Kumra et al., 2002).

Recent etiological explanations have focused on biological factors in schizophrenia. A variety of studies have examined the role of biochemical changes, neurological factors, and other physical agents in the emergence of the disorder (Furlow, 2000; Kumra et al., 2002). Exposure to infection in utero has also been hypothesized as contributing (Brown & Susser, 2002), as has season of birth and complications during pregnancy and birth (Furlow, 2000). Although brain imaging studies fail to show consistent structural abnormalities (Kumra et al., 2002), among the subtle differences identified are increased size of ventricles, smaller cerebral cortex, and smaller limbic region (The Harvard Mental Health Newsletter, 2001). Neurotransmitter irregularities have also been identified. Dopamine transmission has been studied, but it now seems that receptors for N-methyl-D-aspartate, which regulates the release of glutamate, may be abnormal in individuals with schizophrenia (The Harvard Mental Health Newsletter, 2001).

Prevalence of schizophrenia is approximately 0.5% to 1% of the adult population (APA, 2000). Full-blown catatonic schizophrenia is the least common, but catatonic symptoms may be seen in other forms of schizophrenia (McGlashan & Fenton, 1991).

Prognosis

Reviews of literature related to prognosis suggest variable outcomes (Ram, Bromet, Easton, Pato, & Schwartz, 1992). Without drug treatment, the relapse rate is approximately 96%, meaning that individuals with schizophrenia will likely need to remain on medication for long periods of time (Carpenter, 2001). Poor function continues to be a problem, but there may be some slight improvement over time. The individual may have fewer active psychotic episodes and remain in the residual phase for increasingly longer periods of time.

A variety of factors have been examined to determine their value as predictors of outcome. Onset in childhood suggests a more severe course and worse prognosis than is otherwise typical (Eggers et al., 2000). Tsoi and Kua (1992) found that marital status and duration of illness are good predictors; age, sex, and education are somewhat useful predictors; and race and symptoms are poor predictors. Although family history is highly associated with development of schizophrenia, it is not a good predictor of outcome. It appears that prognosis is reasonably good on a first hospital admission and worsens with subsequent admissions (Ram et al., 1992). Subtype may affect outcome, although the research is conflicting, with some researchers finding that paranoid schizophrenia is predictive of better outcome (Tsuang et al., 1999), while others find no difference (Marengo, Harrow, & Westermeyer, 1991). Overall, it appears that about one-third of individuals with schizophrenia have good outcomes, one-third have long-term but moderate symptoms, and one-third continue to have severe symptoms or frequent relapses (Ram et al., 1992). Combined drug treatment and psychotherapeutic interventions are related to better outcomes (Bryden, Carrey, & Kutcher, 2001).

A special problem is the coexistence of secondary depression (Sirls, 1991). There is evidence that this is a fairly common occurrence, and outcomes can be particularly problematic in these cases. Suicide occurs in approximately 10% to 13% of individuals with schizophrenia (Caldwell & Gottesman, 1992). In particular, risk is high when the individual is showing some improvement. Suicide is discussed in greater detail in the next chapter but should be remembered as a significant risk when working with individuals with schizophrenia.

Implications for Function and Treatment

As noted, functional impairment is a defining characteristic of schizophrenia. Performance in all areas—social, vocational, leisure, and self-care—are markedly affected, leading to a global picture of disability. It is important to note, however, that the degree of impairment is variable and depends on the severity, phase, and type of illness.

The prodromal and residual phases are characterized more by functional impairment than by psychological symptoms. Thus, even though delusions and hallucinations disappear, the individual may continue to demonstrate severe social and vocational impairment. This is particularly true for individuals whose premorbid functioning was poor. As was noted above, individuals who develop schizophrenia are often isolated, anhedonic (i.e., lacking the ability to enjoy events), and lacking in motivation prior to the onset of the disorder. An additional factor in probable level of function during the residual phase is the time of onset of the disorder. If the individual develops schizophrenia during childhood or adolescence, he or she may miss important milestones in normal development. This makes it more difficult to function well later, even when acute symptoms abate (Dunn & McDougle, 2001). Individuals with schizophrenia are frequently fearful. Many hallucinations and delusions are quite frightening, as are the reactions of people in the community to these individuals, whose appearance and behavior may seem quite odd.

For some individuals, function during the prodromal and residual phases may be minimally impaired. This is particularly true where supportive treatment, such as out-patient counseling, is available. Individuals who can identify environments in which demand and stress are reduced may do well. They may regain reasonable measures of social and self-care function. In addition, if a supportive work environment with low levels of stress and an understanding supervisor can be found, individuals with schizophrenia may be able to hold jobs.

As an example, a young adult who was isolated and lethargic as a teenager, had few friends, and did poorly in school might develop schizophrenia, continue to have few friends, and find work difficult even during the residual phase. By contrast, someone who held a job, had a social circle, and developed schizophrenia in his or her late 20s would be likely to do much better during residual phases.

For both children and adolescents with schizophrenia, treatment should include medication and psychosocial interventions (Dunn & McDougle, 2001). In addition, educational and vocational habilitation or rehabilitation will be required to improve outcomes.

During active phases of the disease, functional impairment is much more severe. It is rare that individuals can work during this period. They demonstrate very little motivation to engage in other activities, and they tend to be severely withdrawn socially. Personal hygiene suffers, as do other self-care activities.

Deficits occur in performance skills, as well as in performance areas, probably contributing to overall poor function. A whole variety of cognitive deficits have been found, including deficits in communication (Abu-Akel, Caplan, Guthrie, & Komo, 2000), memory (So, Toglia, & Donohue, 1997), and problem solving (Tsuang et al., 1999). Among the other cognitive impairments noted are disturbances of will and volition (Frith, 1987), poor spatial and nonspatial associative learning (Kemali, Majio, Galderisi, Monteleone, & Mucci, 1987), difficulty with color perception (David, 1987), and poverty of written response (Manschreck, Ames, Maher, & Schneyer, 1982). Long-term hospitalization may have an additional negative impact on these skills.

Unfortunately, all of these problems are compounded when tardive dyskinesia appears as a side effect of psychopharmacologic treatment (Gray, 2001). Motor performance, sensory processing, learning, and reasoning are even worse in individuals who have a long history of taking antipsychotic medications. Newer medications may reduce this side effect.

Patterns show severe deficits. Habits are negatively affected by the cyclical nature of the disorder. The typical behavioral and cognitive symptoms make it difficult for individuals to construct and maintain daily routines.

An exception to this picture is noted among individuals with paranoid schizophrenia. These individuals tend to be much better organized and to demonstrate less cognitive impairment even during active phases of the disease. They may be able to work, are usually reasonably competent in self-care activities, and may even have avocational interests (although those activities, for example, might relate to escaping persecution or building "security systems" for the home). Social functioning is impaired as a result of persecutory fears, but superficial social skills are often maintained. Work and social activities are interfered with as a result of suspicions, which often lead to angry exchanges with supervisors and neighbors who are believed to harbor wishes to harm the individual. These fears may be well-masked, however. In some cases, the masking is symptomatic of the disorder, as the individual does not trust anyone enough to confide about his or her concerns. Some research suggests that almost one-half of individuals with paranoid schizophrenia may recover well (Opjordsmoen, 1991), as compared with one-third of schizophrenics overall.

Schizophrenia is generally treated through a combination of modalities. It is a disorder in which psychotropic drugs are clearly effective (Gray, 2001). The older antipsychotic medications, typically referred to as "typical" or "conventional," are most effective in reducing positive symptoms of the disorder, possibly reducing the number of exacerbations, and lengthening the intervals between active periods of the disease. However, these medications do little to ameliorate the negative symptoms and tend to have significant side effects. Newer, "atypical" medications have fewer side effects and show promise in treating negative symptoms. Use of medication for schizophrenia is discussed further in Chapter 11.

Another biological treatment that seems helpful for some individuals with schizophrenia is electroconvulsive treatment (ECT) (Tsuang et al., 1999). Reasons for its effectiveness are not clear, but it can have a substantial impact in reducing symptoms, particularly with older individuals with schizophrenia.

There is clear evidence that biological treatments are most effective when they are combined with psychosocial interventions (Bryden et al., 2001; Hadas-Lidor, Katz, Tyano, & Weizman, 2001), including cognitive, environmental, and social therapies (Beebe, 2002; Hadas-Lidor et al., 2001). During the active period of the disorder, individuals with schizophrenia often require hospitalization. While drug treatment is initiated, the individual may also be placed in a therapeutic milieu or in some sort of behavioral program. Brief hospital stays may be beneficial, particularly if community follow-up is available.

Performance areas may be enhanced through ADL and IADL training (Hamera & Brown, 2000). Vocational assessment and work skills training are also part of intervention, particularly as individuals prepare for discharge in community settings. Work as an activity is clearly important as an intervention (Lloyd & Bassett, 1997; Siu, 1997; Voit, 2001).

Many types of psychotherapy—individual and group—have been attempted with schizophrenics, with reports of varying degrees of success. While Freud suggested that psychoanalysis was not useful with schizophrenics, it has nonetheless been attempted. Other forms of verbal therapy have also been employed, largely as adjuncts to more structured treatments and medication.

In addition, family therapy is often employed, both to assist the family in dealing with the problem and to remediate psychosocial stressors related to family interaction (Wuerker, 2000). Some theorists have suggested that schizophrenia is a rational adaptation to an irrational environment (c.f., Henry, 1972; Laing, 1969). The correlate to this belief is the need to treat the environment as well as the individual. It seems clear that family dynamics are affected by the disorder (Wuerker, 2000), making family therapy a logical choice for intervention. In general, a combination of medication and a variety of psychotherapeutic interventions seems to yield the best outcomes (Birchwood, 1992).

During the prodromal and residual phases of the disease, a variety of approaches are employed to minimize risk of exacerbation. Medications may be continued, though it is not uncommon for the individual to stop taking the drug. Cessation of medication is associated with a high rate of relapse (Carpenter, 2001), so medication patterns must be closely monitored.

A variety of environmental supports have been suggested (Beebe, 2002). Among these are ongoing therapy, medication, and social support provided by community mental health centers. Some schizophrenics do well in sheltered environments, such as group homes and sheltered workshops. Half-way houses in which individuals can live while reintegrating into the community may ease the transition from in-patient care to the community.

Issues relative to management of individuals with schizophrenia in the community have received increasing notice in recent years. In the early '60s, a move began toward deinstitutionalization of individuals with schizophrenia and other chronically mental illnesses. The original intent of this move was quite humane and logical. Prior to that time, long-term institutionalization, often lasting throughout the individual's life, was common. The idea for the change related to a desire to maximize function and quality of life for these patients. The development of community mental health centers, which occurred at the same time, was intended as a means for providing support for these individuals as they returned to their communities.

The realities of deinstitutionalization have proved less satisfactory, however. Funding for community programs has been cut, and other bridges to the community have been slow to develop. Communities have been less than welcoming of these initiatives, as the patients may continue to demonstrate peculiar behaviors. In addition, fears that individuals with schizophrenia may be dangerous are common among the general population. While these fears are not consistent with reality, they have led to resistance to establishment of group homes and half-way houses.

Thus, after being discharged from in-patient care, individuals with schizophrenia or other chronic mental illnesses often end up in boarding houses, nursing homes, or homeless. The growing problem of the homeless is, at least in part, a problem caused by deinstitutionalization (Scott, 1993), as a disproportionate number of homeless individuals have mental disorders of various types. Not only have community supports remained scarce, funds for in-patient treatment have been cut. Length of stay in in-patient settings has been drastically reduced, meaning that some of these individuals may be discharged prematurely. For many, a "revolving door" pattern of admissions is apparent. They are admitted, treated, and discharged; are unable to cope in the community; and must be readmitted.

The problems of deinstitutionalization characterize all chronic mental disorders, not just schizophrenia. Individuals with chronic depression, manic depressive disorders, and substance abuse disorders, among others, may have chronic courses that present intervention difficulties similar to those described above.

Clearly, schizophrenia presents significant treatment dilemmas that have yet to be well-addressed through public policy. Efforts to improve treatment outcomes continue, and certainly the development of more effective psychotropic medications has improved the picture. However, the outlook continues to be bleak for these individuals.

Implications for Occupational Therapy

Like many of the organic mental disorders, schizophrenia affects a broad array of performance areas and skills (Laliberte-Rudman, Yu, Scott, & Pajouhandeh, 2000). Because of this, occupational therapy intervention must be comprehensive. Motor, sensory, sensorimotor, and psychosocial skills must be assessed, and history and current status of performance in self-care, leisure, and work must be considered.

Strengths as well as weaknesses should be assessed. There is a tendency to ignore strengths when dealing with someone who has a disorder with a poor prognosis; however, important assets often exist that can be built upon. For example, one patient was quite artistic and creative. As he improved, he was able to find work as a greeting card artist for a company noted for its somewhat "off the wall" cards.

Another young woman with a long history of psychosis simply decided one day that the other patients on her ward at the state hospital were depressing and that she did not want to be like them. Her recovery was long and arduous, but she eventually went back to school and became an effective psychotherapist. Her case illustrates, among other things, the importance of motivation as a crucial asset (McCann, 2002).

Motivating clients with schizophrenia is no easy matter, as many are quite discouraged. Frequently, careful probing is necessary to uncover activities that have meaning for the person and the ways in which they can be therapeutic. For the woman described above, school was that activity. She wanted to understand as much as possible about her own condition.

Remediating skill deficits through education, behavioral, or sensorimotor approaches is vital. The woman described above had few social skills. She had to learn to make eye contact and engage in social interaction before she could consider going to school. While social skills training has demonstrated effectiveness in the short term, clients may not be able to generalize to new situations (Hayes, Halford, & Varghese, 1991). Therapists should make sure that the individual can function in a variety of settings. Not only must skills and performance be remediated, but self-esteem must be addressed. Performance deficits often lead to negative self-assessment. These individuals may experience poor quality of life (Laliberte-Rudman et al., 2000). Clients indicated that the meaning of quality of life was based on activity, social interaction, time, disclosure, "being normal," finances, and management of illness. Managing time, connecting and belonging, and making choices and maintaining control were themes related to these seven factors. Too often, quality of life is overlooked (Laliberte-Rudman et al., 2000).

Function in the community may require considerable skill training and support for the individual (Hamera & Brown, 2000; Ivarsson, Soderback, & Stein, 2000). Sheltered living may be of value for some. For others, relatively simple strategies are effective. A dentist diagnosed as paranoid schizophrenic was able to return to independent living once he learned, through a behavioral program, to discuss his delusions with only his therapist and family.

Work is often a focus of intervention (Henry & Lucca, 2002; Lloyd & Bassett, 1997; Siu, 1997; Voit, 2001). The occupational therapist should also place particular emphasis on leisure, since individuals with schizophrenia may find unstructured time the hardest to manage. In the hospital, individuals demonstrate a strong focus on the present with little ability to plan ahead (Suto & Frank, 1994), and this may reduce their ability to plan for satisfying activities. One woman whose only leisure activity was watching television had frequent exacerbations of her hallucinations as she came to believe that the TV was talking directly to her and telling her that she was an evil person.

Occupational therapy may be the only discipline to consider and provide sex education for adolescents and young adults with schizophrenia (Penna & Sheehy, 2000). Because individuals so often develop schizophrenia at the time when most young people are developing their social and sexual relationships, this area of performance may be significantly impaired. Sexual behavior is important to self-esteem and identity. Another frequently overlooked concern is physical conditioning. Exercise appears to have beneficial effects (Faulkner & Biddle, 1999) and should be considered as a therapeutic agent.

As with other disorders, differing occupational therapy theories support differing occupational therapy interventions. Therapists who subscribe to the cognitive model (Allen, 1985) will emphasize identification of a specified cognitive level and intervene by adapting tasks and environment to fit the appropriate level. Those who subscribe to the Model of Human Occupation (Kielhofner, 2002) will, instead, emphasize both skills and volition and attempt to assist the individual in enhancing the former and identifying meaningful occupations that are reflected in volition. Differences among theories are considered briefly in Chapter 2 of this text. It is beyond the scope of this text to deal with the subject in detail, however. Therapists should inform themselves about differing theories and research that supports and refutes each. While much research remains to be done to validate specific theories, there is mounting evidence that occupational therapy is helpful in addressing the problems of individuals with schizophrenia (Brown, Harwood, Hays, Heckman, & Short, 1993; Hadas-Lidor et al., 2001; Reisman & Blakeney, 1991).

DELUSIONAL DISORDER

As with paranoid schizophrenia, the primary feature of this disorder is the existence of a persistent, nonbizarre delusion (APA, 2000). The diagnosis is made only in the absence of any identifiable organic problem causing the disorder. The delusion may have any content, with the most prominent being the following:

- Erotomanic, in which the individual believes that he or she is loved by someone else, usually a prominent figure whom the individual does not actually know
- Grandiose, a belief that the individual has some special, great characteristic
- Jealous, in which the individual is convinced that a spouse or lover is unfaithful
- Persecutory, a belief that the individual is being conspired against
- Somatic, a belief that the individual has some gross physical problem.

Persecutory delusions are most common.

The disorder most often occurs in middle or later life and is more common among deaf or immigrant individuals. It is not clear why this might be the case, since the cause of delusional disorder is not known for any group. It is speculated that individuals with hearing impairment or whose English is not good may misunderstand what is occurring around them and come to believe they are being persecuted.

The course of the disease is variable, although most commonly chronic, with exacerbations and remissions. Impairment of vocational, avocational, and self-care is rare, while social impairment is frequent and often severe. Outcome appears worst in cases in which erotomanic or paranoid content is prevalent (Kaschka, Negele-Anetsberger, & Joraschky, 1991).

OTHER PSYCHOTIC DISORDERS

There are several categories of diagnosis that are made when the disorder does not fit the criteria for schizophrenia, paranoid disorder, or mood disorders, which have psychotic features (APA, 2000). In particular, these diagnoses may be made when criteria of duration, symptom constellation, or functional impairment are not met. They include brief reactive psychosis, a label applied when the psychosis clearly relates to a psychosocial stressor and is of brief (1 month maximum) duration. Schizophreniform disorder is identical to schizophrenia without meeting the criterion of duration. Thus, a psychosis that manifests with schizophrenia-like symptoms but lasts from 1 to 6 months will be called schizophreniform. If it persists for more than 6 months, the diagnosis will be changed to schizophrenia.

Schizoaffective disorder does not meet the criteria for either schizophrenia or a psychotic mood disorder but has characteristics of both. In many ways, it represents a hybrid of the two kinds of disorder. For example, the course of the disease is typically chronic, but prognosis is better than that of schizophrenia and worse than that of a mood disorder (Lapensee, 1992a; 1992b).

Finally, shared psychotic disorder (i.e., folie a deux) is a psychosis that occurs as a result of association with someone else who is psychotic. Most typically, an individual will be drawn into the delusional system of a significant other. In these cases, impairment is not as severe as for the first individual, but the disorder is amenable to treatment only if the relationship can be altered.

None of these disorders is well-understood. Etiological factors are not clear, although there is a familiar pattern to most (Kumra et al., 2002). While all have better prognoses than schizophrenia, the course of each is variable. Treatment is employed on the basis of symptoms exhibited, with drugs, hospitalization, psychotherapy, behavioral therapy, etc. being attempted with varying degrees of success.

REFERENCES

Abu-Akel, A., Caplan, R., Guthrie, D., & Komo, S. (2000). Childhood schizophrenia: Responsiveness to questions during conversation. *Journal of the American Academy of Child and Adolescent Psychiatry, 39*, 779-786.

Allen, C. (1985). *Occupational therapy for psychiatric diseases: Measurement and management of cognitive disorders.* Boston: Little, Brown & Co.

American Psychiatric Association. (2000). *Diagnostic and statistical manual of mental disorders* (4th ed., text revision). Washington, DC: Author.

Beebe, L.H. (2002). Problems in community living identified by people with schizophrenia. *Journal of Psychosocial Nursing and Mental Health Services, 40*(2), 34-38, 52-53.

Birchwood, M. (1992). Early intervention in schizophrenia: Theoretical background and clinical strategies. *The British Journal of Clinical Psychology, 31*, 257-278.

Brown, A.S., & Susser, E.S. (2002). In utero infection and adult schizophrenia. *Mental Retardation and Developmental Disability Research Reviews, 8*, 51-57.

Brown, C., Harwood, K., Hays, C., Heckman, J., & Short, J.E. (1993). Effectiveness of cognitive rehabilitation for improving attention in patients with schizophrenia. *Occupational Therapy Journal of Research, 13*, 71-86.

Bryden, K.E., Carrey, N.J., & Kutcher, S.P. (2001). Update and recommendations for the use of antipsychotics in early-onset psychoses. *Journal of Child and Adolescent Psychopharmacology, 11*, 113-130.

Caldwell, C.B., & Gottesman, I.I. (1992). Schizophrenia: A high-risk factor for suicide: Clues to risk reduction. *Suicide & Life-Threatening Behavior, 22*, 479-493.

Carpenter, W.T. (2001). Evidence-based treatment for first-episode schizophrenia. *American Journal of Psychiatry, 158*, 1771-1773.

Citrone, L. (1998). The nursing home patient with schizophrenia: Diagnosis and management. *Annals of Long-Term Care, 6*, 347-351.

David, A.S. (1987). Tachistoscopic tests of colour naming and matching in schizophrenia: Evidence for posterior callosum dysfunction? *Psychological Medicine, 17*, 621-630.

Dunn, D.W., & McDougle, C.J. (2001). Childhood-onset schizophrenia. In A. Breir, P.V. Tran, J.M. Herrera, G.D. Tollefson, & F.P. Bymaster (Eds.), *Current issues in the psychopharmacology of schizophrenia* (pp. 375-388). Philadelphia: Lippincott, Williams & Wilkins.

Eggers, C., Bunk, D., & Krause, D. (2000). Schizophrenia with onset before the age of eleven: Clinical characteristics of onset and course. *Journal of Autism and Developmental Disorders, 30*, 29-38.

Faulkner, G., & Biddle, S. (1999). Exercise as an adjunct treatment for schizophrenia. *Journal of Mental Health, 8*, 441-457.

Fink, M., & Taylor, M.A. (1991). Catatonia: A separate category in DSM-IV. *Integrative Psychiatry, 7*, 2-10.

Frith, C.D. (1987). The positive and negative symptoms of schizophrenia reflect impairments in the perception and initiation of action. *Psychological Medicine, 17,* 631-648.

Furlow, B. (2000). Radiologic assessment of schizophrenia. *Radiologic Technology, 71,* 463-476.

Gray, R. (2001). Medication for schizophrenia. *Nursing Times, 97*(31), 38-39.

Grothe, D.R., Calis, K.A., Jacobsen, L., Kumra, S., DeVane, C.L., Rapoport, J.L., et al. (2000). Olanzapine pharmacokinetics in pediatric and adolescent in-patients with childhood-onset schizophrenia. *Journal of Clinical Psychopharmacology, 20,* 220-225.

Hadas-Lidor, N., Katz, N., Tyano, S., & Weizman, A. (2001). Effectiveness of dynamic cognitive intervention in rehabilitation of clients with schizophrenia. *Clinical Rehabilitation, 15,* 349-359.

Hamera, E., & Brown, C.E. (2000). Developing a context-based performance measure for persons with schizophrenia: The test of grocery shopping skills. *The American Journal of Occupational Therapy, 54,* 20-25.

The Harvard Mental Health Newsletter. (February, 2001). *How schizophrenia develops: New evidence and new ideas. 17*(8), 1-4.

Harvey, P.D. (2001). Vulnerability to schizophrenia in adulthood. In R.E. Ingram & J.M. Price (Eds.), *Vulnerability to psychopathology: Risk across the lifespan* (pp. 355-381). New York: Guilford Press.

Hayes, R.L., Halford, W.K., & Varghese, F.N. (1991). Generalization of the effects of activity therapy and social skills training on the social behavior of low functioning schizophrenic patients. *Occupational Therapy in Mental Health, 11,* 3-20.

Henry, A.D., & Lucca, A.M. (2002). Contextual factors and participation in employment for people with serious mental illness. *Occupational Therapy Journal of Research, 22*(suppl), 83S-84S.

Henry, J. (1972). *Pathways to madness.* New York: Vintage Press.

Howard, R. (1996). Schizophrenia and delusional disorder in late life. *Review in Clinical Gerontology, 6,* 63-73.

Ivarsson, A., Soderback, I., & Stein, F. (2000). Goal, intervention and outcome of occupational therapy in individuals with psychosis. Content analysis through a chart review. *Occupational Therapy International, 7*(1), 21-41.

Kaschka, W.P., Negele-Anetsberger, J., & Joraschky, P. (1991). Treatment outcome in patients with delusional (paranoid) disorder. *European Journal of Psychiatry, 5,* 30-34.

Keks, N., Mazumdar, P., & Shields, R. (2000). New developments in schizophrenia. *Australiam Family Physician, 29,* 129-146.

Kemali, D., Majio, M., Galderisi, S., Monteleone, P., & Mucci, A. (1987). Conditional associative learning in drug-free schizophrenic patients. *Neuropsychobiology, 17,* 30-34.

Kielhofner, G. (Ed.). (2002). *A model of human occupation: Theory and application* (3rd ed.). Philadelphia: Lippincott, Williams and Wilkins.

Kumra, S., Nicolson, R., & Rapoport, J.L. (2002). Childhood-onset schizophrenia: Research update. In R.B. Zipursky & S.C. Schulz (Eds.), *The early stages of schizophrenia* (pp. 161-190). Washington, DC: American Psychiatric Publications.

Laing, R.D. (1969). *The politics of the family.* New York: Vantage Press.

Laliberte-Rudman, D., Yu, B., Scott, E., & Pajouhandeh, P. (2000). Exploration of the perspectives of persons with schizophrenia regarding quality of life. *The American Journal of Occupational Therapy, 54,* 137-147.

Lapensee, M.A. (1992a). A review of schizoaffective disorder: I. Current concepts. *Canadian Journal of Psychiatry, 37,* 335-346.

Lapensee, M.A. (1992b) A review of schizoaffective disorder: II. Somatic treatment. *Canadian Journal of Psychiatry, 37,* 347-349.

Levitt, J.G., Blanton, R.E., Caplan, R., Asarnow, R., Guthrie, D., Toga, A.W., et al. (2001). Medial temporal lobe in childhood-onset schizophrenia. *Psychiatry Research: Neuroimaging, 108,* 17-27.

Lloyd, C., & Bassett, J. (1997). Life is for living: A pre-vocational programme for young people with psychosis. *Australian Occupational Therapy Journal, 44,* 82-87.

Manschreck, T.C., Ames, D., Maher, B.A., & Schneyer, M.L. (1987). Impoverished written responses and negative features of schizophrenia. *Perceptual and Motor Skills, 64,* 1163-1169.

Marengo, J.T., Harrow, M., & Westermeyer, J.F. (1991). Early longitudinal course of acute-chronic and paranoid-undifferentiated schizophrenia subtypes and schizophreniform disorder. *Journal of Abnormal Psychology, 100,* 600-603.

McCann, T.V. (2002). Uncovering hope with clients who have psychotic illness. *Journal of Holistic Nursing, 20*(1), 81-99.

McGlashan, T.H., Fenton, W.S., & Wayne, S. (1991). Classical subtypes for schizophrenia: Literature review for DSM-IV. *Schizophrenia Bulletin, 17*, 609-632.

Opjordsmoen, S. (1991). Paranoid (delusional) disorders in the light of a long-term follow-up study. *Psychopathology, 24*, 287-292.

Penna, S., & Sheehy, K. (2000). Sex education and schizophrenia: Should occupational therapists offer sex education to people with schizophrenia? *Scandinavian Journal of Occupational Therapy, 7*, 126-131.

Ram, R., Bromet, E.J., Easton, W.W., Pato, C., & Schwartz, J.E. (1992). The natural course of schizophrenia: A review of first-admission studies. *Schizophria Bulletin, 18*, 185-207.

Reisman, J.E., & Blakeney, A.B. (1991). Exploring sensory integrative treatment in chronic schizophrenia. *Occupational Therapy in Mental Health, 11*, 25-44.

Scott, J. (1993). Homelessness and mental illness. *British Journal of Psychiatry, 162*, 314-324.

Sirls, S.G. (1991). Diagnosis of secondary depression in schizophrenia: Implications for DSM-IV. *Schizophrenia Bulletin, 17*, 75-98.

Siu, A.M. (1997). Predicting employment outcomes for people with chronic psychiatric illness. *Occupational Therapy in Mental Health, 13*(4), 45-58.

So, Y.P., Toglia, J., & Donohue, M. (1997). A study of memory functioning in chronic schizophrenia patients. *Occupational Therapy in Mental Health, 13*(2), 1-23.

Suto, M., & Frank, G. (1994). Future time perspective and daily occupations of persons with chronic schizophrenia in a board and care home. *The American Journal of Occupational Therapy, 48*, 7-18.

Tsoi, W.F., & Kua, E.H. (1992). Predicting the outcome of schizophrenia ten years later. *Australian and New Zealand Journal of Psychiatry, 26*, 257-261.

Tsuang, M.T., Faraone, S.V., & Green, A.I. (1999). Schizophrenia and other psychotic disorders. In A.M. Nicholi (Ed.), *The new Harvard guide to psychiatry* (3rd ed., pp. 240-280). Cambridge, MA: Harvard University Press.

Tsuang, M.T., Stone, W.S., & Faraone, S.V. (2000). Toward reformulating the diagnosis of schizophrenia. *American Journal of Psychiatry, 157*, 1041-1050.

Voit, S. (2001). Intervention options: Participation in work activities for people with schizophrenia. *Work, 16*, 139-151.

Wuerker, A.K. (2000). The family and schizophrenia. *Issues in Mental Health Nursing, 21*, 127-141.

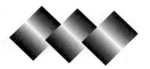 # Mood Disorders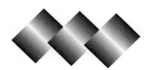

The disorders in this group are characterized by a disturbance of mood: excessive elation, depression, or some combination of these. Some reflect a single episode; others, periodic changes in a single direction or fluctuating between the two extremes. Still others reflect a chronic pattern of affect disturbance. Because mood impacts one's world view, these disorders tend to affect functional ability in global fashion.

Mood disorders are usually categorized as either depressive or bipolar. The depressive disorders are the most common of all psychiatric disorders. They may be either chronic or episodic and may or may not be associated with seasonal changes or stressful events. The bipolar disorders fluctuate between mania and depression. It is rare to find an individual whose mood disorder is characterized only by manic episodes (i.e., episodes of extreme elation). When this occurs, it is diagnosed as a manic episode.

DSM-IV-TR (APA, 2000) groups the various mood disorders into three categories: mood episodes, depressive disorders, and bipolar disorders. This chapter will discuss the more severe mood disorders (i.e., major depressive episode, manic episode, and bipolar disorder), as well as the less severe forms of mood disorder (i.e., hypomanic disorder, dysthymic disorder, and cyclothymic disorder). The first group will be discussed in detail; the second, more briefly. Table 7-1 shows the main diagnoses in this group and the relationship between more severe and less severe forms of the disorders.

MOOD EPISODES

Major Depressive Episode

This disorder represents an episode of extreme depressed mood. To be given this diagnosis, an individual must exhibit at least five symptoms of depressed mood (APA, 2000). Possible symptoms include irritability, anhedonia (i.e, the inability to experience pleasure), unintentional weight loss or gain, insomnia or hypersomnia (i.e., excessive sleeping), psychomotor agitation or retardation, fatigue, feelings of guilt or worthlessness, and poor concentration. Frequent thoughts of death or suicidal ideation may occur. As with a manic episode, hallucinations or delusions may be present, although they are not typical in the majority of cases. With or without psychotic signs, the diagnosis is made only in the presence of depressed mood. In cases in which psychotic symptoms appear without depressed mood, a diagnosis of schizophrenia or some other psychotic disorder would be considered.

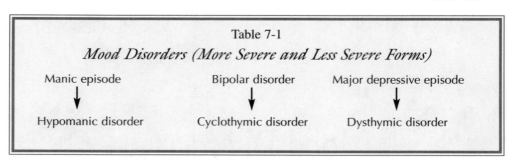

Table 7-1
Mood Disorders (More Severe and Less Severe Forms)

Manic episode	Bipolar disorder	Major depressive episode
↓	↓	↓
Hypomanic disorder	Cyclothymic disorder	Dysthymic disorder

This diagnosis is made only in the absence of obvious organic causes (e.g, anemia or hypothyroidism) and must be distinguished from bereavement. In cases where an individual has recently lost a loved one, it would be considered normal to demonstrate the symptoms listed above. However, the therapist may need to identify a time period beyond which major depressive episode as a diagnosis would be considered. This is somewhat problematic, as a wide range of opinion exists with regard to the "normal" duration of bereavement. The most typical view is that bereavement following a significant loss lasts approximately 1 year, but there is a great deal of individual variation.

Early editions of the DSM distinguished between reactive depressions (i.e., those that had a clear situational precursor [e.g., a significant loss or psychosocial stressor such as divorce or loss of a job]). Endogenous depressions were thought to be those in which no clear and immediate cause for the depression was evident. It is now thought that this distinction is inaccurate, since many depressions appear to have some identifiable major precipitating stressor (Farrell, 2000) and many also have some identifiable biological component (Beats, 1991; Bolwig, 1993; Grahame-Smith, 1992). Thus, the diagnostic distinctions among various kinds of depression are now made on the basis of specific symptoms and the pattern of appearance of depression in the individual's life.

Some major depression has a seasonal pattern of recurrent major depressive episodes (sometimes referred to as seasonal affective disorder, or SAD) (Faedda et al., 1993). In these cases, there is a specific pattern to depressive, and sometimes manic, episodes. Typically, these individuals become depressed in the fall and improve in the spring. This pattern must occur for several years before the SAD diagnosis will be made. If regular seasonal changes in life circumstances, such as regular winter unemployment or return to school in the fall, accompany the mood change, SAD will usually not be diagnosed. One treatment for this type of depression is phototherapy (Rosenthal et al., 1993), in which the individual is exposed to light for specified periods of time during the winter when natural daylight is minimal.

Major depressive episodes may be accompanied by tearfulness, phobias, panic attacks, or excessive brooding. In addition, there may be somatic complaints. Major depressive episodes may occur in individuals of any age (Salzhauer & Setzer, 2001) and have somewhat different characteristics among different age groups. Children often have accompanying somatic complaints and psychomotor agitation, while adolescents often engage in substance abuse or antisocial behavior. In elderly individuals, depression may present with symptoms of dementia, an important issue for differential diagnosis.

One or more major depressive episodes in the absence of any manic or hypomanic episode is labeled a major depression, either single episode or recurrent. Some individuals have only one episode, while others have periodic episodes, sometimes developing into bipolar disorder. While most individuals with depressive disorders return to their prior level of function between episodes, some have a chronic form that is reflected by continuing low-level depression and mild functional impairment between episodes (Howland, Shelton, & Trivedi, 2000).

Etiology and Incidence

The precise etiology of depression is poorly understood, but as noted above, it does appear that there is a biological component (Farrell, 2000; Martin, 2000). There is some argument whether biological patterns noted are a cause or a result of the depressive episode. As with mania, there is a familial pattern to depression, arguing for a genetic component (APA, 2000; Endicott, 1998). Other biological explanations focus on sensory changes (Amsterdam, Settle, Doty, Abelman, & Winokur, 1987), and on other CNS factors, including abnormalities in electroencephalograms (APA, 2000). It appears, for instance, that depression is a common consequence of stroke and that this type of depression is identical to other major depressive episodes (Allman, 1991).

It is also apparent, however, that depressive episodes correlate with psychosocial stressors (Farrell, 2000). Chronic physical illness (Penninx et al., 1997); substance abuse; and stressors, such as divorce and childbirth (Beck, 2001), have all been associated with depression. Recently publicized events surrounding postpartum depression have made it clear that this can be a very serious form of the disorder, with potentially lethal consequences for the child and/or the mother (Beck, 2001). Early stressors, such as childhood sexual abuse (Lesser & Koniak-Griffin, 2000), are also predictive of later depression.

There is a reasonable amount of support for the notion of stress as a risk/precipitant of depression in general (Farrell, 2000), particularly for "undesirable" life events. However, life events alone do not cause depression. There seems to be an interaction between undesirable life events and inadequate coping responses in people who are biologically depression-prone (Martin, 2000). For example, individuals with biological predisposition to depression with high stress levels and poor personal resources (e.g., few social contacts) may be most likely to develop depression.

Other explanations of depression are behavioral and cognitive (Peden, 2000). It is possible that peculiar perceptions of the world, faulty interpretations of those perceptions, or an inadequate repertoire of responses may figure in the disorder.

Major depressive episodes occur in roughly 5% of adults in a given year (National Institute of Mental Health [NIMH], 2001). It is much more likely that an individual will have only major depressive episodes than only manic episodes. The disorder, as with all types of depression, is twice as common in women, a difference that has been explained as resulting from a number of biological (e.g., hormonal) causes or from psychosocial differences in life course (Endicott, 1998; Farrell, 2000). Average age of onset is the mid-20s (NIMH, 2001).

Prognosis

Prognosis for a specific depressive episode is generally good. Since Eysenck (1952) published his landmark work on the effectiveness of psychotherapy, it has been understood that some depressions will resolve within several months, with or without treatment. However, recent reports suggest that less than 40% of depressive episodes resolve spontaneously within 1 year (Nierenberg, 2001). Some episodes persist for years. Onset of an episode may be gradual over several days or weeks, or it may be sudden. Some individuals may have one episode without recurrence, but about 50% of individuals will have recurring episodes

(Endicott, 1998), each of which resolves with return to premorbid function. The episodes may vary in frequency or may be quite predictable in frequency, severity, and duration, as is the case with SAD. Of individuals treated successfully, 28% had a relapse within 1 year, 62% within 5 years, and 75% within 10 years (Howland et al., 2000).

More chronic patients had longer illness prior to treatment, other in-patient hospitalizations, low income, and other psychiatric disorders. Family history is one predictor of prognosis (Endicott, 1998) (i.e., if relatives had the disorder, their course suggests what will happen to the individual). Other factors associated with risk of recurrence include presence of psychotic symptoms, previous episodes of major depression, earlier age of first episode, presence of other psychiatric diagnoses, and life stresses (Endicott, 1998). Among individuals with a more chronic course, significant impairment is more likely to persist between episodes (Howland et al., 2000).

Implications for Function and Treatment

Function in depressed individuals is greatly dependent on the severity of each specific episode. Some individuals may be able to manage nearly normal activity, while others may be totally unable to function. Vocational and social dysfunction are defining characteristics of the diagnosis. Of individuals treated for chronic depression, up to 20% have been reported to be unemployed, with another 31% reporting that they are employed below their level of education and training (Howland et al., 2000). Individuals who have creative jobs or jobs that require high degrees of motivation, such as sales, may find that they lack the energy and drive necessary to complete their required functions. In addition, cognitive and social impairment may interfere with their completion of tasks.

Another performance area likely to be impaired is leisure. Depressed individuals take little pleasure in activity and thus avoid hobbies, social occasions, and other activities that they formerly enjoyed. They may be unable to concentrate long enough to read or to enjoy television, movies, or other performances. They typically lack the energy and motivation needed in physical activities.

ADLs and IADLs may also be affected. In some individuals, this is primarily a matter of "not caring" about appearance or hygiene. In others, irritability, psychomotor retardation, lethargy, and loss of appetite may combine, resulting in greatly diminished function, sometimes to the extent that the individual takes no care at all of him- or herself and may not even get out of bed.

Depression has been defined as a combination of skill and habit deficits (Rogers & Holm, 2000). At the level of specific skills, cognition is almost always impaired. Concentration and problem-solving ability are diminished. Sensation is usually not affected, except in the presence of hallucinations, but psychomotor activity is often either slowed or speeded. Social skills are often poor, leading to significant interpersonal difficulty. Those around the individual may become more hostile, anxious, and rejecting in response to the behavior of the depressed individual. Thus, the behavior of the depressed individual sets a cycle of disturbed interaction.

Coping and problem-solving skills of depressed individuals appear to be worse than those of nondepressed individuals (Farrell, 2000; Peden, 2000). There has been some speculation that perceived lack of control over life events is an important factor, though this "learned helplessness" hypothesis is the subject of much controversy (Farrell, 2000).

Habit deficits include problems with IADLs and with personal care (Rogers & Holm, 2000). It may be that depressed individuals lack motivation and interest in these activities, or that they are too fatigued to complete them. In any case, they often fail to complete these tasks at an adequate level of independence.

While depression is the most common of psychiatric diagnoses, it is also one of the most readily treatable (Howland et al., 2000). There is a vast array of psychotropic medications that are quite useful in resolving a depressive episode. Many of them have undesirable side-effects that make them unappealing over long periods of time, but they can shorten individual episodes and reduce their severity. Some of these medications may be taken on a maintenance basis to prevent recurrence. In general, medications to treat depression have improved over the last two decades. However, recent reports suggest that psychotropic medications alone are insufficient to adequately treat depression (Nierenberg, 2001). They are not effective for everyone (Kocsis & Miller, 1998). Approximately 55% of patients respond to medication alone (Howland et al., 2000)

For some individuals, ECT may be quite effective (Nierenberg, 2001). Generally speaking, when such treatment is applied, it is done for brief periods in the presence of specific sets of symptoms. This is quite unlike earlier forms of ECT, which were given for a wide array of psychiatric disorders and often for courses of dozens (or even hundreds) of treatments. ECT is particularly helpful for the most severe forms of depression and for older adults.

In addition, psychotherapy of various forms, both group and individual, is helpful for depression (Kocsis & Miller, 1998; Nierenberg, 2001). Approximately 55% of individuals respond to psychotherapy alone, comparable to the rate for medication (Howland et al., 2000). A combination of medication and psychotherapy increases the response rate to 80%.

Cognitive therapy has gained popularity as an intervention for depressed individuals (Nierenberg, 2001), leading to improvement in approximately 40% to 50% of those treated. This therapy is based on the notion that depressed individuals inaccurately interpret events around them and that they can learn new and more helpful interpretations (Beech, 2000). Behavior modification and psychoanalysis, as well as a variety of group and family approaches, have all been reported to be successful with depressed individuals.

Special note should be made about depression in children/youth. While there is some debate on the subject, depression is quite common in children and adolescents (Cronin, 2001). Symptoms may differ somewhat from those described for adults and usually reflect developmental stage. Anxiety, school refusal or school problems, and negative behavior are all common. As with adults, low self-esteem is common.

In children, school and social function are likely to be impaired. It may be difficult for the child to articulate the problem (or even to state that a problem exists). Teens often become sullen and withdrawn, behavior that should not be written off as "just a phase," as adolescents are at considerable risk for depression (Cronin, 2001). Thus, intervention must be sensitive to the age and stage of the individual child.

Implications for Occupational Therapy

Occupational therapists may focus on assisting the individual with finding gratifying activities that improve self-esteem and increase motivation. In addition, activities that provide opportunities for self-expression are valuable, since individuals who are depressed may be reluctant or unable to put their feelings into words. Art or other creative activities can provide a valuable outlet for such emotions. One very timid woman was asked to work on a woodworking project. After a few timid taps, she began to pound the hammer, shouting with great enthusiasm, "This is for my husband, this is for my boss, this is for the dog..." She was then better able to express her rage about feeling taken advantage of by those around her. Neville (1986) has suggested four major valuable goals of treatment: re-engaging in valued activities, setting realistic goals for the future, re-establishing routines and habits, and experiencing success and feelings of competence.

Since most individuals who are depressed do not lack the skills to do a variety of activities, motivation is often the key to improvement. These individuals may be extremely reluctant to engage in activity and may sit passively throughout the day. A cognitive behavioral approach has been suggested as a strategy for remediating these problems (Yakobina, Yakobina, & Tallant, 1997). Social skills training may be helpful to individuals who are depressed, particularly those who never acquired social skills because of prolonged, early-onset depression. In addition, activities that ensure positive reinforcement from others can be of great value. One woman spent a week baking cookies every day for the other patients. She thoroughly enjoyed their appreciation. At the end of the week, she was able to say, "Now I think I'll do something for me," and she began to knit a scarf for herself. She chose a bright cheery yellow that was in marked contrast to the drab browns and grays she had been wearing.

Manic Episode

These episodes are severe, usually of abrupt onset, and are characterized by major changes in attitude and behavior. Most prominent is an elevated or irritated mood, with at least three of the following characteristic behaviors: grandiosity, decreased need for sleep, talkativeness, flight of ideas, distractibility, increased activity, and excessive involvement in pleasurable activities with disregard for the consequences. For example, individuals experiencing a manic episode may spend money wildly or become involved in inappropriate sexual activities. Functioning is impaired in all spheres, with marked deficits in occupational and social functioning. Hospitalization is often required.

As with all psychiatric diagnosis, part of the diagnostic process is the exclusion of other possible disorders. If hallucinations and delusions are present, they must be accompanied by alterations in mood. Schizophrenia; other psychotic disorders; and organic factors, such as intoxication, must be ruled out. While thought disorders may be present in individuals experiencing manic episodes, mood alterations are the most prominent feature of the symptom constellation.

Another characteristic is emotional lability. The individual may be expansive and grandiose one minute, angry and hostile the next. There are frequent rapid shifts from mania to depression and occasionally, the symptoms of the two appear together. Furthermore, the individual may be oblivious to his or her behavior, totally unaware that there is a problem.

Manic episodes may be preceded by a prodromal period (George, 1998) during which early symptoms emerge. Insomnia, excessive energy, difficulty concentrating, and other manic symptoms may appear. Approximately 75% of individuals experiencing repeated manic episodes can identify prodromal changes (George, 1998).

Etiology and Incidence

Mania most often appears in individuals in their 20s, though it may have later onset (NIMH, 2001). The most characteristic pattern of appearance is a rapid, abrupt onset. It is not precisely clear what causes the disorder, although family studies have established that there is a familial pattern (APA, 2000). This pattern has appeared even when family members have been raised in different environments and is thus a strong argument for some sort of genetic component to the disorder.

Pure manic episodes, without accompanying depression, are rare. Bipolar disorders (mania and depression in combination) are discussed following.

Prognosis

Prognosis for specific manic episodes is good. Duration of episodes is variable, although if untreated, they may last for a month or more. However, often there is a pattern of recurring episodes, meaning that without maintenance treatment, it is probable that the individual will have manic episodes on a periodic basis. In some individuals, the episodes follow a particular pattern (e.g., appearing each spring) (Faedda et al., 1993), while in others, they may appear unpredictably. In still others, there may be a single episode, with no recurrence. Long-term treatment involves use of medication (Baker, 2001). In order to prevent recurrence, however, it must be continued in maintenance doses for long periods of time, and recent research questions earlier reports that medication is highly effective in most cases (Baker, 2001). Medication presents a set of problems related to the potential for toxicity from the drug and the possible unwillingness of these individuals to follow the prescribed regimen. The nature of the disorder itself, and the tendency toward impulsive acts, leads to frequent failure to take medication as prescribed (George, 1998). As a manic episode develops, judgment and self-control are reduced, and the individual may stop taking the medication. Further, there are some individuals who do not respond (Baker, 2001). Even among responders, psychosocial consequences continue after individual episodes resolve (George, 1998). About half of individuals who experience one manic episode have repeated episodes (Tohen, Waternaux, Tsuang, & Hunt, 1990)

Because of the severity of manic episodes, hospitalization, often involuntary, is frequently warranted (Baker, 2001). Manic individuals demonstrate extremely poor judgment and must often be protected from a tendency to engage in illegal or imprudent acts or to abuse drugs.

Implications for Function and Treatment

As with schizophrenia, function is severely impaired. This is, in fact, a defining characteristic of the disorder. Judgment is extremely poor, and individuals tend to engage in acting-out behaviors. For example, the individual may begin to gamble wildly, take drugs, abuse alcohol, argue with colleagues at work, or become involved in promiscuous sexual activity. Impulsiveness and grandiosity interfere with vocational and social activities, alienating co-workers and friends (Coryell et al., 1993) and decreasing the individual's ability to complete tasks. There are changes in cognition and perception. Motor skill does not change, but hyperactivity is almost always present; in fact, a diagnosis of ADHD may be made in children when the actual problem is repeated manic episodes (Akin, 2001). It appears that there are changes in CNS function that contribute to the characteristic symptom constellation (Klerman, 1988).

Individuals with manic disorder may be able to function reasonably normal between episodes. Depending on the frequency and duration of the manic periods, it is possible that they may hold jobs, have families, and carry on other activities much of the time. However, all of these functions are impaired during episodes, often resulting in loss of job and in family disruption. In individuals who have reasonable levels of function between episodes, maintenance treatment with drugs, as well as family therapy to assist others to understand the disorder, may be quite effective. However, recent research suggests that at least some psychosocial impairment persists even when the disorder is in remission (Baker, 2001).

When hospitalization is part of the treatment, it is usually brief. The primary objective is to protect the individual from harming him- or herself or others as a result of poor judgment and impulsivity. Once medications have begun to ameliorate the symptoms, hospitalization is no longer necessary.

Implications for Occupational Therapy

During the acute episode, an important role for the occupational therapist is monitoring behavior changes and providing a structured environment in which behavior can be managed. A typical manic patient might breeze into the clinic to begin "building a castle," switch to "creating a new Mona Lisa" after the first two nails are in place, then to making a leather coat after the first stroke of paint is on the canvas, etc. Setting limits is important. Signs of behavior change as medication is introduced are important to decision-making about long-term treatment. These signs are often best identified in the context of activity.

Between episodes, the occupational therapist may assist the individual in coping with the possibility of a chronic illness. The individual needs to learn the signs of an impending episode in order to seek help. In addition, activity patterns may need to be examined to determine whether some stressful activities should be stopped or changed. If onset was early, assessment of skills and remediation of skill deficits may be needed, since skill acquisition can be impaired if manic episodes are frequent (Baker, 2001). Function in all areas of performance should be assessed to determine how stress can be managed and how quality of life can be maximized.

For most individuals who have manic episodes, performance and skills are unimpaired between episodes. However, behavior during episodes may have long-term consequences in terms of lost friends, family disputes, lost jobs, and financial difficulties. Clients need to learn how to avoid or manage these difficulties by altering lifestyle, monitoring symptoms, and getting family members involved (Baker, 2001; George, 1998). One woman recognized that she'd begin to have problems as soon as the lilacs bloomed each spring. Her husband learned to put away the credit cards then, and she learned to go see her physician immediately.

Hypomanic Episode

Hypomanic episode is the diagnosis made when an individual shows signs similar to those in a manic episode, but with symptoms that are less severe and disabling (APA, 2000). The distinction between a major manic episode and a hypomanic episode is one of degree. While major episodes are quite striking, hypomanic episodes are less so and are sometimes written off as excess energy. As with ADHD in children, the disorder is, to some extent, in the eye of the beholder. However, in many instances, judgment is impaired, and irritability leads to fights with spouses, employees, etc. The individual may have rapid mood swings from euphoria to irritability; sleep less than usual; start a wide variety of projects, none of which are finished. Hallucinations and delusions are not present, and the individual does not become disoriented to time and place.

DEPRESSIVE DISORDERS

DSM-IV-TR (APA, 2000) lists two main types of depressive disorder. The first of these is major depressive disorder, characterized by one or more major depressive episodes. The diagnosis is made only if there are no manic, mixed, or hypomanic episodes. The second is dysthymic disorder, which is described below. A common pattern is a dysthymic disorder that ultimately develops into a major depressive disorder.

Dysthymia

This is a depressive disorder in which the individual has some symptoms of depression most of the time. For the diagnosis to be made, symptoms must be ongoing for at least 2 years, with periods of no more than 2 months at a time symptom-free. As hypomanic episode is a less severe form of manic episode, dysthymia is a less severe (though more chronic) form of depression. The symptoms are milder, but much more persistent than in a major depressive episode. Dysthymia may precede a major depressive episode, leading to so-called "double depression." These are cases in which a major depressive episode is superimposed on a chronic minor depression (APA, 2000; Keller et al., 1995). This is a particularly pernicious depression with poor prognosis.

Dysthymia often coexists with other Axis I or Axis III disorders, in which case it is referred to as secondary. For example, many individuals who are anorexic are depressed, as are some individuals with arthritis. Secondary depression occurs when there is a clear precipitating event, but normal bounds of the mourning process have been passed. For example, job loss or physical illness may lead to an on-going secondary depression.

This is a very common disorder, although diagnosis may be difficult, as the boundary between dysthymia and major depressive episode is not clear. While DSM-IV lists specific criteria, these characteristics are largely a matter of degree. A moderate depression might be diagnosed by one practitioner as dysthymia, by another as major depressive episode. Dysthymia is notable primarily for its chronicity and for the absence of some of the more severe depressive symptoms (e.g., hallucinations and delusions).

Function is generally impaired to a mild or moderate degree in individuals with dysthymia. While they typically hold jobs and have social relationships and interests, these are not maintained at optimal levels because of lethargy and lack of interest. Their constant depression wears on those around them, and they may lose friends as a result of their inability to enjoy activities or take pleasure in people. The chronicity of the disorder is a problem, as individuals tend to feel bad for long periods of time without relief.

Dysthymia has apparent biological origins. Changes in rapid eye movement (REM) sleep, thyroid functioning, and electroencephalogram (EEG) readings have all been found (APA, 2000). These differences are not the same as those found during major depressive episodes.

Treatment for dysthymia is somewhat more problematic than for major depressive episodes. Medication has been used with some success (Kocsis & Miller, 1998), although the widely touted SSRIs have side effects, including sexual dysfunction, that make them less than ideal for some individuals. In addition, recent evidence suggests they may be less effective than initially thought. In any case, some experimentation is required to find the right drug and dose, a process that can take time and be frustrating to the individual. Cognitive therapy and psychotherapy have both been reported as somewhat helpful. A mixture of these therapies may be most effective. However, dysthymic disorder is more intractable than major depression.

Children are also at risk for dysthymia. They may present with anxiety, school phobias, or difficulty sleeping. School refusal or negative behavior are also common signs of depression. School and social function are likely to be impaired. At the same time, it may be difficult for them to articulate the problem (or even state that it exists). Intervention must be sensitive to the age and stage of the individual child. Play therapy may help the child express feelings nonverbally.

BIPOLAR DISORDERS

These disorders are characterized by fluctuations in mood, with episodes of both mania and depression. Three main types of bipolar disorder have been included in DSM-IV-TR (APA, 2000). Bipolar disorder I is characterized by intermittent manic and major depressive episodes. Bipolar disorder II is characterized by intermittent hypomanic and major depressive episodes with no occurrence of manic episodes (Baker, 2001). The third type of bipolar disorder, cyclothymia, is discussed separately on pp. 119 and 120.

Etiology and Incidence

There is a clear familial pattern in the appearance of bipolar disorder. This finding, combined with the fact that psychotropic medications are effective, suggests a biological basis for the disorder. One research report describes the case of an older client whose bipolar disorder was caused by hyperthyroidism (Nath & Sagar, 2001) and suggests that late onset bipolar disorder is quite likely to be organic in nature. However, although many researchers feel that the disorder is primarily biological, the failure of psychotropic medications leads others to feel that alternative explanations are needed (George, 1998).

The disorder is not uncommon, with an estimated occurrence of 1% of the adult population of the United States (George, 1998; NIMH, 2001).

Prognosis

While single manic or depressive episodes may resolve relatively quickly, bipolar disorder is most often chronic (George, 1998). An estimated 95% of those with bipolar disorder will experience recurrent episodes. Some individuals experience what is called "rapid cycling," which is defined as having at least four affective episodes within a year (Goodwin & Jamison, 1990).

Implications for Function and Treatment

For specific episodes, functional decrements are the same as those described above for manic episodes and major depressive episodes. Between episodes, function may be quite normal. The individual will be able to work, engage in social and avocational activities, and perform self-care. This is particularly true for individuals who have long periods between exacerbations. However, as noted, some individuals have chronic problems, either because of the frequency of manic or depressive episodes or because of the consequences of the dysfunctional behavior in which they engage during the episodes (Baker, 2001).

All performance areas can be affected. Self-care may deteriorate, and leisure interests can be affected. Although the employment rate for individuals with bipolar disorder is better than that of those with schizophrenia, many individuals are still unable to work or to work at their level of premorbid ability (Tse & Walsh, 2001). Work is particularly difficult for those individuals whose onset of illness was in their 20s (NIMH, 2001). Skill acquisition may not occur, meaning problems continue even when the individual is symptom-free (Tse & Walsh, 2001). Social functioning is also affected significantly (Baker, 2001).

Skills and habits are likewise affected. Perception is distorted, and insight tends to be poor (Pollack & Cramer, 2000); 25% of individuals could not identify prodromal signs of depression (George, 1998). Another study (Perkins & Moodley, 1993) found that more than 55% of subjects in a study of psychiatric in-patients with bipolar disorder did not think they had psychiatric problems. Because manic and depressive episodes cause so much behavioral disruption, habits and patterns are hard to form and maintain.

Treatment almost always includes medication. When taken as advised, lithium can minimize symptoms and prevent recurrences, although early reports of its effectiveness may have been overstated (Baker, 2001; Clinical Courier, 2001; George, 1998). Lithium has a number of problematic side effects and must be carefully monitored. Antidepressant medications are also prescribed in some cases. Effective medication is dependent on accurate and early diagnosis, and this often is a problem (Clinical Courier, 2001). Group psychotherapy, family therapy, educational approaches, and behavioral interventions have all had some effectiveness, particularly in combination with medication (Baker, 2001; George, 1998).

Implications for Occupational Therapy

Interventions for individual manic and depressed episodes in those with bipolar disorder are identical to those described in previous sections. Manic phase and depressed phase are no different for bipolar disorder than for major episodes. However, bipolar disorder tends to be chronic, with problems in all areas of function lasting for years (Pollack & Cramer, 2001). Intervention must address the pervasiveness and persistence of functional deficits. Because of the severity of symptoms, including the high risk of suicidal behavior, treatment may well be provided in an in-patient setting (Pollack, Harvin, & Cramer, 2001).

Two important considerations apply. First, self-esteem and self-concept are likely to be damaged by both the chronic nature of the disorder and the enormous fluctuations in personality that characterize it (Baker, 2001). When an individual is sometimes withdrawn, sad, and lethargic and other times energetic and effervescent, it is difficult for him or her to form a clear picture of his or her abilities or even desires. It is also difficult to feel good about one's performance when it is so unstable.

Medication may help the individual reach a more even keel, but it cannot repair the damage to self-concept done by these mood swings. The occupational therapist must help the individual identify strengths, weaknesses, likes, and dislikes through exposure to a wide range of activities.

A second consideration is that needed skills may have been lost or may never have been acquired. One young mother had fluctuated between withdrawal from her two preschool children and extreme irritability with them. She needed a good bit of training in parenting skills to resolve this and to begin to repair the damage done by her inconsistent and unpredictable behavior. This is fairly typical of individuals with long-standing bipolar disorder, particularly those who have not had adequate diagnosis and treatment.

Educational approaches are particularly needed with individuals with bipolar disorder. These individuals must learn to recognize prodromal signs, and develop management strategies for coping with remissions (Baker, 2001; George, 1998; Pollack & Cramer, 2001). Social skills require particular attention, as deficits in social skills have been associated with poor ability to manage the disorder (Pollack & Cramer, 2001).

Cyclothymia

This is a chronic disorder in which episodes of hypomania and depressed mood (but not major depressive episode) are interspersed. It is a less severe form of bipolar disorder. In order for the diagnosis to be made, there must be at least a 2-year period during which the individual is symptom-free for no more than 2 months at a time. Some theorists believe that cyclothymia is simply a less severe form of bipolar disorder. In fact, the boundary between the two is indistinct. It is not unusual for cyclothymia to eventually develop into bipolar disorder.

Because cyclothymia is less severe than bipolar disorder, functional capacity is less impaired. In fact, some individuals report that they are unusually productive during hypomanic episodes. Vocational function is affected during depressed periods. Social function is often impaired, as the wide, unpredictable mood swings may cause difficulty for those around the individual. Substance abuse may become a problem as the individual attempts to deal with the depressed episodes or loses capacity for good judgment during hypomanic episodes.

Implications for Occupational Therapy

For all of the less severe mood disorders (i.e., hypomanic episode, dysthymia, and cyclothymia), principles discussed for the more severe disorders can be applied. While the functional impact of these disorders is less, they can be very frustrating because of their chronicity. This alone can enhance the depression and irritability that characterize the disorders. Thus, the individual may benefit from support in coping with chronic illness, education and information, and assistance in clarifying valued goals and activities.

Individuals who tend to be hypomanic often have difficulty with time management. They may be overcommitted and may create interpersonal friction by being unable to meet their commitments. Effective use of time and realistic self-appraisal are important goals for occupational therapy.

Dysthymia presents an opposite problem, although the consequences are somewhat similar. The individual has extremely low motivation that may be quite irritating to others. These individuals are the "Eeyores" (Milne, 1947) of the world, constantly seeing the gloomy side of life (Munoz, personal communication, August, 1988). In their interactions with others, nothing is ever enough to help them feel loved and happy. These individuals need to discover activities that will be satisfying and motivating to them.

Cyclothymic disorder requires a combination of approaches, much like those suggested for bipolar disorder. While the functional impairments are less extreme, their impact on self-esteem should not be minimized. Table 7-2 shows the symptoms and functional deficits of the most frequently diagnosed mood disorders.

SUICIDE

Suicide is a particular concern related to mood disorders (Nierenberg, 2001). The rate of suicide in the United States is 11.2 per 100,000 people (Hamilton, 2000), with the rate of suicidal behavior much higher. Rates are particularly high among older adults and adolescents. Approximately 60% of all suicides are associated with depression. Many depressed individuals contemplate suicide, and those who appear to have active suicidal intent may require hospitalization to prevent them from harming themselves (Karasu et al., 1993). The problem is complicated by the fact that some antidepressant medications can be lethal if abused, thus requiring careful monitoring, especially before they have the opportunity to take effect in elevating mood, a process that can take several weeks.

Professionals who work with depressed individuals must be aware of the potential for suicide, note the presence of suicidal potential in these individuals, and take necessary precau-

Table 7-2

Mood Disorders

Disorder	Symptoms	Functional Deficits
Major depressive episode	1. Depressed mood 2. Anhedonia 3. Appetite/weight change 4. Insomnia/hypersomnia 5. Lack of energy 6. Feelings of worthlessness/ guilt 7. Possible suicidal ideation 8. Impaired function	Social, work, leisure Possibly ADLs and IADLs Habits, roles, routines deteriorate during episode Motor, process, and communication slowing All improve between episodes
Manic episode	1. Abnormally elevated or irritable mood 2. Grandiosity 3. Decreased sleep 4. Distractibility, flight of ideas 5. Poor judgment 6. Impaired function 7. May be delusions or hallucinations	Work, social, leisure habits, roles, and routines deteriorate during episodes Motor hyperactivity Process deficits Communication not severely affected Function tends to improve between episodes
Bipolar disorder	1. Recent alternating symptoms of both manic and major depressive episodes	As above
Dysthymia	1. Same as major depressive, but less severe 2. Duration at least 2 years (1 year for children)	Same as major depressive, but less severe More chronic
Hypomanic episode	1. Same as manic, but less severe	Same as manic, but less severe
Cyclothymia	1. Fluctuating hypomanic periods and periods of depressed mood 2. Duration at least 2 years (1 year for children) Symptom free for no more than 2 months	Same as bipolar but less severe

tions (Hamilton, 2000). They should directly ask the individual if he or she is suicidal and determine whether a plan of action has been developed. Because many suicidal individuals are actually looking for an "avenue of escape" (Tummey, 2001, p. 41), they are likely to answer these questions honestly and accept assistance in finding other, less damaging, methods to resolve their difficulties.

While responsibility for assessing suicidal ideation falls primarily to the main therapist (i.e., team leader, psychiatrist, etc.), other professionals must also be alert to suicide risk in clients (Tummey, 2001). Individuals with a clear and feasible plan must be considered at high risk for suicide. In addition, individuals whose depression appears to resolve suddenly are considered high risks, as this may signify that they have made a decision to act. Depressed individuals are at greatest risk during the period when the depression is just beginning to lift because they have increased energy to act on their suicidal thoughts.

Precautions include careful monitoring, often in in-patient settings, and removal of means to cause death until the individual is clearly no longer actively suicidal (Hamilton, 2000; Tummey, 2001). Contracting with the patient (i.e., having the patient agree he or she will not make any suicide gesture) is also helpful (Drew, 2001). While most suicide attempts are made with drugs and guns, access to other lethal substances and sharp implements, as well as carbon monoxide, should be monitored as well. Occupational therapists should be sensitive to use of sharp implements and toxic solvents by suicidal patients in their care. There is a belief that some single car accidents are, in fact, suicide attempts, so it may be necessary to monitor driving, especially when accompanied by drinking, in these individuals.

Children and adolescents who are depressed are at risk of suicide, as well as adults (Pfeffer, 2000). A wish to reunite with a loved one or to punish an adult is a common motivation for suicide attempts in this age group. Teens who become sullen and withdrawn should be watched carefully (McIntosh, 1991). It should not be assumed that the adolescent is just "going through a phase."

Suicide risk is also high among individuals with HIV or at high risk of acquiring HIV (e.g., homosexuals and intravenous drug users) (Starace, 1993). Another high-risk group is older adults, among whom the suicide rate is almost twice what it is for younger adults (Lester & Yang, 1992). It is hypothesized that stressors such as loss of spouse, retirement, and reduced economic circumstances contribute to this risk. Individuals with physical illnesses that cause significant pain are at high risk for suicide as well (Rao, 1990).

Staff in in-patient settings will need to deal with feelings of other patients, as well as their own, when a suicide attempt or completed suicide occurs on the unit (Little, 1992). While precautions can reduce the incidence, individuals who are determined to complete a suicide are quite difficult to stop. However, the vast majority of suicide attempts are a cry for help. Careful attention to warning signs can reduce the incidence of both attempts and completed suicides.

REFERENCES

Akin, L.K. (2001). Pediatric and adolescent bipolar disorder: Medical resources. *Medical Reference Services Quarterly, 20*(3), 31-44.

Allman, P. (1991). Depressive disorder and emotionalism following stroke. *International Journal of Geriatric Psychiatry, 6,* 377-383.

American Psychiatric Association. (2000). *Diagnostic and statistical manual of mental disorders* (4th ed., text revision). Washington, DC: Author.

Amsterdam, J.D., Settle, R.G., Doty, R.L., Abelman, E., & Winokur, A. (1987). Taste and smell perception in depression. *Biological Psychiatry, 22,* 1477-1481.

Baker, J.A. (2001). Bipolar disorders: An overview of the current literature. *Journal of Psychiatric and Mental Health Nursing, 5,* 437-441.

Beats, B.C. (1991). Structural imaging in affective disorder. *International Journal of Geriatric Psychiatry*, 6, 419-422.

Beck, C.T. (2001). Predictors of postpartum depression: An update. *Nursing Research*, 50, 275-285.

Beech, B.F. (2000). The strengths and weaknesses of cognitive behavioural approaches to treating depression and their potential for wider utilization by mental health nurses. *Journal of Psychiatric and Mental Health Nursing*, 7, 343-354.

Bolwig, T.G. (1993). Regional cerebral blood flow in affective disorder. *Acta Psychiatrica Scandinavica*, 371, 48-53.

Clinical Courier. (2001). *New advances in bipolar disorder*. 19(3), 1-8.

Coryell, W., Scheftner, W., Keller, M., Endicott, J., Maser, J., & Klerman, G.L. (1993). The enduring psychosocial consequences of mania and depression. *American Journal of Psychiatry*, 150, 720-727.

Cronin, A.F. (2001). Psychosocial and emotional domains. In J. Case-Smith (Ed.), *Occupational therapy for children* (4th ed., pp. 413-452). St. Louis, MO: Mosby.

Drew, B.L. (2001). Self-harm behavior and no-suicide contracting in psychiatric in-patient settings. *Archives of Psychiatric Nursing*, 15(3), 99-106.

Endicott, J. (1998). Gender similarities and differences in the course of depression. *The Journal of Gender-Specific Medicine*, 1(3), 40-43.

Eysenck, H.J. (1952). The effects of psychotherapy: An evaluation. *Journal of Consulting Psychology*, 16, 219-324.

Faedda, G.L., Tondo, L., Teicher, M.H., Baldessarini, R.J., Gelbard, H.A., & Floris, G.F. (1993). Seasonal mood disorders. Patterns of seasonal recurrence in mania and depression. *Archives of General Psychiatry*, 50, 17-23.

Farrell, A. (2000). Psychosocial aspects of depression in women. *British Journal of Therapy and Rehabilitation*, 7, 215-220.

George, S. (1998). Towards an integrated treatment approach for manic depression. *Journal of Mental Health*, 7, 145-156.

Goodwin, F.K., & Jamison, K.R. (1990). *Manic-depressive illness*. Cambridge, England: Oxford University Press.

Grahame-Smith, D.G. (1992). Serotonin in affective disorders. *International Clinical Psychopharmacology*, 6, 5-13.

Hamilton, N.G. (2000). Suicide prevention in primary care. *Postgraduate Medicine*, 108(6), 81-84, 87, 109-110.

Howland, R.H., Shelton, R.C., & Trivedi, M.H. (2000). Chronic depression: Now a treatable condition. *Patient Care for the Nurse Practitioner*, 54-71.

Karasu, T.B., Docherty, J.P., Gelenberg, A., et.al. (1993). The American Psychiatric Association practice guideline for major depressive disorder in adults. *American Journal of Psychiatry*, 150, 1-26.

Keller, M.B., Klein, D.N., Hirschfield, R.M., Koscis, J.H., McCullough, J.P., Miller, I., et al. (1995). Results of the DSM-IV field trial. *American Journal of Psychiatry*, 52, 843-849.

Klerman, G.L. (1988). Depression and related disorders of mood (affective disorders). In A.M. Nicholi (Ed.), *The new Harvard guide to psychiatry* (pp. 309-336). Cambridge, MA: Belknap Press.

Kocsis, J.H., & Miller, N.L. (1998). Looking at chronic depression and dysthymia. *Journal of the California Alliance for the Mentally Ill*, 9(4), 31-33.

Lesser, J., & Koniak-Griffin, D. (2000). The impact of physical or sexual abuse on chronic depression in adolescent mothers. *Journal of Pediatric Nursing*, 16, 378-387.

Lester, D., & Yang, B. (1992). Social and economic correlates of the elderly suicide rate. *Suicide & Life-Threatening Behavior*, 22, 36-47.

Little, J.D. (1992). Staff response to in-patient and out-patient suicide: What happened and what do we do? *The Australian and New Zealand Journal of Psychiatry*, 26, 162-167.

Martin, A.C. (2000). Major depressive illness in women: Assessment and treatment in the primary care setting. *Nurse Practitioner Forum*, 11, 179-186.

McIntosh, J.L. (1991). Epidemiology of suicide in the United States. In A.A. Leenaars (Ed.), *Life span perspectives of suicide*. New York: Plenum Press.

Milne, A.A. (1947). *The world of Pooh*. London: Linder.

Nath, J., & Sagar, R. (2001). Hyperthyroidism-induced bipolar disorder. *Nurses' Drug Alert*, 25(11), 82.

National Institute of Mental Health. (2001). *The numbers count*. Retrieved June 5, 2002, from http://www.nimh.nih.gov/publicat/numbers.cfm.

Neville, A. (1986). *Depression and the model of human occupation: Theory and research. Depression: Assessment and treatment update* (pp. 14-21). Rockville, MD: American Occupational Therapy Association.

Nierenberg, A.A. (2001). Current perspectives on the diagnosis and treatment of major depressive disorder. *American Journal of Managed Care*, 7(suppl.), S353-S366.

Peden, A.R. (2000). Negative thoughts of women with depression. *Journal of the American Psychiatric Nurses Association, 6*(2), 41-48.

Penninx, B.W.J., van Tilburg, T.G., Deeg, D.J.H., Kriesgsman, D.M.W., Boeke, A.J.P., & van Eijk, J.T.M. (1997). Effects of social support and personal coping resources on mortality in older age: the longitudinal study of Amsterdam. *American Journal of Epidemiology, 146*, 510-519.

Perkins, R.E., & Moodley, P. (1993). Perception of problems in psychiatric in-patients: Denial, race and service usage. *Social Psychiatry and Psychiatric Epidemiology, 28*, 189-193.

Pfeffer, C.R. (2000). Suicidal behavior in prepubertal children from the 1980s to the new millennium. In R.W. Maris, S.S. Canetto, & M.M. Silverman (Eds.), *Review of suicidology: An official publication of the American Association of Suicidology* (pp. 159-169). New York: Guilford Press.

Pollack, L.E., & Cramer, R.D. (2000). Perceptions of problems in people hospitalized for bipolar disorder: Implications for patient education. *Issues in Mental Health Nursing, 21*, 765-778.

Pollack, L.E., Harvin, S., & Cramer, R.D. (2001). In-patient group therapies for people with bipolar disorder: Comparison of a self-management and an interactional model. *Journal of the American Psychiatric Nurses Association, 7*, 179-187.

Rao, A.V. (1990). Physical illness, pain, and suicidal behavior. *Crisis, 11*, 48-56.

Rogers, J.C., & Holm, M. B. (2000). Daily-living skills and habits of older women with depression. *Occupational Therapy Journal of Research, 20*(Supplement 1), 68S-85S.

Rosenthal, N.E., Moul, D.E., Hellekson, C.J., Oren, D.A., Frank, A., Brainard, G.C., et al. (1993). A multicenter study of the light visor for seasonal affect disorder: no difference in efficacy found between two different intensities. *Neuropsychopharmacology, 8*, 151-160.

Salzhauer, A., & Setzer, N. (2001). Childhood depression: How do you know and how can you help? *School Nurse News, 18*(5), 20-23.

Starace, F. (1993). Suicidal behavior in people infected with human immunodeficiency virus: A literature review. *International Journal of Social Psychiatry, 39*, 64-70.

Tohen, M., Waternaux, C.M., Tsuang, M.T., & Hunt, A.T. (1990). Four-year follow-up of twenty-four first-episode manic patients. *Journal of Affective Disorders, 19*, 79-86.

Tse, S.S., & Walsh, A.E.S. (2001). How does work work for people with bipolar affective disorder? *Occupational Therapy International, 8*, 210-225.

Tummey, R. (2001). A collaborative approach to urgent mental health referrals. *Suicide Prevention, 15*(52), 39-42.

Yakobina, S., Yakobina, S., & Tallant, B.K. (1997). I came, I thought, I conquered: Cognitive behavior approach applied in occupational therapy for the treatment of depressed (dysthymic) females. *Occupational Therapy in Mental Health, 13*(4), 59-73.

Chapter 8

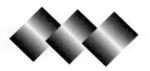 # Anxiety Disorders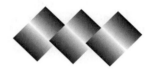

This group of disorders is characterized by the presence of anxiety and behavior intended to avoid the feeling of anxiety. Disorders in this category include panic attack, panic disorder, agoraphobia, specific phobia, obsessive-compulsive disorder, post-traumatic stress disorder, and acute stress disorder. Generalized anxiety disorder, a milder and less disabling disorder will be described only briefly, since it is not seen frequently in occupational therapy settings. Occupational therapy intervention for all the anxiety disorders will be considered at the end of the chapter. Table 8-1 lists the main diagnoses in this cluster.

PANIC ATTACK

A single panic attack is not diagnosed as a psychiatric disorder. Occurrence of panic attacks is characteristic of a number of anxiety disorders, so DSM-IV-TR (APA, 2000) lists the criteria for determining whether one has occurred.

Panic attacks are characterized by the presence of at least four symptoms from the following list: palpitations, increased heart rate, sweating, trembling, shortness of breath, a choking sensation, chest pain, nausea, dizziness or faintness, fear of dying, and chills. The symptoms of panic attacks can be provoked in a laboratory through chemical means, including excessive caffeine (Nutt & Lawson, 1992). Hyperventilation can also produce a panic attack (Mehta, Sutherland, & Hodgkinson, 2000). Regardless of their source, panic attacks are accompanied by an intense state of fear (Reiss, 1991).

A panic attack may be perceived by the individual as a heart attack, so it is not unusual for the individual to present in the emergency room (Potokar & Nutt, 2000). Physicians may be able to identify panic attacks because of subtle differences in presentation as compared with coronary events. Distinguishing features of a panic attack include relatively young age, feelings of fear or apprehension before the attack, and atypical presentation of chest pain. Panic attacks usually end within minutes or, rarely, as long as hours, but a person who has experienced such an episode may well develop anxiety about the potential for other attacks. It is the fear of recurrence, not the attack itself, that characterizes anxiety disorders (Beck, 1996). Three percent to 4% of the population can be expected to experience at least one panic attack (Korbett & St. John, 1999).

```
┌─────────────────────────────────────────────────────────────────────────┐
│                                                                           │
│                               Table 8-1                                   │
│                           Anxiety Disorders                               │
│                                                                           │
│     • Panic attack                      • Specific phobia                 │
│     • Panic disorder                    • Obsessive-compulsive disorder   │
│     • Agoraphobia                       • Post-traumatic stress disorder  │
│                                                                           │
└─────────────────────────────────────────────────────────────────────────┘
```

PANIC DISORDER

This diagnosis is made when the primary symptom is recurrent unexpected panic attacks (Schweitzer, Nesse, Fantone, & Curtis, 1995). These may result in agoraphobia, an extreme fear of going into new or unfamiliar situations. Sometimes, however, panic disorder occurs in the absence of agoraphobia, and agoraphobia, as noted below, may occur in the absence of panic attacks.

Each panic attack is characterized by severe anxiety and feelings of panic that may be accompanied by apprehension, shortness of breath, dizziness, nausea, chest pain, hot flashes, numbness, and fear of doing something uncontrolled. These attacks appear unpredictably, particularly at first, and the individual may develop fear about the possibility of having a panic attack. This fear is ongoing between attacks (Reiss, 1991). Typically, the individual begins to associate these attacks with specific situations, which are then avoided, or begins to fear being anywhere where help might not be readily available, thus developing avoidance of any new situation (i.e., agoraphobia).

The attacks may be relatively frequent, occurring several times a day for example, or rare. Occasionally, the disorder is limited to one attack, or to a brief period during which the attacks occur, followed by a complete disappearance of symptoms of panic attack. More typically, there is a chronic pattern, with some periods of relative freedom from attacks, others during which the attacks become more frequent or more severe (Korbett & St. John, 1999).

Etiology and Incidence

Panic disorder is quite common but not well-explained. Between 1% and 3% of the population meets the criteria for panic disorder (Korbett & St. John, 1999). It may occur in the presence of some form of depression, although the most common pattern is for depression to occur later (Boulenger & Lavallee, 1993), probably because the panic attacks can be so demoralizing. Another commonly-occurring comorbid condition is substance use disorder, possibly the result of attempts to self-sedate during panic attacks (Korbett & St. John, 1999).

The disorder may have a biological basis, specifically, serotonin dysregulation (Glod & Cawley, 1997). It may also be a learned response or some combination of biological and learned (Rapee, 1991). Separation from family or disruption of important relationships during childhood is a predisposing factor (Rapee, 1991), as are presence of avoidance behavior in childhood and stressful life events.

Prognosis

Prognosis is variable, depending on severity and on unknown and unpredictable factors. Approximately 39% of individuals experience remission within 1 year (Korbett & St. John, 1999). Others have relatively chronic courses, particularly those who develop agoraphobia. There is a marked excess mortality from other causes, including heart disease and suicide.

Implications for Function and Treatment

Function is dependent on the severity of the disorder. In some individuals, functional impairment is minimal. While they experience extreme discomfort during attacks, they may be relatively symptom-free between attacks and have long periods without problems. In other instances, function is severely impaired, particularly occupational and social function (Agras, 1993). Generally speaking, ADLs remains intact, although IADLs may be impaired by an unwillingness to leave the house. Some of these individuals, for example, experience panic attacks while driving and, as a result, refuse to drive.

The most effective treatment is a combination of psychotropic medications and cognitive behavioral treatment (Schweitzer et al., 1995). The most effective medications include some of the tricyclic antidepressants, SSRIs, and antianxiety agents. Behavioral interventions include systematic desensitization, which is useful but sometimes quite stressful to the individual. This involves pairing of increasingly anxiety-provoking stimuli with relaxation methods to reduce the incidence of panic and to provide the individual with a sense of control of the symptoms. Relaxation therapy is also an effective behavioral intervention. Overall, treatment is relatively effective (Korbett & St. John, 1999) even when accompanied by coexisting depression.

AGORAPHOBIA

Agoraphobia is diagnosed in the context of panic attacks, fear of having panic attacks, or of being in unfamiliar situations. It is not an independently coded diagnosis. Individuals who are agoraphobic are fearful of leaving a familiar environment, usually the house or even a specific room in the house. When the fear of panic attacks is based on prior experience of having the attacks, the diagnosis is agoraphobia with panic disorder. Some individuals fear panic attacks but have never had them. In this case, a diagnosis of agoraphobia without panic disorder is made.

Etiology and Incidence

This can be a very severe condition, but its origin is not well-understood. Incidence is roughly 3% in community populations (Franklin, 1991), and it is somewhat more common in women. Risk factors include early experiences of loss, childhood separation or school anxiety, and recent experiences of loss. Family history of anxiety disorders is also predictive.

The prognosis is variable, as agoraphobia tends to represent a long-term pattern of maladaptation. However, some individuals find that symptoms wax and wane (Schweitzer et al., 1995). They may also find that as one situation becomes less anxiety-provoking, another replaces it. Antianxiety medications and behavior modification have been employed with some degree of success, but the disorder can be intractable. In particular, comorbidity with other mental disorders is prognostic of poor outcome (Brown & Barlow, 1992).

Implications for Function and Treatment

Agoraphobia can be extremely disabling (Hoffart, 1993). While underlying skills (cognitive, sensory, motor) appear to be intact, the interaction of the disorder with skills is not well-understood. It is possible that some sort of sensory change may occur, but this is not well-researched. Performance is severely impaired in those areas requiring movement to public places, like grocery stores, offices, and shopping malls. Individuals with agoraphobia have difficulty with most occupations. They often cannot work because they fear leaving the house. Their social lives may become quite circumscribed, and they are fearful of any activity that requires them to be in new situations, although they may be able to maintain ADLs and those IADL functions that do not require them to go out. Their families may be involved in the condition as well. In one extreme case, the individual's husband reported that no one in the family was allowed to use the upstairs portion of the house, as this would precipitate a panic attack for the individual. Since the bedrooms were all upstairs, the family had to move beds into the living room. In some instances, the individual may be able to go out with one trusted companion (e.g., a friend or spouse). Performance patterns are excessively entrenched, as these patterns are experienced by the individual as reducing anxiety. The patterns are typically avoidant (i.e., the individual has a routine that reduces new or unfamiliar experiences).

Treatments include behavioral fear reduction and avoidance reduction procedures (Otto, Pollack, Jenike, & Rosenbaum, 1999). Cognitive behavioral treatments are of value as are psychotropic medications that reduce anxiety (Schweitzer et al., 1995). Overall, treatment is effective in somewhere between 20% and 60% of cases (O'Sullivan & Marks, 1991).

SPECIFIC PHOBIA

This is a condition in which excessive, persistent fear is caused by presence of a specific and limited object. In social phobia (which is separately diagnosed but typical of specific phobias), for example, it is social situations that evoke the response. Specific phobias are often related to a stimulus that has evoked the panic response in the past (e.g., snakes, enclosed spaces, high places, driving, flying, etc.). Unlike panic attack disorder, however, the source of the fear is identifiable, and the individual typically recognizes that it is unreasonable.

Specific phobia diagnoses are not made unless the individual alters his or her behavior in some way as a result. Someone who is afraid of flying but does so regardless would not be diagnosed, while someone who avoided flying at all costs would be given a simple phobia diagnosis. In children, crying or tantrums may occur instead of panic attacks. Children, unlike adults, may not recognize that the fear is unreasonable.

Etiology and Incidence

Phobias seem to develop through conditioning (i.e., an individual will have an experience with the stimulus that is anxiety provoking and then associate other similar experiences with the feeling of fear) (Rogers & Gournay, 2001). A child who is frightened by a spider while playing outside may develop a feeling of panic in other circumstances in which spiders are present. Alternatively, individuals may be taught their phobias or model on parent fears. In such a case, a parent's fear of spiders might be conveyed to a child who then exhibits the fear as well. These phobias may persist for long periods of time. If they begin in adulthood, they will generally continue unless they are treated. Individuals whose phobias began in childhood and persisted into adulthood tend to have worse outcomes than those whose phobias emerged in adulthood (Keller et al., 1992).

Social phobia may be the most common phobia, with estimates as high as 13% of the population (Otto et al., 1999). Other phobias are also extremely common, occurring in approximately 7% of the general population (Rogers & Gournay, 2001). Almost all individuals experience fear related to specific stimuli, and while most do not have panic attacks as a result, large numbers of people do.

Implications for Function and Treatment

Functional impact is largely dependent on the nature of the feared stimulus. Social phobias may be relatively disabling, as they lead people to avoid any situation in which new people will be present. However, many feared stimuli can be readily avoided without undue impact on the individual's life. Fear of snakes may be managed by avoiding most outdoor activity, a limitation that some individuals would not consider too great a hardship. Among the individuals most likely to seek treatment are those who have relatively late onset of symptoms that do interfere with function (e.g., a traveling salesman who develops fear of flying). Another particularly troubling phobia is school phobia, which is not uncommon in children. This phobia may develop as a result of a frightening or anxiety-provoking experience at school, although in some instances it is unexplained. One child became sick every morning for weeks until it was discovered that she was afraid of the computer room at school—a small, windowless, rather dark space. Her symptoms abated when the computers were moved. In some cases, the child refuses to go to school; in others, he or she is too anxious to perform well while there.

Treatment usually involves some sort of behavior modification. Systematic desensitization has been found to be effective. Occasionally, antianxiety agents will be used, but this is not common, since the phobias tend to be circumscribed and self-limiting. Many individuals, in fact, find ways to alter their routines to avoid the feared stimulus entirely and never seek other treatment. The most effective treatment appears to be a combination of behavioral and physiological methods (e.g. biofeedback) (Rogers & Gournay, 2001). Treatment is clearly effective (Chapman, Fyer, Mannuzza, & Klein, 1993). At least 60% of individuals treated with behavioral methods have reduced phobic reactions (O'Sullivan & Marks, 1991).

It is noteworthy that there is a familial pattern to anxiety disorders, meaning that children whose parents have anxiety disorders are more likely to develop them as well (Bernstein & Borchardt, 1991). For this reason, family therapy is often recommended when the client is a child (Dadds, Heard, & Rapee, 1992).

OBSESSIVE-COMPULSIVE DISORDER

Obsessions are thoughts or ideas that are intrusive and anxiety-provoking. Most common are obsessions with violence or contamination. The individual may recognize that these ideas are internally-derived (i.e., not based on any external event), but he or she is unable to control them and finds that the thoughts intrude while he or she is attempting to do something else. The individual often knows that the obsessive thoughts are unreasonable (Eddy & Walbroehl, 1998).

Compulsions are repetitive, purposeful behaviors performed in response to an obsession with the goal of preventing the discomfort caused by the obsession. The activity is, however, either excessive or not realistically helpful in resolving the obsession. For example, someone with an obsession about contamination may engage in ritual handwashing (Glod & Cawley, 1997) or laundering of clothing, even though this cannot eliminate all possible contaminants in the environment.

Many obsessive-compulsive individuals recognize the nature of the obsession and the futility of the compulsion, but experience great anxiety or tension when attempting to resist them. Over time, the individual may become increasingly unwilling to experience the anxiety, and thus stop resisting the compulsion.

Depression, anxiety, and avoidance of anxiety-provoking situations are commonly seen. Thus, in addition to engaging in ritual handwashing, an individual may begin to avoid unfamiliar situations that he or she may view as providing further risk of contamination.

Etiology and Incidence

Obsessive-compulsive disorder (OCD) has a clear biological component. Serotonin disregulation is well-documented, as are brain changes, including increased blood flow to the orbital-frontal lobes and the basal ganglia (Glod & Cawley, 1997). Heredity may play a role (Khouzam, 1999).

The disorder in its most severe form is rare, but it appears that many individuals have mild forms of OCD. Lifetime occurrence in the general population is between 2% and 3% (Khouzam, 1999). Rasmussen and Eisen (1992) have suggested that OCD is substantially underdiagnosed because of shame on the part of the individual, as well as lack of awareness on the part of health care providers. An example they provide is of an individual presenting to a dermatologist with a skin rash, which is not recognized as being the result of excessive washing in a compulsive effort to remove germs. OCD is considered one of the five major causes of disability in the world, as the fourth most common psychiatric condition after phobias, substance abuse disorders, and major depressive disorder (Olfson et al., 1997).

Prognosis

It has been suggested that OCD has as many as eleven subtypes (Rosario-Campos et al., 2001). One subtype is early onset, characterized by a higher rate of comorbid tic disorders, more frequent occurrence in males, and greater familial association. This type appears to have a worse prognosis than other forms of the disorder, with as many as 71% having some form of psychiatric disorder at follow-up 11 years after first diagnosis, and 36% still showing signs of OCD (Wewetzer et al., 2001).

For adults, the course is variable (Rasmussen & Eisen, 1992). Some do quite well, eventually returning to normal function. In others, it may be constant and chronic (Wever & Rey, 1997). The course of recovery is typically marked by exacerbations and remissions. In recent years, the prognosis has improved considerably, perhaps because of the effectiveness of psychotropic medications (Khouzam, 1999).

Implications for Function and Treatment

Depending on the compulsion, function may not be impaired or may be severely impaired. Many individuals have some ritualistic, almost superstitious, behavior that is not disruptive (e.g., wearing a particular set of clothing when taking a test, or checking the door lock exactly seven times before leaving home) (Gournay, 1998). However, in some cases, the compulsion may become the central focus of life (as in the case of a individual who must wash clothing 13 times before wearing it). Some of these individuals may be unable to maintain jobs or social relationships or have any activity other than the compulsion (Khouzam, 1999). This is true in spite of the individual's recognition of the disabling nature of the compulsion.

Obsessive compulsiveness may lead to social isolation. Many of the fears of these individuals do not materialize, however. They are, for example, not likely to commit suicide, engage in criminal behavior, or become addicted to drugs, even though these are common obsessional worries. While the incidence of suicide and drug abuse is higher in these individuals than in the general population, neither is frequent.

In the area of skills, cognition is the most obviously affected function. Individuals with OCD have distorted perceptions that may even include psychotic features (Razali, 2000). Performance patterns are seriously affected. Unlike those psychiatric disorders in which patterns are disrupted, patterns are rigid, well-established, and highly dysfunctional in OCD.

The most effective treatment involves the use of psychotropic medication in combination with cognitive-behavioral therapy (Glod & Cawley, 1997; Khouzam, 1999; Wever & Rey, 1997). In some cases, treatment is highly effective, but this is not a consistent outcome. The disorder is considered difficult to treat, although combination treatment can reduce symptoms significantly (Wever & Rey, 1997). In one study of 54 children and adolescents with OCD, 70% were taking maintenance medication at the 2 to 5 year follow-up (Leonard et al., 1997). Children can have a longer course and worse outcomes than adults, however (Wewetzer et al., 2001).

POST-TRAUMATIC STRESS DISORDER

By definition, the emergence of this disorder always follows an event that was a major life stress, one that must be more severe and unusual than those found in everyday life. Distress following a divorce would not be considered post-traumatic stress disorder (PTSD), while distress following a life-threatening fire might. The trauma may involve threat to one's life or the lives of one's family, destruction of home, victimization during a crime, or seeing someone else severely injured or killed. The trauma may be something that occurs only to the individual (e.g., cases of sexual or physical abuse in children) or to groups of individuals (e.g., holocaust survivors).

PTSD was identified following the Vietnam war as a result of the large numbers of combat veterans who had extreme difficulty readapting to civilian life. It should be noted, however, that the syndrome certainly existed prior to this time (e.g., as "shell shock" during World War I) (Tierney, 2000). World War II veterans who were prisoners of war showed signs of psychological distress long after the event (Tennant, Goulston, & Dent, 1986).

The trauma is usually accompanied by extreme feelings of terror and helplessness, and a primary characteristic of PTSD is a re-experiencing of both the event and these feelings that are recurrent and intrusive. The individual may have bad dreams or experience these feelings at unpredictable times and in unpredictable places. As this occurs, the individual begins to avoid the situations that seem to stimulate it or to develop a diminished ability to respond to the world as a mechanism for avoiding the unpleasant emotions.

Individuals who have this disorder have disturbed sleep, exaggerated startle reflexes, poor concentration, and extreme irritability often accompanied by aggression. It frequently occurs in conjunction with depression or anxiety. Substance abuse is also a commonly-co-existing condition, perhaps as the individual attempts to self-medicate to reduce symptoms (Miller, 2000).

Etiology and Incidence

A traumatically stressful event is a necessary precondition to the emergence of this disorder. It is not clear, however, why some individuals are susceptible while others who have similar experiences may not develop PTSD. For example, not all war veterans develop PTSD (Murray, 1992), although most report some change in outlook as a result of their experiences. There has been some speculation that individuals who develop the disorder had pre-existing psychopathology (Choy & DeBosset, 1992; Keane & Wolfe, 1990), but this is not well-established. It may emerge immediately after the trauma or after a period of months or years (Miller, 2000).

As the disorder has gained wider attention, the number of individuals diagnosed with PTSD has increased dramatically and it is now considered relatively common. It is estimated that 85% of holocaust survivors and 30% of auto accident and crime victims have PTSD (Choy & DeBosset, 1992). It is also thought to be common among victims of physical or sexual abuse (Woods, 2000). As increasing numbers of refugees enter the United States, PTSD associated with war or refugee experiences is also being seen more often in medical situations (D'Avanzo & Barab, 1998). Practitioners working with immigrant groups should be alert to the possibility of PTSD, as well as to the potential for its expression in somewhat varied form in some cultural groups. For example, for some groups, overt expression of anxiety may be unacceptable, leaving them to demonstrate their worries through withdrawal or excessive lethargy instead.

An important factor for occupational therapists is the increasing recognition that PTSD may occur in individuals who have experienced a traumatic injury. Burn victims (Ehde, Patterson, Wiechman, & Wilson, 2000; Robert et al., 1999), children treated for cancer (Tierney, 2000), and individuals with spinal cord injuries (Boyer, Tollen, & Kafkalas, 1998) often show evidence of PTSD. This can complicate recovery from the physical injury. For example, individuals remembering the experience of being burned may have agitated movement that can compromise skin grafts.

Prognosis

Because this disorder has been identified so recently, prognosis is not well-known. It appears that some individuals have a relatively time-limited disorder, while others develop chronic symptoms. By definition, it must last at least 1 month, but it may persist for long periods of time. It appears, for example, that World War II prisoners of war showed high levels of depression 40 years after the war (Tennant et al., 1986).

Good prognosis is predicted by healthy premorbid function, less severe and briefer trauma, and good social support, according to some reports (Miller, 2000). There is some dispute on this subject, though, with other researchers reporting that PTSD emerges unpredictably (Resnick, 1993). The acute form may be somewhat more responsive to treatment than more chronic forms (Miller, 2000). Children with PTSD as a result of abuse, invasive medical procedures (e.g., cancer treatment), or refugee experiences often show later signs of personality disorder (Tierney, 2000).

Implications for Function and Treatment

Depending on the severity of the disorder, function may be minimally or severely impaired. Some individuals continue to hold jobs and to maintain social and avocational activities. Because a defining characteristic of PTSD is the avoidance of any stimulus that might cause the individual to remember the event, some individuals find their function circumscribed. If the trauma occurred in a place that is difficult to avoid, the resultant PTSD may be quite disabling. Similarly, some individuals find that the re-experience of the event is frequent, and that the accompanying fears are severe, leading to significant disability.

Children who have experienced trauma may have difficulty with school function (Driver & Beltran, 1998). Skill areas, such as cognition, are impaired as intrusive thoughts affect concentration. Social and academic performance areas are also affected.

Where the trauma has been severe and prolonged, rage, depression, and humiliation may persist for years (Herman, 1992). For example, abused children may show signs of trauma throughout adulthood. More than one-third of abused women in a homeless shelter had symptoms of PTSD (Humphreys, Lee, Neylan, & Marmar, 2001), suggesting these women were unable to manage work and daily life performance in multiple areas.

Effective treatment is not well-understood, although it appears that group therapy, particularly in which the individual can talk with others who have had similar experiences, may be of value. Antianxiety or antidepressant medication may be employed, although one of the concerns related to the disorder is the possible emergence of a substance abuse disorder as the individual seeks to relieve tension (Miller, 2000). Behavioral and cognitive interventions are preferred for this reason as well because they appear to be somewhat more effective (Miller, 2000). Hypnosis may also be helpful (Degun-Mather, 2001).

In cases of sexual or physical abuse, remediation of the situation that led to the disorder is an important component of treatment. The abuser must be treated or the child removed from his or her presence, sometimes by removal from the family. In cases of natural disasters, children who receive supportive intervention immediately tend to have improved better outcomes than when treatment is delayed (Deering, 2000). Similarly, women who are in abusive relationships do best when they can escape the situation and learn adaptive mechanisms for coping with their anxiety and their life situations (Woods & Isenberg, 2001).

Implications for Occupational Therapy

Occupational therapists employ a variety of approaches when working with individuals with anxiety disorders. Several goals are prominent. First, anxiety management is essential (Rosier, Williams, & Ryrie, 1998). Relaxation, either by diverting attention or through relaxation training, is one strategy. The therapist might, for example, help the individual identify a pleasurable activity that requires attention (e.g., writing a poem, playing chess). This approach requires that the therapist be sensitive to the possibility that such activity could increase anxiety for some people. Activities that require gross motor action to the point of fatigue may also promote relaxation. Once the client is relaxed, it may be possible to draw this to the individual's attention so that he or she knows what this state feels like.

Alternatively, it may be possible to use this relaxed state as a component of a systematic desensitization program. The relaxing activity can be paired with anxiety-provoking stimuli until relaxation can be maintained.

For individuals with PTSD, opportunities to express emotion can be valuable. These individuals often benefit from talking with others who have had the experience and from nonverbal expressive activities. One such client, a rape victim, progressed over time from drawing horrible monsters in stormy skies to drawing pleasant pastoral scenes. She found the activity both relaxing and cathartic. In situations of abuse, enhancement of independent living skills may promote a sense of control and self-esteem for women who are homeless (Davis & Kutter, 1998).

As anxiety is resolved, attention must be paid to substituting new activities that are satisfying. An individual with agoraphobia who is increasingly able to leave the house must find new and enjoyable ways to spend time formerly spent worrying. Individuals may need help re-establishing social ties, work activities, or leisure pursuits.

GENERALIZED ANXIETY DISORDER

This disorder is characterized by a generalized state of anxiety or worry in the absence of specific reason to do so. The individual may worry excessively about the state of his or her health or about finances when there is no realistic basis for the concern. The diagnosis is not made if substance abuse or depression might cause the anxiety, although mild depressive symptoms may be present. This is usually a chronic disorder, although any functional impairment is mild (Otto et al., 1999). Lifetime prevalence is approximately 5%, although individuals with the disorder typically experience exacerbations and remissions depending on the level of stress in their lives at a given point in time. This disorder is unpleasant for the individual but not typically disabling. Occupational therapists may see individuals with this disorder in the context of treatment for other conditions and should be aware that even low levels of anxiety can interfere with motivation and with ability to comprehend and follow instructions. Table 8-2 shows the main symptoms and functional deficits that occur with anxiety disorders.

Table 8-2
Anxiety Disorders

Disorder	Symptoms	Functional Deficits
Panic disorder	1. Panic attacks 2. Attacks include feelings of panic, sweating, dizziness, nausea, chest pain, and intense fear	Work, leisure, and ADLs during attacks Fear of attack may impact on any function Affects routines and habits as individual attempts to avoid panic attacks
Agoraphobia	1. Fear of being in situations in which escape is not possible 2. Avoidance of such situations	May be mild to severe If mild, often no impairment If severe, global impairment
Specific phobia	1. Intense fear of specific stimulus 2. Avoidance of stimulus	Dependent on stimulus, may or may not limit any sphere
OCD	1. Obsessions are intrusive ideas that may be distressing and cannot be suppressed, but are recognized as only ideas (i.e., not delusions) 2. Compulsions are repetitive, purposeful actions intended neutralize upsetting aspects of obsessions 3. Obsessions and compulsions cause distress	May be mild to severe Work, leisure, and social ADLs/IADLs Dysfunctional roles, habits, and routines Impaired process skills Motor skills and communication are not affected
PTSD	1. Experience outside the normal range of experience, which is distressing 2. Recurrent distressing recollection/dreams about the event 3. Avoidance of stimuli related to the event 4. Insomnia, irritability 5. Physiological signs of fear 6. Minimum 1 month duration	May be mild to marked Most typical deficits are in social, work, and leisure Habits, routines, and roles are affected by periodic exacerbations and anxiety Process skills are affected by intrusive thoughts Motor and communication skills are intact

REFERENCES

Agras, W.S. (1993). The diagnosis and treatment of panic disorder. *Annual Review of Medicine, 44*, 39-51.

American Psychiatric Association. (2000). *Diagnostic and statistical manual of mental disorders* (4th ed., text revision). Washington, DC: Author.

Beck, C.T. (1996). A concept analysis of panic. *Archives of Psychiatric Nursing, 10*, 265-275.

Bernstein, G.A., & Borchardt C.M. (1991). Anxiety disorders of childhood and adolescence: A critical review. *Journal of the American Academy of Child and Adolescent Psychiatry, 30*, 519-532.

Boulenger, J.P., & Lavallee, Y.J. (1993). Mixed anxiety and depression: Diagnostic issues. *Journal of Clinical Psychiatry, 54*, 3-8.

Boyer, B.A., Tollen, L.G., & Kafkalas, C.M. (1998). A pilot study of posttraumatic stress disorder in children and adolescents with spinal cord injury. *SCI Psychosocial Process, 11*(4), 75-81.

Brown, T.A., & Barlow, D.H. (1992). Comorbidity among anxiety disorders: Implications for treatment and DSM-IV. *Journal of Consulting and Clinical Psychology, 60*, 835-844.

Chapman, T.F., Fyer, A.J., Mannuzza, S., & Klein, D.F. (1993). A comparison of treated and untreated simple phobia. *American Journal of Psychiatry, 150*, 816-818.

Choy, T., & DeBosset, F. (1992). Post-traumatic stress disorder: An overview. *Canadian Journal of Psychiatry, 37*, 578-583.

Dadds, M.R., Heard, P.M., & Rapee, R.M. (1992). The role of family intervention in the treatment of child anxiety disorders: Some preliminary findings. *Behavior Change, 9*, 171-177.

D'Avanzo, C.E., & Barab, S.A. (1998). Depression and anxiety among Cambodian refugee women in France and the United States. *Issues in Mental Health Nursing, 19*, 541-556.

Davis, J., & Kutter, C.J. (1998). Independent living skills and posttraumatic stress disorder in women who are homeless: Implications for future practice. *The American Journal of Occupational Therapy, 52*, 39-44.

Deering, C.G. (2000). A cognitive developmental approach to understanding how children cope with disasters. *Journal of Child and Adolescent Psychiatric Nursing, 13*(1), 7-16.

Degun-Mather, M. (2001). The value of hypnosis in the treatment of chronic PTSD with dissociative fugues in a war veteran. *Contemporary Hypnosis, 18*(1), 4-13.

Driver, C., & Beltran, R.D. (1998). Impact of refugee trauma on children's occupational role as students. *Australian Occupational Therapy Journal, 45*, 23-38.

Eddy, M.F., & Walbroehl, G.S. (1998). Recognition and treatment of obsessive-compulsive disorder. *American Family Physician, 57*, 1623-1628.

Ehde, D.M., Patterson, D.R., Wiechman, S.A., & Wilson, L.G. (2000). Post-traumatic stress symptoms and distress 1 year after burn injury. *The Journal of Burn Care & Rehabilitation, 21*, 105-111.

Franklin, J.A. (1991). Agoraphobia. *International Review of Psychiatry, 3*, 151-162.

Glod, C.A., & Cawley, D. (1997). The neurobiology of obsessive-compulsive disorder. *Journal of the American Psychiatric Nurses Association, 3*(4) 120-122.

Gournay, K. (1998). Obsessive compulsive disorder: Nature and treatment. *Nursing Standard, 13*(10), 46-54.

Herman, J.L. (1992). Complex PTSD: A syndrome in survivors of prolonged and repeated trauma. *Journal of Traumatic Stress, 5*, 377-391.

Hoffart, A. (1993). Cognitive treatments of agoraphobia: A critical evaluation of theoretical basis outcome evidence. *Journal of Anxiety Disorders, 7*, 75-91.

Humphreys, J., Lee, K., Neylan, T., & Marmar, C. (2001). Psychological and physical distress of sheltered battered women. *Health Care for Women International, 22*, 401-414.

Keane, T.M., & Wolfe, J. (1990). Comorbidity in post-traumatic stress disorder: An analysis of community and clinical studies. *Journal of Applied Social Psychology, 20*, 1776-1788.

Keller, M.B., Lavori, P.W., Wunder, J., Beardslee, W.R., Schwartz, C.E., & Roth, J. (1992). Chronic course of anxiety disorders in children and adolescents. *Journal of the American Academy of Child and Adolescent Psychiatry, 31*, 595-599.

Khouzam, H.R. (1999). Obsessive-compulsive disorder. *Postgraduate Medicine, 106*(7), 133-141.

Korbett, A.B., & St. John, D. (1999). Panic disorder: Workup, management, and referral. *Journal of the American Academy of Physician Assistants, 12*(2), 62-64, 67-68, 71-72.

Leonard, H.L., Swedo, S.E., Lenane, M.C., Rettew, D.C., Hamburger, S.D., Bartko, J.J., et al. (1993). A 2- to 7-year follow-up of 54 obsessive-compulsive children and adolescents. *Archives of General Psychiatry, 50*, 429-439.

Mehta, T.A., Sutherland, J.G., & Hodgkinson, D.W. (2000). Hyperventilation: Cause or effect? *Journal of Accident and Emergency Medicine, 17*, 376-377.

Miller, J.L. (2000). Post-traumatic stress disorder in primary care practice. *Journal of the American Academy of Nurse Practitioners, 12*, 475-485.

Murray, J.B. (1992). Post-traumatic stress disorder: A review. *Genetic, Social, and General Psychology Monographs, 118*, 313-338.

Nutt, D., & Lawson, C. (1992). Panic attacks: A neurochemical overview of models and mechanisms. *British Journal of Psychiatry, 160*, 165-178.

Olfson, M., Fireman, B., Wiessman, M.M., Kathol, R.G., Farber, L., Sheehan, D., et al. (1997). Mental disorders and disability among patients in a primary care group practice. *American Journal of Psychiatry, 154*, 1734-1740.

O'Sullivan, G., & Marks, I. (1991). Follow-up studies of behavioral treatment of phobic and obsessive compulsive neuroses. *Psychiatric Annals, 21*, 368-373.

Otto, M.W., Pollack, M.H., Jenike, M.A., & Rosenbaum, J.F. (1999). Anxiety disorders and their treatment. In A.M. Nicholi (Ed.), *The Harvard guide to psychiatry* (3rd ed., pp. 220-239). Cambridge, MA: Belknap Press.

Potokar, J.P., & Nutt, D.J. (2000). Chest pain: Panic attack or heart attack? *International Journal of Clinical Practice, 54*, 110-114.

Rapee, R.M. (1991). Panic disorder. *International Review of Psychiatry, 3*, 141-149.

Rasmussen, S.A., & Eisen, J.L. (1992). The epidemiology and differential diagnosis of obsessive compulsive disorder. *The Journal of Clinical Psychiatry, 53*, 4-10.

Razali, S.M. (2000). Obsessive-compulsive psychosis. *Australian and New Zealand Journal of Psychiatry, 34*, 530-531.

Reiss, S. (1991). Expectancy model of fear, anxiety, and panic. *Clinical Psychology Review, 11*, 141-153.

Resnick, P.A. (1993). The psychological impact of rape. *Journal of Interpersonal Violence, 8*, 223-255.

Robert, R., Meyer, W.J., Villarreal, C., Blakeney, P.E., Desai, M., & Herndon, D. (1999). An approach to the timely treatment of acute stress disorder. *Journal of Burn Care & Rehabilitation, 20*, 250-258.

Rogers, P., & Gournay, K. (2001). Phobias: Nature, assessment and treatment. *Nursing Standard, 15*(30), 37-43.

Rosario-Campos, M.C., Leckman, J.F., Mercadante, M.T., Shavitt, R.G., Prado, H.S., Sada, P., et al. (2001). Adults with early-onset obsessive-compulsive disorder. *American Journal of Psychiatry, 158*, 1899-1903.

Rosier, C., Williams, H., & Ryrie, I. (1998). Anxiety management groups in a community mental health team. *British Journal of Occupational Therapy, 61*, 203-206.

Schweitzer, P.B., Nesse, R.M., Fantone, R.F., & Curtis, G.C. (1995). Outcomes of group cognitive behavioral training in the treatment of panic disorder and agoraphobia. *Journal of the American Psychiatric Nurses Association, 1*(3), 83-91.

Tennant, C.C., Goulston, K.J., and Dent, O.F. (1986). The psychological effects of being a prisoner of war: Forty years after release. *American Journal of Psychiatry, 143*, 618-621.

Tierney, J.A. (2000). Post-traumatic stress disorder in children: Controversies and unresolved issues. *Journal of Child and Adolescent Psychiatric Nursing, 13*(4), 147-158.

Wever, C., & Rey, J.M. (1997). Juvenile obsessive-compulsive disorder. *Australian and New Zealand Journal of Psychiatry, 31*, 105-113.

Wewetzer, C., Jans, T., Muller, B., Neudorfl, A., Bucherl, U., Remschmidt, H., et al. (2001). Long-term outcome and prognosis of obsessive-compulsive disorder with onset in childhood or adolescence. *European Child & Adolescent Psychiatry, 10*, 27-46.

Woods, S.J. (2000). Prevalence and patterns of post-traumatic stress disorder in abused and postabused women. *Issues in Mental Health Nursing, 21*, 309-324.

Woods, S.J., & Isenberg, M.A. (2001). Adaptation as a mediator of intimate abuse and traumatic stress in battered women. *Nursing Science Quarterly, 14*, 215-221.

Chapter 9

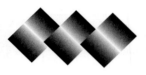 Personality Disorders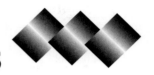

Personality disorders are identified as Axis II labels according to the DSM-IV (APA, 1994) system. Remember that this axis is specifically for disorders that are life-long patterns of adaptation. A defining characteristic of all the personality disorders is that they emerge no later than adolescence. In general, they are less severe than Axis I diagnoses (with the exceptions of borderline, antisocial, and possibly schizotypal personality disorders), but they also tend to be longer-lasting, with no periods of remission, and are generally thought to be resistant to intervention.

The personality disorders are also among the more controversial diagnoses for a number of reasons (Gunderson, 1999; Shedler & Weston, 1998). First, reliability is a concern. To some extent, this is because the personality disorders represent exaggerations of traits evident in people without psychiatric disturbance (Divac-Jovanovic & Lecic-Tosevski, 1994; Shedler & Weston, 1998). In addition, life-long patterns are difficult to clearly establish in clinical settings. As Gunderson (1988) points out, "traits are identifiable as disorders only when they become so prominent and rigid as to cause dysfunction" (p. 337). When these individuals come into treatment, it is rarely because of the personality disorder, but rather because of depression or anxiety as a consequence of disturbed interpersonal relationships caused by their problematic personality traits (Turner, 1994).

Some of the diagnostic criteria for these disorders have been described as unclear or overlapping (Gunderson, 1999). There is a high rate of comorbidity with other psychiatric disorders that may reflect dilemmas in making distinctions between them (Crawford, Cohen, & Brook, 2001a). Further, there is inconsistency about placement of some disorders on Axis I or Axis II. For example, schizotypal personality is presumably a mild, nonpsychotic relative of schizophrenia and is found in the personality disorder section. Dysthymic disorder, which seems to be at a similar point on the affective disorder continuum (i.e., a mild, nonpsychotic relative of major depression) is an Axis I diagnosis.

Adding to the dilemma presented by these diagnoses is the fact that they are most often self-diagnosing (i.e., they are labeled only if the individual comes for help [or is sent by someone else]). Many individuals who would otherwise be diagnosed never feel sufficiently bad or behave peculiarly enough to enter therapy. In some instances, it is the development of a coexisting Axis I disorder, most typically an affective or anxiety disorder, that brings these individuals into treatment (Turner, 1994).

The personality disorders typify the kinds of issues that were considered when revising the DSM. Several new personality disorders that appeared in the appendices of DSM-III-R (APA, 1987) were considered for inclusion among the personality disorders. These included SDPD (Fiester, 1991), sadistic personality disorder (SPD) (Fiester & Gay, 1991), and

```
+----------------------------------------------------------------------+
|                          Table 9-1                                   |
|                      Personality Disorders                           |
|                                                                      |
|   Cluster A              Cluster B              Cluster C            |
|  ----------             ----------             ----------           |
|                                                                      |
|   • Paranoid             • Antisocial           • Avoidant          |
|   • Schizoid             • Borderline           • Dependent         |
|   • Schizotypal          • Histrionic           • Obsessive-compulsive |
|                          • Narcissistic                             |
+----------------------------------------------------------------------+
```

depressive personality disorder (Phillips, Hirschfeld, Shea, & Gunderson, 1993). Arguments for and against each focused on reports of clinicians and research evidence of validity and reliability, particularly issues of overlap with other personality disorders. Some of the arguments for and against reflected concerns about potential for abuse of labels, as well as the scientific data. For example, there was concern that a diagnosis of SDPD might be used to "blame the victim" in abusive relationships (Fiester, 1991) and SPD to excuse the perpetrator (Fiester & Gay, 1991).

In another instance, a personality disorder found in DSM-III-R was considered for elimination (Gunderson, 1999). Passive-aggressive personality disorder was the most controversial personality disorder in that edition because of its reliance on a single trait as a diagnostic marker. Ultimately, depressive personality disorder and passive-aggressive personality disorder were placed in the appendices, among the list of disorders requiring further research. SDPD and SPD were both eliminated entirely.

DSM-IV-TR (APA, 2000) identifies three clusters of personality disorders, which are grouped according to common symptomatology. Paranoid, schizoid, and schizotypal personality disorders (cluster A) are characterized by odd or peculiar behavior. Cluster B—antisocial, borderline, histrionic, and narcissistic personality disorders—present with flamboyant or dramatic behavior. The third category, cluster C, is characterized primarily by anxiety or fear. Table 9-1 summarizes the personality disorders and the clusters in which they are categorized. They will be grouped in this way for discussion in this chapter, even though the clusters are somewhat subjective (Gunderson, 1999). Occupational therapy intervention for all the personality disorders will be discussed at the end of the chapter.

PARANOID PERSONALITY DISORDER

This disorder is identified by the individual's tendency to experience a sense of being threatened or persecuted. Associates and coworkers will be suspected of intent to harm the individual, and jealousy and suspicion characterize most relationships. The individual is typically isolated, with few friends or close relationships. The individual relates to others in a fashion that is withdrawn, suspicious, and frequently hostile (Shopshire & Craik, 1996). Paranoid personality disorder is less severe than paranoid schizophrenia and is characterized more by misinterpretation of input rather than by outright delusions. For example, someone who has a paranoid personality disorder may interpret a minor reprimand from a boss as "he's never liked me; he wants to fire me; everyone here hates me." Someone with paranoid schizophrenia might interpret the same reprimand as part of a CIA or mafia plan to kill him or her.

Typically, such individuals are argumentative and withdrawn, with little sense of humor and a "chip on their shoulders." They look for slights and frequently find them, tend to bear grudges, and may be litigious. They are hypercritical of others, while accepting criticism of themselves poorly. They tend to be excessively self-sufficient and quite egocentric. One such individual had constant trouble at work because he routinely violated company rules, reasoning that they had been instituted only to harass him.

Etiology and Incidence

The etiology of this personality disorder is not clear, but it is estimated to affect 0.5% to 2.5% of the general population (APA, 2000). One explanation that has been advanced about its origin is that this is a learned pattern of behavior. Others feel that it is the result of some sort of CNS disturbance (Gunderson, 1999). As with many of the personality disorders, there is some speculation about a familial link, but the data to confirm or refute this suspicion do not exist (Widiger & Bornstein, 2001).

Implications for Function and Treatment

The characteristic behavior pattern of individuals with paranoid personality disorder creates considerable difficulty. Performance areas affected are primarily work and social as a result of interpersonal difficulties. The suspiciousness and irritability of these individuals, coupled with their tendency to believe others are plotting against them, makes for troubled interactions, often resulting in lost jobs, divorce, and so on. In particular, relationships with authority figures tend to be problematic. Leisure interests may be few and often of a solitary nature. ADL, IADL, and work functions other than relationships with coworkers are maintained at acceptable levels. One man worked as a painter for a large corporation, moving from area to area to repaint walls. He worked mostly alone and was reported to be a good worker but hard to get along with. He ultimately lost his job, not because of poor painting skills but because of frequent fights with coworkers in the lunchroom.

Skills remain largely intact. Motor and sensory skills, sensory integration, and cognition are, for the most part, unaffected except for the inaccurate processing of social cues from others. Patterns are problematic because of the habitual tendency to attribute bad motives to others. Treatment, through behavior modification, medication, education, or psychotherapy is not notably successful with these individuals (Gunderson, 1999). Their personality pattern tends to be intractable, although some individuals can be taught how to interact more effectively.

SCHIZOID PERSONALITY DISORDER

This personality disorder is defined by an absence or indifference to social activity and a restricted range of emotion (Gunderson, 1999). These are individuals often identified as "loners" who have no interest in friendships, appear aloof and withdrawn, and demonstrate little emotion. They may seem self-absorbed and vague. One such woman rarely spoke to coworkers, but often had what others described as a "peculiar smile" on her face.

Etiology and Incidence

The cause of schizoid personality disorder is not well-established. As with paranoid personality disorder, the major theories about its emergence are that it is a learned pattern of behavior and that it is due to some sort of CNS dysfunction (Divac-Jovanovic & Lecic-Tosevski, 1994). The latter explanation seems more likely. The disorder is more common in men, and incidence is estimated at 1% to 2% of the general population (APA, 2000). This is a rough estimate at best, since these individuals are unlikely to seek treatment (Kalus, Bernstein, & Siever, 1993).

Implications for Function and Treatment

As with paranoid personality disorder, the primary functional impairment is in the area of social relationships. Unlike those with paranoid personality disorder, however, these individuals tend to display little aggression, making work situations easier to maintain. They do well in jobs that require little social interaction (Gunderson, 1999). They have few social relationships, however, and rarely marry or have close friends. Other skills and performance areas are unimpaired, meaning that these individuals are functional but lead lives restricted by the absence of meaningful friendships. The disorder persists throughout life, although some changes in specific characteristics may occur (e.g., the symptoms may come to more closely mirror narcissistic personality) (Gunderson, 1999).

When such individuals come into treatment, it is often because they are depressed about their isolation. Social skills training may provide a mechanism for helping them to establish relationships, although their interactions tend to remain stilted, awkward, or distant. Psychotherapy is sometimes attempted, as is psychotropic medication, particularly the antipsychotics and antidepressants (Millon, 1995).

SCHIZOTYPAL PERSONALITY DISORDER

Individual with schizotypal personalities have peculiar thought patterns, behaviors, and appearance (Gunderson, 1999). This may include bizarre fantasies, beliefs about special senses or powers, or odd patterns of speaking. Typically, odd perceptual experiences are present as well. Affect is either inappropriate or flat, and social isolation is common. It is differentiated from schizophrenia largely by matter of degree; the symptoms are not severe enough to fit the criteria for schizophrenia, although the disorders are related (Shedler & Weston, 1998). Such individuals are often described by neighbors as strange and as loners. If they have friends, their friends are often rather odd too.

Etiology and Incidence

As with the other personality disorders in this cluster, etiology is unclear but suspected to be the result of either CNS dysfunction or learning. Incidence is unknown, although the disorder is more common in family members of individuals who are schizophrenic (Siever, Bernstein, & Silverman, 1991). The diagnostic category is relatively new, so data are sparse, but there is speculation that this disorder differs only in degree from schizophrenia (Tsuang, Stone, & Faraone, 2000).

Implications for Function and Treatment

It is unclear whether there is some dysfunction at the skill level. It is possible that CNS function is impaired, particularly the ability to accurately process sensory input. Characteristic cognitive-perceptual deficits have been identified, a finding that is helpful when making the diagnosis (Gunderson, 1999). Such deficits may be the cause of some of the peculiar ideas held by these individuals.

At the performance level, function is distinctly impaired. Social function is particularly poor. Odd ideas held by these individuals make it difficult for others to understand them. The individual may avoid others because of discomfort in social situations and because they misperceive the social environment (Gunderson, 1999). Vocational function is impaired to the extent that social skills are required to do a job. As is true of those with schizoid personalities, these individuals may do best at jobs that require little social interaction. Actual work performance may also be poor, however, lending credence to the speculation that there is some underlying CNS or cognitive dysfunction. ADLs performance is impaired, and these individuals tend to be unkempt or to dress peculiarly.

Efforts at intervention are similar to those used for other disorders in this cluster, including medication, skill training, behavioral interventions, and verbal therapies (Millon, 1995).

ANTISOCIAL PERSONALITY DISORDER

Of all the personality disorders, this is most likely to be brought to the attention of health care professionals by someone other than the individual. The individual him- or herself (this diagnosis is much more common in males) tends not to be concerned about the behavior problems that create serious problems for others. This is also the personality disorder with the clearest diagnostic criteria (Widiger, 1992), making its diagnosis more clear-cut than many of the others.

The diagnosis is made in individuals who are at least 18 years old; prior to this, a conduct disorder would be diagnosed, since antisocial personality is characterized by a long-standing pattern of behavior. The individual has a pattern of antisocial behavior prior to age 15 (e.g., truancy, fighting, cruelty to animals or people, or stealing). In addition, this behavior continues after age 15, with the addition of problems in work settings (e.g., loss of jobs, unemployment, absence from work), illegal activity, aggressiveness, impulsivity, lying, recklessness, and inability to function responsibly in significant relationships (e.g., parenting). A significant characteristic is the lack of remorse for any of these behaviors (APA, 2000).

It is important to distinguish antisocial personality from other disorders, especially mania, since many behaviors typical of antisocial personality also occur during manic episodes. The long-standing pattern of antisocial behavior makes it noticeably different, as does the absence of periods of remission. The tendency to engage in criminal behavior is unique to this diagnosis. There is a common misperception that individuals with psychiatric disorders are prone to criminal behavior, but the data support this only for individuals with antisocial personality disorder (Gunderson, 1999).

Etiology and Incidence

Among the beliefs about the origin of antisocial personality is the theory that it is learned behavior, the result of overprotective or inconsistent parenting that does not allow the individual to learn that actions have consequences (Gunderson, 1999). There is also speculation about a biochemical etiology, supported by research showing neurotransmitter alterations and by family research suggesting genetic links (Reiss et al., 1995). None of the research is definitive. This disorder is more common in men and is found in 2% to 3% of the general population (APA, 2000). There is some concern that the disorder is overdiagnosed in criminal justice settings and underdiagnosed elsewhere (Widiger, 1992). In addition, this disorder has an extremely high rate of comorbidity with substance abuse (Gunderson, 1999).

Implications for Function and Treatment

Performance is impaired primarily in social and work spheres. ADLs are intact with the exception of management of finances. Typically, money is a serious problem, with stealing a common solution. Social relationships are impaired by the lack of depth and conscience displayed by these individuals. One individual who was imprisoned for armed robbery and murder explained that he had to kill the security guard because the guard got in the way, and therefore, deserved to die. In work situations, the belligerence and aggressiveness of these individuals is problematic. They may be quite able to perform the tasks required but are not able to maintain acceptable relationships with coworkers and supervisors, as they misinterpret some social situations, responding with excessive anxiety or anger. One man, during his short tenure on a construction job, routinely punched new employees just to "let them know who the real boss is!"

There has been some speculation that antisocial individuals have sensory impairments. Some research suggests that a large percentage of the prison population shows signs of learning disabilities linked to sensory processing problems, but this remains unproven. Habits and patterns are problematic in the individual's tendency to focus energy on behaviors that are illegal and harmful to self and others.

In general, these individuals do not respond well to treatment. Psychotherapy and in-patient and out-patient milieu therapy have all been shown to have some value. Milieu therapy is an in-patient intervention in which the entire environment is carefully structured to assure that actions have specific and predictable consequences, thereby, at least theoretically, remediating previous faulty learning. Psychotropic medications do not seem beneficial.

BORDERLINE PERSONALITY DISORDER

The diagnosis of borderline personality disorder (BPD) has become increasingly common in the last decade, a source of dispute since some do not believe it exists as a clinical entity (Gunderson, Zanarini, & Kisiel, 1991). Recent research suggests a significant overlap with other personality disorders, especially histrionic personality disorder (Crawford et al., 2001a). BPD is marked by instability of mood, relationships, and self-image, usually appearing during early adulthood. Relationships and affect tend to be unstable. Affect may also be inappropriate, in particular reflected by poor control of anger. Suicidal ideation and self-mutilation may also occur, and these individuals tend to be quite impulsive. These individuals fear abandonment and have self-image problems characterized by uncertainty about sexual orientation, long-term goals, or values. It is common to find depression and/or substance abuse coexisting in these individuals and to find a family history of alcoholism. A distinguishing characteristic, added in DSM-IV (APA, 1994) to help clarify diagnosis, is occurrence of transient psychotic-like or dissociative episodes (Gunderson, Zanarini, et al., 1991).

One borderline client had achieved a relatively stable work situation but found herself in great difficulty with social life. Her boyfriends, all short-term, routinely abandoned her and roommates moved out. Much of this was due to the extreme instability of her behavior toward them. One day she would be quite enamored and invested, bringing daily gifts and writing long letters about how close she felt to them. Within hours or days of this behavior, she would write angry, spiteful letters; splatter their clothes with ink; and scream obscenities at them.

Etiology and Incidence

It is possible that genetics contribute to occurrence of this disorder (Livesley, Jang, Jackson, & Vernon, 1993). However, it is also possible that borderline behaviors are learned from these dysfunctional relatives (Gunderson, 1999). The contribution of CNS dysfunction to the emergence of the disorder is not known, although individuals with BPD do have cognitive-perceptual problems (Gunderson, Zanarini, et al., 1991). It occurs in about 2% of the population (APA, 2000). Both men and women are diagnosed with BPD, although the presentation differs somewhat based on gender (Zlotnick, Rothschild, & Zimmerman, 2002). Men with BPD had more substance abuse disorders and concurrent antisocial and explosive tendencies, while women reported more concurrent eating disorders. It is noteworthy that cluster B disorders, including borderline, histrionic, and narcissistic personality disorders, appear to be quite common, with overall prevalence possibly as high as 17% (Crawford et al., 2001a). There is also clear evidence that these disorders do, indeed, emerge in adolescence and persist throughout life (Crawford, Cohen, & Brook, 2001b)

Implications for Function and Treatment

As with other personality disorders, function seems to be impaired at the level of performance of self-care, work, and leisure tasks as opposed to motor, sensory, and other skills. Vocational and social function are markedly impaired. Relationships tend to be unstable, with these individuals fluctuating wildly between excessive involvement with others and devaluation of friends. These relationship difficulties are the most consistent diagnostic criterion (Gunderson, 1999). Impulsiveness and difficulty handling anger magnify interpersonal difficulties, as does a feeling of depersonalization that arises for many individuals with BPD. Similar problems affect work; however, work problems are not solely the result of interpersonal difficulties. Since these individuals have problems identifying and maintaining a set of values and goals, they are unable to select and pursue career goals. Work history is unstable as they move from job to job or miss work because of substance abuse or suicide gestures.

ADLs are unimpaired at a basic level (i.e., these individuals are able to dress, maintain hygiene, cook and eat, and so on). However, their impulsivity may lead them to ignore their ADL needs, manage money poorly, drive recklessly, and so on. A particular issue with borderline personality is the tendency to "split," to see him- or herself and others as either "all good" or "all bad," and to fluctuate rapidly between these poles. These rapid shifts in attitude have an impact on both self-concept and relationships with others.

The evidence regarding impaired skills is somewhat equivocal (Millon, 1995). It is wide-ly believed that some level of CNS dysfunction affects individuals with BPD. Motor skills are unaffected. Establishment and maintenance of patterns is quite problematic for these individuals, as their rapid mood changes and impulsive nature impede orderly progression of activity.

Treatments recommended include long-term psychotherapy (Millon, 1995). In addition, a combination of short-term hospitalization, family education, and low-dose neuroleptics seems effective. Prognosis is fair. In one study, 75% of BPD patients followed for an average of 15 years were no longer diagnosable and showed functional improvement (Paris, Brown, & Nowlis, 1987). However, there was also a high risk for completed suicide.

HISTRIONIC PERSONALITY DISORDER

Individuals with histrionic personality disorder (HPD) demonstrate excessive emotional-ity or theatricality and attention-seeking behavior (Crawford et al., 2001a). They tend to need a great deal of approval or reassurance, which they may seek by being sexually seduc-tive, excessively concerned with physical attractiveness, and attempting to be the center of attention in all situations. Self-centeredness is extreme, and emotions are exaggerated. At the same time, emotions shift rapidly and are quite shallow. Descriptors that are considered prototypical are "self-dramatizing" and "vain" (Shopshire & Craik, 1996). These individu-als have low thresholds for frustration and are unable to delay gratification.

Etiology and Incidence

Etiology is unclear. At least some evidence exists for the possibility of a genetic link, as well as hyper-responsivity of the noradrenergic system (Widiger & Bornstein, 2001). In addition, cognitive problems, as well as problem relationships with family members, have been implicated as fostering the insecurity that is notable in these individuals. Incidence is estimated at about 2% of the general population (APA, 2000). It is diagnosed much more frequently in women, and there is some speculation that HPD and antisocial personality dis-order are gender-differentiated manifestations of a similar psychopathology (Cale & Lilienfeld, 2002). Alternatively, it may be that HPD and narcissistic personality disorder are the female and male counterparts in this cluster (Widiger & Bornstein, 2001).

Implications for Function and Treatment

Skills, including motor and process abilities, do not appear impaired in HPD. This disor-der impairs function at the performance level, specifically in social situations. Friendships are superficial and focus on the individual. People with HPD are unable to respond with gen-uine emotion to the needs of others. They romanticize relationships and respond with exces-sive disappointment to disagreements. One such young woman arrived at work to announce loudly and tearfully that she would have to "end it all" because her boyfriend had to cancel a date because he had the flu.

Such individuals are unpleasant to be around, but they are typically able to function at work. They may, however, have problems with coworkers or supervisors and are prone to quit unpredictably in fits of pique or when they become bored. ADLs are usually not impaired; in fact, such individuals may spend a great deal of time on hygiene and grooming in order to be attractive to others. They often dress quite seductively, then act puzzled when others respond to the apparent seduction.

Some of these individuals are able to learn new behaviors, often through behavior modification, and to develop insight into their behavior through psychotherapy (Gunderson, 1999). Making the changes tends to be quite difficult, however. Most often, when they seek treatment, these individuals want a "quick fix" for an immediate crisis rather than any major change in their attitudes or behaviors. One woman came into therapy because her father had "disowned" her and she was "now an orphan." It turned out he had stopped her allowance when she got her first job at age 25. Her wish for therapy was that the therapist call her father and tell him to resume the allowance.

NARCISSISTIC PERSONALITY DISORDER

Grandiosity is the defining feature of this disorder (APA, 2000). This is accompanied by a lack of empathy for others and excessive need for attention. Individuals with narcissistic personality disorder (NPD) identify themselves as special, exaggerate accomplishments, and feel entitled to recognition and special attention. However, these feelings fluctuate with feelings of insecurity and unworthiness. Self-esteem is poor but masked by expressions of superiority. There is focus on fantasies of power and success, accompanied by feelings of envy for those who have accomplished more (Widiger & Bornstein, 2001).

Etiology and Incidence

NPD is not well-researched, given that it was added to the diagnostic list only in DSM-III (Gunderson, Ronningstam, & Smith, 1991). Like HPD, NPD may be a learned pattern of adaptation, the result of disordered family life (Widiger & Bornstein, 2001). These individuals may get conflicting messages from parents, feel undervalued, and as a result, come to undervalue themselves. At the same time, their grandiosity is an attempt to win approval that may not have been forthcoming in their homes. There is also speculation that NPD is uniquely related to U.S. culture in which material possessions are so highly valued (Widiger & Bornstein, 2001). There is no compelling evidence of a genetic or familial pattern to NPD. NPD, diagnosed primarily in men, is thought to be relatively rare, occurring in less than 1% of the general population (APA, 2000).

Implications for Function and Treatment

This disorder does not appear to cause dysfunction at the skill level. Process skills and motor function are intact. Primary dysfunction is noted in interpersonal relationships. These individuals are self-centered and unable to display empathy for others, making friendships difficult. They charm others briefly until their disregard for others' feelings becomes obvious. Thus, relationships tend to be brief and often contentious. This pattern of relationships is also problematic in work situations where relationships with supervisors may be difficult. In some situations, vocational performance may be unusually good as the individual strives for great success, while in others, performance is poor as the individual becomes resentful of expectations of others. Good performance rarely lasts. One man had a long work history of jobs, each of which lasted no more than 6 months. As each new job began, he had "great new plans to save the company." As each ended, he excoriated his coworkers for failing to recognize his "genius." ADLs are usually unimpaired, although money management may become an issue. In an attempt to impress others, these individuals may spend to excess. Patterns can also be problematic, as the individual's social interactions are extremely unstable, reducing the ability to arrange consistent work and social habits.

When these individuals present for treatment, it is usually for depression as a result of their social isolation (Millon, 1995). It is rare that they are able to develop insight or to change behaviors, as they tend to blame others for their problems and to be impatient with the therapeutic process. In most instances, the depression rather than the personality disorder is the focus of treatment.

AVOIDANT PERSONALITY DISORDER

Social discomfort and avoidance of interpersonal relationships is the primary characteristic of this disorder (APA, 2000). Individuals with avoidant personality disorder fear that others will disapprove of them. As a result, they avoid interaction.

Etiology and Incidence

This is probably a learned pattern of behavior. It appears to result from poor early experiences with relationships. Incidence is estimated at 0.5% to 1% of the general population (APA, 2000).

Implications for Function and Treatment

Most function is intact in these individuals at the level of performance but affected by the inability to form relationships. These individuals work and care for themselves but have emotionally and socially restricted lives. Skills are unimpaired, with exception of social skills. Even in this sphere, superficial relationships may be adequate. One client was a university professor who managed brief casual interactions with students, as well as the more formalized classroom relationships. His personal life, however, was barren of friends or close family ties; four marriages had ended in divorce because of his inability to sustain close relationships.

As with NPD, these individuals often seek treatment as a result of depression (Gunderson, 1999). Treatment may focus on insight, behavior change, or a combination of the two. Unlike individuals with NPD, these individuals may be able to make a commitment to treatment and to benefit from it.

DEPENDENT PERSONALITY DISORDER

Individuals with avoidant personality disorder avoid relationships; individuals with dependent personality disorder feel they cannot survive without them. They are dependent and submissive in an attempt to win approval and to avoid abandonment (APA, 2000).

They have difficulty making decisions and look to others to tell them what to do. As a result, they are unable to successfully initiate activity. They fear being alone.

Etiology and Incidence

As with other disorders in this cluster, this is probably a learned behavioral pattern (Hirschfeld, Shea, & Weise, 1991). It is a commonly reported personality disorder in clinical settings (APA, 2000). However, this may be an artifact, given that these individuals may be more likely to seek treatment than others with personality disorders.

There is some concern about diagnosis of dependent personality disorder in individuals from other cultures. In Japanese and Indian cultures, for example, dependent characteristics may be considered more socially-appropriate (Widiger & Bornstein, 2001). This fact suggests that the disorder is a result of social learning or specific parenting messages.

Implications for Function and Treatment

Performance is intact in these individuals, although they are limited by their need for approval and advice from others. In social situations, friends are granted excessive control; in work situations, they are unable to progress because of their inability to take initiative and function independently. One woman refused to buy new clothes without approval from her husband and her mother. Work performance can be compromised by the inability to make decisions independently or by the excessive need for approval.

Individuals with dependent personality disorder often come into treatment as a result of depression or anxiety resulting from fear of abandonment. In some instances, the abandonment is real, as their dependency needs can be quite draining to others. This is a difficult disorder to treat, although psychotherapy and behavior modification can be of value in some instances.

OBSESSIVE-COMPULSIVE PERSONALITY DISORDER

This is potentially the most disabling of the cluster C personality disorders, as these individuals are perfectionistic and rigid and engage in ritualistic behavior. Defining descriptors are "perfectionistic," "methodical," and "serious" (Shopshire & Craik, 1996). These individuals never feel they have done well enough, and they focus on minor detail, wasting time that could be better spent. Decision-making is difficult, since these individuals are unable to evaluate choices and act. They are judgmental and moralistic, often quite stingy, and have difficulty expressing warmth. It has been theorized that these individuals have an extreme need for acceptance, causing conflicts about autonomy (Gunderson, 1999).

Etiology and Incidence

Etiology is not well established. It is possible that the same CNS dysfunction that seems to contribute to OCD may also contribute to obsessive-compulsive personality disorder, making it simply a less severe manifestation of the same problem. It is also possible that this is a learned problem or evidence of developmental delay, as many young children demonstrate obsessive compulsive behavior (e.g., "step on a crack, break your mother's back" leads to careful avoidance of cracks in the sidewalk in many 8 year olds). Most children outgrow these compulsions rather quickly, but there is speculation that perhaps these individuals do not for some reason. Prevalence is estimated at 1% in the adult population (APA, 2000).

Implications for Function and Treatment

Primary impairments resulting from this disorder are social and vocational. The rigidity and moralistic nature of these individuals makes it difficult for them to form warm relationships. Their perfectionism, difficulty making decisions, and inability to use time well make work performance less than optimal. Task completion, in particular, is problematic. One individual, a bookkeeper, was unable to complete any page that had an erasure and, as a result, was frequently unable to complete assigned tasks.

Treatment of obsessive-compulsive personality disorder is difficult. Intervention most often focuses on depression. These individuals tend to be aware of their behavior and the problems it causes, leading to considerable depression or anxiety.

IMPLICATIONS FOR OCCUPATIONAL THERAPY

Although the manifestations of various personality disorders differ, the underlying issues are similar:

- Inaccurate perceptions of self and others
- Inadequate social skills
- Poorly developed personal values and goals
- Poor self-esteem (Ward, 1999).

For some, particularly the cluster A disorders, inaccurate perceptions extend to many situations. This cluster may also be characterized by subtle neurological deficits in addition to the faulty learning that has been implicated as an etiological factor for all the personality disorders.

Because of the commonality of issues, some approaches to occupational therapy intervention may be suitable for all the personality disorders. Opportunities for group interaction with clear, consistent feedback may be quite valuable. A variety of group/cooperative activities may be helpful, from planning a social event to social skills training. A particular goal is interpreting accurately what others say and developing empathy; consistent, clear, and nonjudgmental feedback from the therapist and from other group members may assist in accomplishing this goal. It is fairly characteristic that individuals with personality disorders show little regard for or understanding of the feelings of others, and they must learn to make an active effort to do so. One histrionic client, a young female college student, was quite astonished to learn that other females resented her tendency to flirt with their boyfriends. It had never occurred to her to consider their feelings, even though she felt unhappy about her lack of girlfriends.

Realistic appraisal of self is similarly problematic. Provision of a range of activities may be useful as a mechanism for exploration and for learning strengths and weaknesses. Both successes and failures must be analyzed. This not only enhances self-awareness, but also is a way to explore values and goals. Activities that build self-esteem through experiences of success and the appreciation of others may help convince these individuals of their worth. The insecurity tends to be so deep, however, that it is quite problematic to provide them with all the reassurance they need.

The three clusters present with somewhat differing characteristics that must also be addressed. Cluster A personality disorders may respond to sensory integrative/sensory-motor interventions because of the suspected neurological component. Cluster B may benefit from behavioral approaches because of the probability that they reflect deficits in early learning. For example, a work experience might be structured in the clinic, with reinforcement for desired behaviors. Individuals with cluster C personality disorders may be particularly amenable to social skills training since this is the predominant deficit for these individuals. Behavior modification may be helpful in reducing anxiety for these individuals.

All the personality disorders are somewhat intractable. While change is possible, it requires considerable motivation, something often lacking in these individuals. Even those who are motivated may find change frightening and will certainly find ingrained habits hard to alter. Table 9-2 summarizes the main symptoms of each personality disorder and the most common functional deficits that occur.

REFERENCES

American Psychiatric Association. (1987). *Diagnostic and statistical manual* (3rd ed.). Washington, DC: Author.

American Psychiatric Association. (1994). *Diagnostic and statistical manual of mental disorders* (4th ed.). Washington, DC: Author.

American Psychiatric Association. (2000). *Diagnostic and statistical manual of mental disorders* (4th ed., text revision). Washington, DC: Author.

Cale, E.M., & Lilienfeld, S.O. (2002). Histrionic personality disorder and antisocial personality disorder: Sex-differentiated manifestations of psychopathy? *Journal of Personality Disorders, 16*, 52-72.

Crawford, T.N., Cohen, P., & Brook, J.S. (2001a). Dramatic-erratic personality disorder symptoms: I. Continuity from early adolescence into adulthood. *Journal of Personality Disorders, 15*, 319-335.

Crawford, T.N., Cohen, P., & Brook, J.S. (2001b). Dramatic-erratic personality disorder symptoms: II. Developmental pathways from early adolescence into adulthood. *Journal of Personality Disorders, 15*, 336-350.

Divac-Jovanovic, M., & Lecic-Tosevski, D. (1994). Personality disorders revisited. *Psihijatrija Danas, 26*(1), 37-48.

Fiester, S.J. (1991). Self-defeating personality disorder: A review of data and recommendations for DSM-IV. *Journal of Personality Disorders, 5*, 194-209.

Fiester, S.J., & Gay, M. (1991). Sadistic personality disorder: A review of data and recommendations for DSM-IV. *Journal of Personality Disorders, 5*, 376-385.

Gunderson, J.C. (1988). Personality disorders. In A.M. Nicholi (Ed.), *The new Harvard guide to psychiatry* (pp. 337-357). Cambridge, MA: Belknap Press.

Gunderson, J.C. (1999). Personality disorders. In A.M. Nicholi (Ed.), *The Harvard guide to psychiatry* (3rd ed., pp. 308-327). Cambridge, MA: Harvard University Press.

Gunderson, J.G., Ronningstam, E., & Smith, L.E. (1991). Narcissistic personality disorder: A review of data on DSM-III-R descriptions. *Journal of Personality Disorders, 5*, 167-177.

Gunderson, J.G., Zanarini, M.C., & Kisiel, C.L. (1991). Borderline personality disorder: A review of data on DSM-III-R descriptions. *Journal of Personality Disorders, 5*, 340-352.

Hirschfeld, R.M.A., Shea, M.T., & Weise, R. (1991). Dependent personality disorder: Perspectives for DSM-IV. *Journal of Personality Disorders, 5*, 135-149.

Kalus, O., Bernstein, D.P., & Siever, L.J. (1993). Schizoid personality disorder: A review of current status and implications for DSM-IV. *Journal of Personality Disorders, 7*, 43-52.

Livesley, W.J., Jang, K.L., Jackson, D.N., & Vernon, P.A. (1993). Genetic and environmental contributions to dimensions of personality disorder. *American Journal of Psychiatry, 150*, 1826-1831.

Table 9-2

Personality Disorders

Disorder	Symptoms	Functional Deficits
Cluster A		
Paranoid personality disorder	1. Tendency to suspect others and to interpret their actions as hostile	Work, leisure, social, and all patterns Process and communication skills
Schizoid	1. Lack of interest in social relationships 2. Restricted emotional range	Work, leisure, social, and all patterns Process and possibly communication skills
Schizotypal	1. Poor relationships 2. Restricted emotional range 3. Odd perceptual experiences 4. Odd appearance and speech 5. Inappropriate affect	Work, leisure, social, and ADL/IADL patterns Process skills
Cluster B		
Antisocial	1. At least 18 years old 2. Previous conduct disorder 3. At least four types of antisocial behavior (e.g., theft, lying, child abuse, etc.) that occur in a persistent pattern 4. Lacks remorse/guilt 5. Inability to sustain relationships	Work, leisure, social, and IADLs (especially financial) Process and motor are not affected Habits/roles emphasize illegal behaviors
Borderline	1. Relationships fluctuate between intense involvement and devaluation 2. Impulsiveness and instability 3. Lack of control of anger 4. Suicide gestures or self-mutilation	Work, leisure, social, and ADLs/IADLs Process/communication skills impaired, as are roles, habits, and routines
Histrionic	1. Excessive concern with appearance; seductive 2. Excessive need for praise and reassurance 3. Self-centered; lack of empathy for others 4. Exaggerated expression of emotion, with rapid mood shifts and shallow emotion 5. Need for constant attention	Work, leisure, social, and communication skills impaired Patterns may or may not be affected

(continued)

Table 9-2 (Continued)

Disorder	Symptoms	Functional Deficits
Cluster C Avoidant	1. Discomfort with social relationships 2. Avoidance of social relationships and activities	Social, possibly work and leisure skills not impaired, although communication may be poor Patterns not severely affected in most cases
Dependent	1. Excessively dependent and submissive behavior 2. Fear of abandonment 3. Easily hurt by criticism	Social, possibly work and leisure, process, and communication skills impaired
Obsessive-compulsive	1. Perfectionistic 2. Indecisiveness 3. Preoccupation with detail 4. Lack of generosity, empathy 5. Excessively moralistic, conscientious	Work, leisure, and social skills Excessively patterned, rigid Skills not severely affected
Narcissistic	1. Sense of self-importance 2. Preoccupied by fantasies of success 3. Belief he or she is special, arrogance 4. Sense of entitlement, exploits others, requires admiration 5. Lacks empathy	Social, work, and sometimes leisure roles impaired by grandiosity

Millon, T. (1995). *Disorders of personality: DSM-IV and beyond.* New York: Wiley.

Paris, J., Brown, R., & Nowlis, D. (1987). Long-term follow-up of borderline patients in a general hospital. *Comprehensive Psychiatry, 28,* 530-535.

Phillips, K.A., Hirschfeld, M.A., Shea, M.T., & Gunderson, J.G. (1993). Depressive personality disorder: Perspectives of DSM-IV. *Journal of Personality Disorders, 7,* 30-42.

Reiss, D., Hetherington, E.M., Plomin, R., Howe, G.W., Simmens, S.J., O'Connor, T.J., et al. (1995). Genetic questions for environmental studies: Differential parenting and psychopathology in adolescence. *Archives of General Psychiatry, 52,* 925-936.

Shedler, J., & Weston, D. (1998). Refining the measurement of Axis II: A Q-sord procedure for assessing personality pathology. *Assessment, 5,* 333-353.

Shopshire, M.S., & Craik, K.H. (1996). An act-based conceptual analysis of the obsessive-compulsive, paranoid, and histrionic personality disorders. *Journal of Personality Disorders, 10,* 203-218.

Siever, L.J., Bernstein, D.P., & Silverman, J.M. (1991). Schizotypal personality disorder: a review of its current status. *Journal of Personality Disorders, 5,* 178-193.

Tsuang, M.T., Stone, W.S., & Faraone, S.V. (2000). Toward reformulating the diagnosis of schizophrenia. *American Journal of Psychiatry, 157,* 1041-1050.

Turner, R.M. (1994). Borderline, narcissistic, and histrionic personality disorders. In R.T. Ammerman & M. Herson (Eds.), *Handbook of prescriptive treatments for adults* (pp. 393-420). New York: Plenum Press.

Ward, J.D. (1999). Psychosocial dysfunction in adults. In M.E. Neistadt & E.B. Crepeau (Eds.), *Willard and Spackman's occupational therapy* (9th ed., pp. 716-740). Philadelphia: Lippincott, Williams & Wilkins.

Widiger, T.A. (1992). Antisocial personality disorder. *Hospital and Community Psychiatry, 43*, 6-8.

Widiger, T.A., & Borstein, R.F. (2001). Histrionics, dependent, and narcissistic personality disorders. In H.E. Adams & P.B. Sutker (Eds.), *Comprehensive handbook of psychopathology* (pp. 509-531). New York: Kluwer Academic Publishers.

Zlotnick, C., Rothschild, L., & Zimmerman, M. (2002). The role of gender in the clinical presentation of patients with borderline personality disorder. *Journal of Personality Disorders, 16*, 277-282.

Chapter 10

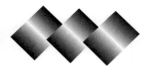 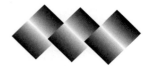

Other Disorders

A large number of disorders have not been discussed in previous chapters either because they are uncommon or because they are seen infrequently by occupational therapists. However, it is useful to be familiar with their fundamental characteristics, as they do appear not only in mental health facilities but also in other health care settings.

All categories of diagnosis previously discussed include a "not otherwise specified" (NOS) label. This may be considered a residual category used in situations in which the individual fits most but not all of the criteria or when presentation is in some way atypical. There are also labels for deferred diagnoses or for those situations in which there is an Axis I but not Axis II disorder, or Axis II without Axis I. For example, an individual may present with clear symptoms of schizophrenia but not fit precisely in one of the subgroups. In this case, NOS would be applied. If someone is diagnosed as having dysthymia, the therapist might defer Axis II diagnosis rather than say none if he or she is uncertain whether or not a personality disorder coexists.

In addition, many of the categories have subheadings that allow for greater specificity where it is possible to make more concrete identification of the symptom constellation. For example, panic disorder may be with agoraphobia or without agoraphobia, major depression may be identified as single episode or recurrent, and so on. Causes of the disorder may be reflected in the diagnostic label, as in the case of dementia due to head trauma. These subheadings, which can be seen in Appendix A, provide clarifying information to assist with treatment decisions.

There are also several groups of disorders that are useful to recognize as they do occur in settings in which occupational therapists work, although relatively infrequently. Because the disorders described in this chapter are not common in occupational therapy practice, description of each will be brief. As with all occupational therapy interventions, when individuals with these disorders are referred to occupational therapy, treatment must be based on a theoretical framework that can guide assessment and intervention, keeping in mind that the goal of occupational therapy is improved ability to accomplish needed and desired activities.

It is also helpful to remember that the incidence of various diagnoses changes over time. As has been discussed in previous chapters, some disorders are being diagnosed with increasing frequency (e.g., autism and ADHD). The eating disorders described in this chapter are examples of disorders that have increased dramatically, either because of real change in frequency or because therapists and others are more aware of their existence. Therapists may encounter individuals with eating disorders not only in mental health practice but also in physical dysfunction settings because of the profound physical consequences of disrupted diet. Thus, while most of the disorders included in this chapter are less common than oth-

---

Table 10-1
Disorders Discussed in This Chapter

- Feeding and eating disorders of infancy and childhood
- Tic disorders
- Elimination disorders
- Other disorders of infancy, childhood, and adolescence
- Mental disorders due to a general medical condition not elsewhere classified
- Somatoform disorders
- Factitious disorders
- Dissociative disorders
- Sexual and gender identity disorders
- Eating disorders (anorexia nervosa and bulimia nervosa)
- Sleep disorders
- Impulse control disorders not elsewhere classified
- Adjustment disorders
- V codes: other conditions that may be a focus of clinical attention

---

ers, individual therapists may actually encounter some of them relatively often. The disorders found in this chapter are summarized in Table 10-1.

FEEDING AND EATING DISORDERS OF INFANCY OR EARLY CHILDHOOD

Occupational therapists frequently treat infants with feeding problems (Case-Smith & Humphry, 2001), although not all feeding problems carry a psychiatric diagnosis. Therapists are well-aware that psychological problems often coexist with feeding problems, however, sometimes as precursors of the problem, sometimes as a consequence. DSM-IV-TR (APA, 2000) reflects the psychological content of feeding disorders and includes pica (i.e., persistent eating of nonnutritive substances), rumination (i.e., long-term chewing of food that is regurgitated by the child), and a more general "feeding disorder" category. The last of these is used in situations of failure to thrive when no medical cause can be identified.

TIC DISORDERS

These include Tourette's syndrome, chronic motor or vocal tic disorder, and transient tic disorder. Tics are involuntary, sudden, stereotyped motor or vocal movements. They may be simple, as an involuntary eye-blinking or neck jerking movement, grunting, or snorting. Complex tics include stereotyped facial gestures, hitting self, touching, or echolalia (Marcus & Kurlan, 2001).

Tourette's syndrome is characterized by numerous motor and vocal tics that occur at varying frequencies and which change over time. Frequently, the head is involved in concert with other parts of the body and almost always accompanied by vocal tics, such as barking, grunting, and coprolalia (i.e., uttering obscenities). This disorder usually appears in childhood (Chouinard & Ford, 2000) and is apparently the result of CNS dysfunction, possibly genetic (Marcus & Kurlan, 2001). It has been associated with learning disorders (Casat, Pearson, & Casat, 2001) and with OCD (Cohen, Riddle, & Leckman, 1992). This finding raises the possibility that all three disorders are the result of similar CNS dysfunction.

Tourette's syndrome is a chronic condition with periods of exacerbation and remission. Severity of the disorder varies. As can be imagined, function in all performance spheres is impaired to a great extent in the most severe cases. However, medication (neuroleptics) in combination with education, psychological counseling, and other support can be valuable (Cohen et al., 1992). One specific caution is that Tourette's syndrome is frequently comorbid with ADHD. In these cases, use of stimulants—a common treatment for ADHD—should be avoided, since this treatment tends to intensify Tourette's syndrome (Casat et al., 2001). Chronic motor or vocal tic disorder is much more limited, usually to a single motor or vocal tic (Chouinard & Ford, 2000). Severity of symptoms and of occupational impairment is much less than with Tourette's syndrome.

Transient tic disorder is most often a single tic, such as eye-blinking or another facial tic. This diagnosis applies to tics that appear during childhood or adolescence, but disappear within 1 year. Tics may be precursors to Tourette's syndrome or disappear completely, or they may be intermittent throughout life. Tics are common among children, and many seem to resolve themselves in time. However, in some instances, tics may emerge in adulthood (Chouinard & Ford, 2000). These tics seem to be part of a continuum of tic disorder and do not differ substantially from those emerging in childhood.

ELIMINATION DISORDERS

This category includes encopresis (i.e., the inability to control feces) and enuresis (i.e., the inability to control urine). The lack of control may be voluntary or involuntary. For the diagnosis to be made, the child must be at least 4 years old (encopresis) or 5 years old (enuresis) years old, with correlating mental age. Thus, it will not be diagnosed in retarded individuals who lack either motor control or intelligence to be readily trained. For both disorders, the problem may be transient (e.g., caused by the stress of a new sibling or hospitalization) or may become chronic. In making this diagnosis, it is vital to rule out possible physical problems, such as urinary tract infections. Behavioral programs can be helpful in remediating these problems.

OTHER DISORDERS OF INFANCY, CHILDHOOD, AND ADOLESCENCE

This category includes five disorders. They are separation anxiety disorder; selective mutism; reactive attachment disorder of infancy or early childhood; stereotypic movement disorder; and disorder of infancy, childhood, or adolescence NOS.

Separation anxiety, a form of anxiety disorder, is discussed in Chapters 3 and 8. Selective mutism is a refusal to talk in one or more specific social situations after it is clear that the child can speak. While it is rare, it can be quite disabling in children in whom it occurs.

Disturbance of social relatedness in early childhood is characteristic of reactive attach-ment disorder. It is believed to be the result of severely inadequate care during infancy and early childhood (Lyons-Ruth, Repacholi, McLeod, & Silva, 1992). Symptoms include fail-ure to initiate or respond in social interaction, diffuse attachments to adults, and pathogen-ic care by caregivers, such as disregard for emotional and physical needs. Failure to thrive may be related to this disorder.

Stereotypic movement disorder is demonstrated by repetitive nonfunctional behaviors, such as head banging. The activities are usually intentional and may cause injury to the child, or interfere with activities.

Mental Disorders Due to a General Medical Condition Not Elsewhere Classified

When a mental disorder is known to be caused by a medical condition, this diagnosis would be used. For example, catatonia and personality change that result from a medical condition would be categorized here. This diagnosis is not used frequently, although it is not uncommon to find medical conditions associated with short- or long-term psychiatric symp-toms. For example, individuals with multiple sclerosis (MS) often experience personality changes associated with changes in their nervous system functioning. They might show signs of personality disorder, depression, or psychosis. In someone with MS and psychotic symp-toms, a diagnosis of schizophrenia would be unlikely; the more likely label would be "men-tal disorder due to a general medical condition not elsewhere classified."

For occupational therapists, the most important factor with regard to this diagnostic cat-egory is the recognition that medical conditions can be associated with psychological symp-toms. When these symptoms interfere with performance, the therapist can assist in modify-ing activity demands or the environment to enable the individual to regain lost or dimin-ished abilities.

Somatoform Disorders

These include body dysmorphic disorder, conversion disorder, hypochondriasis, somatiza-tion disorder, and somatoform pain disorder. These disorders are important to understand, as they frequently present in general medical and rehabilitation settings.

Body dysmorphic disorder reflects an obsessive dissatisfaction with a portion of the body (Hollander, Neville, Frenkel, Josephson, & Liebowitz, 1992). The individual may, for exam-ple, believe that his or her nose is ugly or face too wrinkled. There may, in fact, be some minor anomaly with regard to the feature in question, but this disorder appears in normal-looking individuals. The result is often frequent visits to plastic surgeons, with dissatisfac-tion with surgical outcomes. Extreme functional impairment is rare but may occur when the individual becomes so fixated on the "disfigurement" that other activities are excluded.

Conversion disorder is characterized by a loss of body function or physical impairment that suggests a physical disorder in the absence of physical findings. Psychogenic nonepilep-tic seizures, found in approximately 5% to 33% of patients presenting with seizure disorders, may be a form of conversion reaction (Cragar, Berry, Fakhoury, Cibula, & Schmitt, 2002).

The individual does not intentionally produce the physical symptom, but the symptom will lack some features of the true physical condition (Dhossche, van der Steen, & Ferdinand, 2002). Conversion reactions appear suddenly and often as a result of identifiable psychosocial stressors. They tend to occur in individuals with histrionic personality disorder. In some instances, there is also a lack of concern about the condition (i.e., "la belle indifference") (Nemiah, 1988). This attitude is quite striking, as the individual is apparently unworried by a sudden paralysis, loss of hearing, and so on. Sudden, rapid recovery may occur. It is important to note that the condition is not intentional (i.e., the individual is not consciously and willfully producing a set of symptoms) (Dhossche et al., 2002). When occupational therapists see such individuals, it is typically in the context of a physical dysfunction referral. The obvious problem for occupational therapy intervention is that the individual does not conform to the usual pattern for the diagnosed difficulty, and because the origin is psychogenic, does not respond to the usual interventions.

Obsessive worry about physical condition is the defining feature of hypochondriasis (Hiller, Rief, & Fichter, 2002). The fears are unwarranted by any physical finding, although in the absence of physical findings, the individual is likely to assume the physician has not done enough. The individual makes frequent visits to the physician and changes doctors often as he or she assumes that care is inadequate or improper. This is usually a chronic condition, and it impairs performance in all spheres to some extent. Those around the individual become annoyed by the obsession with physical worries, and the individual misses work because of physical concerns. In severe cases, the individual may decide to become an invalid and refuse to function for fear of "further harm" to physical condition. The condition is significantly worse than the normal subjective complaints found in as many as 75% of nonpsychiatrically involved individuals (Eriksen & Ihlebaek, 2002). It is common to find that individuals with hypochondriasis have long histories of illness, including chronic childhood illness (Hotopf, 2002). Hypochondriasis is strongly associated with anxiety (Hiller et al., 2002), although antianxiety agents are of limited value. Likewise, reassurance that there is no physiological problem is of limited value. The presence of hypochondriasis complicates occupational therapy intervention in every setting, since individuals with the disorder are unlikely to perceive much benefit from intervention.

Somatization disorder is characterized by multiple physical complaints over a period of years with no accompanying physical disorder (Bucholz, Dinwiddie, Reich, Shayka, & Cloniger, 1993). The individual seeks care for the specific disorder, presenting complaints in a vague or dramatic way. There is usually a pattern of intensive investigation of these complaints, with no positive findings. The disorder is entirely unconscious; the individual does not intentionally produce symptoms (Hutchinson, 2001). As with hypochondriasis, physician switching is common. Unlike hypochondriasis, where there is simply generalized fear that "something" may be wrong or go wrong, these individuals have specific, though unwarranted, physical complaints.

Somatoform pain disorder is the preoccupation with pain when there is no physical reason for such pain. It often occurs in individuals with a history of conversion reactions, and, like other disorders in this group, occurs in the absence of any positive physical findings. In some cases, it may develop following a physical trauma but continue once the physical problem is resolved.

FACTITIOUS DISORDERS

These are physical or psychological disorders that are intentionally produced and under the voluntary control of the individual. This is in direct contrast to the somatoform disorders, all of which are unconscious in origin (Hutchinson, 2001). The concept of voluntary control is somewhat problematic here, however. While the individual may actively induce a symptom (e.g., through ingestion of drugs), he or she is not able to control the impulse to do so. This group of diagnoses does not include malingering, in which the individual both produces the symptom voluntarily and wishes to do so at a conscious level.

The best known factitious disorder is Munchausen syndrome (Fliege, Scholler, Rose, Willenberg, & Klapp, 2002). This syndrome is characterized by numerous hospitalizations for a variety of symptoms, with accompanying physical signs, such as nausea and vomiting, rashes, bleeding, all of which have been induced by the individual. Symptoms are dramatic but vague, and the individual has extensive knowledge of hospital routines. This disorder is difficult to manage because the individual is likely to be both noncompliant and demanding. It appears that these individuals are socially isolated and derive most of their social satisfaction by being taken care of in an in-patient setting. When confronted with the real nature of their symptoms, they may leave against medical advice, often to seek readmission elsewhere.

Hutchinson (2001) notes that the somatoform and factitious disorders fit along several continua. One is the degree to which the symptoms emerge as a result of voluntary action on the part of the individual as opposed to involuntary emergence of symptoms. The second continuum relates to the degree to which the individual has conscious awareness of the source of the problem. Somatoform disorders are the result of unconscious motivation producing involuntary physical symptoms, while factitious disorders are the result of unconscious motivation but voluntary production of symptoms. Malingering, by contrast, is both under voluntary control and a conscious effort to appear ill.

An additional interesting condition is factitious disorder by proxy, in which one individual, typically a parent, induces physical illness in another, typically a child, to get attention from the health care system (McNicholas, Slonims, & Cass, 2000). There are reported instances of factitious disorder by proxy being reflected by complaints of educational problems for the child, including learning disorders and ADHD (Ayoub, Schreier, & Keller, 2002). Occupational therapists may be faced with the challenge of determining the reality of the educational concerns, perhaps based on the extent to which they conform to expected patterns of difficulty.

Long-term outcomes for all of these disorders are poor, particularly since many of these individuals have accompanying personality disorders. There is evidence that adults with factitious disorders were children of parents who had factitious disorder by proxy (Libow, 2002). This theory suggests that as the children grow, they learn to participate in the production of symptoms and, as adults, produce them independently.

Factitious disorder and factitious disorder by proxy are difficult to diagnose because of the accuracy with which individuals are able to produce symptoms and the frequency with which they switch providers (Fliege et al., 2002). However, estimates suggest that approximately 0.3% to 0.5% of medically ill individuals have one of these conditions.

DISSOCIATIVE DISORDERS

Dissociative identity disorder (DID) (formerly multiple personality disorder), dissociative fugue, dissociative amnesia, and depersonalization disorder are included in this group. Interest in this category of diagnoses has clearly escalated (Spiegel & Cardena, 1991). They are striking and have frequently been portrayed in movies and television programs as "mental illness" in a global sense. Individuals with DID typically have at least two personalities and may have many, some more fully developed than others (Ross, 1997). The personalities may not be aware of each other; one personality may not remember an anxiety-provoking event that is "managed" by another, or one may express anger that is frightening to the dominant persona. Personalities seem to reflect different facets of the individual that are split or dissociated from the primary personality.

Rate of occurrence is not well-established, although there are reports of an increase in prevalence (APA, 2000). There is a familial pattern.

A common thread in DID is a history of psychological trauma. Histories of childhood physical, emotional, and sexual abuse are extremely common (Ross, 1997; Saxe, Chawla, & Van der Kolk, 2002). Function depends on the extent and frequency with which dissociative reactions occur in the individual. There is a high prevalence of self-injurious or self-destructive behavior associated with the disorder (Saxe et al., 2002).

The goal of treatment is most often unification (i.e., reintegration of the separate personalities into one functional whole) (Ross, 1997). Hypnotherapy and cognitive therapy are among those reported effective. Group therapy seems helpful to some individuals. Expressive therapy and psychoeducation (Richert & Bergland, 1992) have sometimes been used with success. Occupational therapists who work with individuals with DID may want to emphasize sensorimotor activities that allow the person to experience a sense of control that might otherwise be absent (Waid, 1993).

SEXUAL AND GENDER IDENTITY DISORDERS

There are two main groups of sexual disorders: paraphilias and sexual dysfunctions. Paraphilias are characterized by sexual arousal in response to objects or situations that are not normally part of sexual activity, with accompanying problems relating in normal sexual activity. These include pedophilia, sexual sadism and masochism, transvestic fetishism, and others. Sexual dysfunctions represent problems in engaging in sexual relationships, including sexual aversion, inhibited orgasm, dyspareunia, premature ejaculation, and so on. Functional impairment is primarily in the area of sexual relationships but may extend to heterosexual relationships more generally if the sexual problem begins to generalize to feelings of low self-esteem or anxiety.

Gender identity disorders reflect conflict between assigned sex and gender identity. Specifically, they reflect extreme discomfort with assignment as male or female, and a conviction that the individual should be the other sex (Diamond, 2002). This may be manifested as a generalized sense of dissatisfaction with assigned sex or a more specific sense that one should be of the other gender.

In the most extreme form, this is reflected as transsexualism, in which the individual may simply choose to live as the other sex and possibly have hormonal and surgical treatment to allow reassignment (Dean et al., 2000). Transsexualism is quite rare and is not to be confused with tomboyishness in girls, "feminine" behavior in boys, or anxiety about living up to sex role expectations. It reflects a profound belief that the individual was born in the wrong body. This belief is most often present in childhood, where the child is distressed about his or her sex and insistent that he or she is really the opposite sex.

The cause of these disorders is unknown, with speculation ranging from prenatal hormonal exposure to genetic flaws to learned behaviors (Dean et al., 2000). Research is inconclusive about the roots of the problem, but it does seem to appear early in childhood in most cases. There is evidence of brain abnormality in many of these individuals (Griffiths, 2002). It is a rare phenomenon; a 1993 study in the Netherlands reported prevalence as 1 per 11,900 males and 1 per 30,400 per females (Bakker, van Kesteren, Gooren, & Bezemer, 1993).

Treatment of transsexualism includes two primary alternatives (Dean et al., 2000). One involves sex reassignment, including hormonal treatment and sometimes surgery, to make the body more consistent with gender assumed by the individual. This approach also requires extensive therapy to work through psychological difficulties associated with this kind of dramatic change and to provide training about appropriate gender behavior. However, when handled carefully, outcomes seem to be good, with no evidence of long-term psychopathology beyond that found in the general population (Haraldsen & Dahl, 2000; Smith, Cohen & Cohen-Kettenis, 2002). The other treatment is to help the individual feel more comfortable with existing sex assignment. This second alternative is facilitated through skill training, behavior therapy, and psychotherapy. Evidence about its effectiveness is equivocal, with some suggestion that individuals choosing against surgery are more ambivalent. This ambivalence may result in more problematic long-term consequences (Dean et al., 2000).

EATING DISORDERS

In DSM-III-R (APA, 1987), eating disorders were listed with the disorders of infancy, childhood, and adolescence. Their move to a separate section reflects the fact that while they may occur in children (Hodes, 1993), these disorders may occur at any time during the life span and are most likely to emerge in adolescents and young adults. It is possible for them to emerge in older adults as well (White & Litovitz, 1998), although older adults have better prognoses than those who develop the disorder early. Of the disorders described in this chapter, these are the most commonly occurring and the most likely to be seen by occupational therapists.

Anorexia Nervosa

Anorexia nervosa is characterized by a refusal to gain weight, fear of gaining weight, and belief that one is overweight in individuals who refuse to maintain minimally normal body weight (APA, 2000). In women, amenorrhea is also present.

Bulimia Nervosa

Bulimia is characterized by a binge/purge cycle in individuals who are more likely to be of normal weight or overweight. The purging is accomplished through induced vomiting or the use of laxatives, and the entire cycle is accompanied by a sense of loss of control of eating. Binging and purging occurs frequently, at least twice a week, and must persist over at least 3 months before the diagnosis is made. Individuals with bulimia are excessively concerned about weight.

Etiology and Incidence

To some extent, these disorders are cultural, as thinness is considered desirable in the United States (Andersen, 1999). Anorexia and bulimia are completely absent in cultures with significant food shortages. Vocation also correlates with eating disorders. Ballet dancers, for example, are very likely to suffer from bulimia or anorexia, as are gymnasts and wrestlers. The family has been implicated as the source of the disorder, as well. Some suggest that anorexia is likely to occur in families in which expectations are high for performance (Waller, 1992). Perfectionism and need for control are well-documented personality characteristics, particularly in the case of individuals with anorexia (Andersen, 1999). It has also been suggested that these disorders are related to sexual abuse (Connors & Morse, 1992). Approximately 30% of individuals with eating disorders report earlier sexual abuse. It has been suggested that lesbians have lower rates of anorexia and bulimia than other women, while for men, being gay is associated with an increased risk (Andersen, 1999).

A variety of physiological changes occur in individuals with anorexia and bulimia, leading some to suggest that the cause is biological (Gambill, 1998). It is difficult to know which is cause and which is effect though, since starvation diets can lead to hormonal upset, chemical imbalance, and other physical problems. Menstruation is affected in women with anorexia, and abnormal brain serotonergic metabolism has been found in individuals with both anorexia and bulimia.

Individuals with anorexia have disturbed body image, absence of concern about the problem, overactivity, and inability to recognize hunger. This may suggest perceptual abnormalities in these individuals. Individuals with bulimia nervosa are highly impulsive (Fahy & Eisler, 1993).

It now appears that approximately 5% of American women have anorexia nervosa (Patton, 1992), 1% bulimia nervosa, and another 3%, subclinical cases of one of these disorders. Approximately 90% to 95% of cases occur in women (Gambill, 1998).

Prognosis

It has been estimated that between 5% and 20% of individuals with anorexia ultimately die of the disorder (Gambill, 1998). The death rate goes up with duration of the disorder. Physical consequences include cyanosis; difficult tolerating cold temperatures; bradycardia; hypotension; dental enamel and skin changes; gastrointestinal problems; and heart, thyroid, and renal problems. Severe depression and anxiety are also common and are poor prognostic signs (Gambill, 1998). In some cases, only one period of anorexia or bulimia occurs, after which weight and eating return to normal (Cosford & Arnold, 1992). In others, however, the disorder may be chronic, persisting into late life. Overall, approximately half of individuals with anorexia have good outcomes, 24% have poor outcomes, and 28% have intermediate outcomes with exacerbations and remissions (Gambill, 1998). For individuals with bulimia, the prognosis is better, with as many as 60% having good outcomes. The morbidity estimate for bulimia is 5% at most (Gambill, 1998). However, in the case of both anorexia and bulimia, significant medical complications—including gastrointestinal, cardiac, and kidney dysfunction—can occur.

Implications for Function and Treatment

Individuals with anorexia often have good vocational function. Social functioning, however, tends to be poor, as these individuals are often isolated and asexual. ADLs and IADLs are generally not affected, except in the area of eating and cooking (Ward, 1999). The term *anorexia* is somewhat misleading, as these individuals are often obsessed with food and plan their lives around it.

An obsession with food is the key factor interfering with function in individuals with bulimia. They are so preoccupied with food and eating that their work may suffer, and social activities are often badly affected. One woman with bulimia was fired from her job at a grocery store when it was discovered that she was prolonging her breaks to binge and then purge food she had sneaked from the shelves. Functional problems are the result of the time taken with obsessing about food, as well as the fear that they will be rejected by anyone who learns of the obsession. As with individuals with anorexia, ADL and IADLs are not affected, except as they relate to food and its preparation.

Many forms of treatment have been employed for individuals with both anorexia and bulimia. In some cases, individuals with anorexia require hospitalization, often as the result of life-threatening weight loss, while those with bulimia are almost always treated in outpatient settings. Recommended treatments for both anorexia and bulimia include behavior therapy, individual and family psychotherapy, cognitive therapy, and cognitive-behavior therapy (Gambill, 1998). The use of antidepressant medications sometimes used with individuals with anorexia is somewhat problematic because weight loss can be a side effect (Gambill, 1998). On the other hand, antidepressants seem quite helpful for individuals with bulimia (Gambill, 1998). It appears that men benefit from somewhat different interventions, including both short-term intervention and treatment with testosterone to increase muscle mass and body weight (Andersen, 1999).

Implications for Occupational Therapy

Occupational therapists may contribute to behavioral programs for individuals with anorexia and bulimia (Rockwell, 1990). The occupational therapist may, for example, assist the client in developing acceptable leisure pursuits that de-emphasize food. In addition, the therapist may provide social skills training to remediate difficulties these individuals have in developing and maintaining satisfying relationships. Therapists also offer stress management techniques and opportunities for self-expression through the expressive arts.

Bridgett (1993) recommends that occupational therapists focus on body self-image, time management, and development of a greater sense of internal control through use of activity. In general, interventions that assist the individual in enhancing self-concept and experiencing a sense of control and self-esteem through positive engagement in occupation can be beneficial (Ward, 1999).

SLEEP DISORDERS

Sleep disorders are not diagnosed in situations in which the duration of the problem is brief. Many individuals have periods of sleep disturbance when stressed or ill, but for most people, these are brief and transient. In some cases, though, the problem persists, either in the form of dyssomnia (i.e., difficulty sleeping) or hypersomnia (i.e., excessive sleeping). The DSM-IV-TR (APA, 2000) listing does not include physical disorders such as narcolepsy, but only those that are thought to be psychogenic.

Included in this category are sleep-wake disturbances, in which the normal diurnal cycle of sleep is disturbed, and parasomnias, which are characterized by abnormal events during sleep (e.g., nightmares and sleepwalking). Again, the problem must be of several months duration for a diagnosis to be made, as occasional problems are not unusual. In some instances, the disorder can be tied to work patterns (Akerstedt et al., 2002). In others, disruptions in normal circadian rhythms seem to contribute (Hobson & Silvestri, 1999). Behavioral therapy can be effective in minimizing sleep disturbance in many situations (Hobson & Silvestri, 1999; Owens, Palermo, & Rosen, 2001). Physical activity during the day can help some individuals and is a consideration for occupational therapy intervention for individuals with sleep disorders.

IMPULSE CONTROL DISORDERS NOT ELSEWHERE CLASSIFIED

These include intermittent explosive disorder, kleptomania, pathological gambling, pyromania, and trichotillomania. In each, the individual is driven to engage in a behavior that is damaging to self or others that he or she is unable to control (Lesieur & Rosenthal, 1991). Origin of the disorders is not well-understood, but interference with function is common. Explosive disorder, kleptomania, and pyromania may ultimately result in imprisonment, while pathological gambling is damaging to social and work relationships. Trichotillomania (i.e., pulling out one's own hair) is the least damaging of these disorders, although it may indicate poor self-esteem that is reflected in other performance.

Pathological gambling is often compared to substance abuse and is, in fact, often comorbid with alcoholism (Lesieur & Rosenthal, 1991). Individuals who are pathological gamblers often suffer from vocational and social difficulties, particularly marital difficulties, as gambling takes increasing amounts of their time and financial resources. Treatment reflects a belief that it is an addictive behavior, as 12-step programs such as Gamblers Anonymous are often suggested (Murray, 1993). Two examples of impulse control disorder that seem to be increasing are compulsive shopping (Hartston & Koran, 2002) and compulsive Internet use (Treur, Fabian, & Furedi, 2001). Among the helpful interventions are short-term therapy and behavioral therapy (Pollard, 2001). Substitution of positive activities is important to long-term recovery.

ADJUSTMENT DISORDERS

These disorders may appear at any time in life, but usually occur within 3 months of a stressful event. By definition, function is impaired, as the individual has difficulty with social, vocational, school, or leisure activities. Stressors include such things as divorce, loss of a job, physical illness, or natural disaster. The severity of the disorder is not necessarily in proportion to the severity of the stressor, but rather a reflection of the individual's ability to cope. Anxiety, depression, and physical complaints may accompany the disorder. These symptoms are self-limiting, occurring within 3 months of the stressor, with a duration of no more than 6 months following the stressor.

In most instances, adjustment disorder can be resolved through supportive therapy and intervention to teach new coping skills. Outcomes tend to be worse for children (Newcorn & Strain, 1992).

V CODES: OTHER CONDITIONS THAT MAY BE A FOCUS OF CLINICAL ATTENTION

There are times when individuals enter treatment for specific problems that are not directly tied to psychiatric disorders. Academic problems, marital problems, uncomplicated bereavement, occupational (vocational) problems, and parent-child problems are among those on this list. While individuals seeking treatment for these problems may have accompanying disorders, the difficulty may not have resulted from the mental disorder. As an example, an individual who has had anxiety problems may still experience uncomplicated bereavement as a result of loss of a spouse.

IMPLICATIONS FOR OCCUPATIONAL THERAPY

For each of the disorders described in this chapter, occupational therapy may be warranted if the disorder impacts negatively on function, the disorder impacts negatively on self-esteem, or remediation requires learning a new set of performance skills. As an example, transsexual individuals may have performed quite adequately in both work and social spheres but have suffered severe difficulty in terms of self-esteem and self-concept. Should they opt for sex reassignment, a whole new set of skills will be needed. A male who decides on sex-reassignment as female will need to learn behaviors considered socially-appropriate for women, including modes of dress, walk, and talk. Many physicians and psychiatrists require the individual to live as the other gender for at least 1 year prior to surgery, during which time the occupational therapist may assist the individual in developing behaviors consistent with his or her new gender.

A more commonly encountered example would be individuals with hypochondriasis. Function is typically impaired, as the individual worries about health and takes to bed with every real or imagined ailment. Self-esteem is likely to be impaired, either as a precursor to the disorder or as a consequence of the inability to function and the inevitable annoyance of others. These individuals clearly need a new set of behaviors that can provide a source of satisfaction and improved self-esteem. In the absence of such learning, remediation of symptoms is difficult. This is because hypochondriasis is so often a plea for attention from individuals who have very low self-regard. For many of the disorders in this chapter, as with those described in previous sections of the book, occupational therapists must be concerned with assisting the individual to create a meaningful constellation of valued activities that can provide a sense of satisfaction and serve as a source of self-esteem.

Review of disorders in this chapter provides an opportunity to restate the occupational therapy view of dysfunction. This view cuts across lines drawn by medical diagnosis. Issues of self-esteem, self-concept, and performance appear almost regardless of diagnosis. While the degree of impairment and the specific nature of the impairment differ, these themes are consistent and primary to the occupational therapist. Occupational therapists should be alert to the fact that psychiatric diagnosis can provide only the most general information about performance deficits and should emphasize assessment and intervention focused on ensuring that every individual can accomplish needed and desired daily occupations, regardless of psychiatric diagnosis.

REFERENCES

Akerstedt, T., Knutsson, A., Westerholm. P., Theorell, T., Alfredsson, L., & Kecklund, G. (2002). Sleep distur-bances, work stress and work hours: A cross-sectional study. *Journal of Psychosomatic Research, 53*, 741-748.

American Psychiatric Association. (1987). *Diagnostic and statistical manual of mental disorders* (3rd ed.). Washington, DC: Author.

American Psychiatric Association. (2000). *Diagnostic and statistical manual of mental disorders* (4th ed., text revi-sion). Washington, DC: Author.

Andersen, A.E. (1999). Gender-related aspects of eating disorders: A guide to practice. *Journal of Gender Specific Medicine, 2*(1), 47-54.

Ayoub, C.C., Schreier, H.A., & Keller, C. (2002). Munchausen by proxy: Presentations in special education. *Child Maltreatment, 7*, 149-159.

Bakker, A., van Kesteren, P., Gooren, L., & Bezemer, P. (1993). The prevalence of transsexualism in the Netherlands. *Acta Psychiatrica Scandinavica, 87*, 237-238.

Bridgett, B. (1993). Occupational therapy evaluation for patients with eating disorders. *Occupational Therapy in Mental Health, 12*, 79-89.

Bucholz, K.K., Dinwiddie, S.H., Reich, T., Shayka, J.J, & Cloniger, C.R. (1993). Comparison of screening propos-als for somatization disorder empirical analyses. *Comprehensive Psychiatry, 34*, 49-64.

Casat, C.D., Pearson, D.A., & Casat, J.P. (2001). Attention-deficit/hyperactivity disorder. *Clinical Assessment of Child and Adolescent Behavior, 16*, 263-306.

Case-Smith, J., & Humphry, R. (2001). Feeding interventions. In J. Case-Smith (Ed.), *Occupational therapy for chil-dren* (4th ed., pp. 453-488). St. Louis, MO: Mosby.

Chouinard, S., & Ford, B. (2000). Adult onset tic disorders. *Journal of Neurology, Neurosurgery, and Psychiatry, 68*, 738-743.

Cohen, D.J., Riddle, M.A., & Leckman, J.F. (1992). Pharmacotherapy of Tourette's Syndrome and associated dis-orders. *Pediatric Psychopharmacology, 15*, 109-129.

Connors, M.E., & Morse, W. (1992). Sexual abuse and eating disorders: A review. *International Journal of Eating Disorders, 13*, 1-11.

Cosford, P., & Arnold, E. (1992). Eating disorders in later life: A review. *International Journal of Geriatric Psychiatry, 7*, 491-498.

Cragar, D.E., Berry, D.T.R., Fakhoury, T.A., Cibula, J.E., & Schmitt, F.A. (2002). A review of diagnostic techniques in the differential diagnosis of epileptic and nonepileptic seizures. *Neuropsychology Review, 12*, 31-64.

Dean, L., Meyer, I.H., Robinson, K., Sell, R.L., Sember, R., Silenzio, V.M.B., et al. (2000). Lesbian, gay, bisexual, and transgender health: Findings and concerns. *Journal of the Gay and Lesbian Medical Association, 4*(3), 102-151.

Dhossche, D., van der Steen, F., & Ferdinand, R. (2002). Somatoform disorders in children and adolescents: A comparison with other internalizing disorders. *Annals of Clinical Psychiatry, 14*, 23-31.

Diamond, M. (2002). Sex and gender are different: Sexual identity and gender identity are different. *Clinical Child Psychology and Psychiatry, 7*, 320-334.

Eriksen, H.E., & Ihlebaek, C. (2002). Subjective health complaints. *Scandinavian Journal of Psychology, 43*, 101-103.

Fahy, T., & Eisler, I. (1993). Impulsivity and eating disorders. *British Journal of Psychiatry, 162*, 193-197.

Fliege, H., Scholler, G., Rose, M., Willenberg, H., & Klapp, B.F. (2002). Factitious disorders and pathological self-harm in a hospital population: An interdisciplinary challenge. *General Hospital Psychiatry, 24*, 164-171.

Gambill, C.L. (1998). Anorexia and bulimia in girls and young women. *Physician Assistant, 18*, 20, 25-27, 31-32, 37-38, 41-42, 44, 47, 51-52, 54.

Griffiths, M. (2002). Invisibility: The major obstacle in understanding and diagnosing transsexualism. *Clinical Child Psychology, 7*, 493-496.

Haraldsen, I.R., & Dahl, A.A. (2000). Symptom profiles of gender dysphoric patients of transsexual type compared to patients with personality disorders and healthy adults. *Acta Psychiatrica Scandinavica, 102*, 276-281.

Hartston, H.J., & Koran, L.M. (2002). Impulsive behavior in a consumer culture. *International Journal of Psychiatry in Clinical Practice, 6*(2), 66-69.

Hiller, W., Rief, W., & Fichter, M.M. (2002). Dimensional and categorical approaches to hypochondriasis. *Psychological Medicine, 32*, 707-718.

Hobson, J.A., & Silvestri, R. (1999). Sleep and its disorders. In A.M. Nicholi (Ed.), *The Harvard guide to psychiatry* (3rd ed., pp. 155-167). Cambridge, MA: Harvard University Press.

Hodes, M. (1993). Anorexia nervosa and bulimia nervosa in children. *International Review of Psychiatry, 5*, 101-108.

Hollander, E., Neville, D., Frenkel, M., Josephson, S., & Liebowitz, M.R. (1992). Body dysmorphic disorder: Diagnostic issues and related disorders. *Psychosomatics, 33*(2), 156-165.

Hotopf, M. (2002). Childhood experience of illness as a risk factor for medically unexplained symptoms. *Scandinavian Journal of Psychology, 43*, 139-146.

Hutchinson, G.L. (2001). *Disorders of simulation: Malingering, factitious disorders, and compensation neurosis.* New York: Psychosocial Press.

Lesieur, H.R., & Rosenthal, R.J. (1991). Pathological gambling: A review of the literature (prepared for the American Psychiatric Association Task Force on DSM-IV Committee on Disorders of Impulse Control not Elsewhere Classified). *Journal of Gambling Studies, 7*, 5-37.

Libow, J.A. (2002). Beyond collusion: Active illness falsification. *Child Abuse & Neglect, 26*, 525-536.

Lyons-Ruth, K., Repacholi, B., McLeod, S., & Silva, E. (1992). Disorganized attachment behavior in infancy: Short-term stability, maternal and infant correlates, and risk-related subtypes. *Developmental Psychopathology, 3*, 377-396.

Marcus, D., & Kurlan, R. (2001). Tics and its disorders. *Movement Disorders: Official Journal of the Movement Disorder Society, 19*, 735-758.

McNicholas, F., Slonims, V., & Cass, H. (2000). Exaggeration of symptoms or psychiatric Munchausen's syndrome by proxy? *Child Psychology & Psychiatry Review, 5*(2), 69-75.

Murray, J.B. (1993). Review of research on pathological gambling. *Psychological Reports, 72*, 791-810.

Nemiah, J.C. (1988). Psychoneurotic disorders. In A.M. Nicholi (Ed.), *The new Harvard guide to psychiatry* (pp. 208-233). Cambridge, MA: Belknap.

Newcorn, J.H., & Strain, J. (1992). Adjustment disorder in children and adolescents. *Journal of the American Academy of Child and Adolescent Psychiatry, 31*, 318-326.

Owens, J.A., Palermo, T.M., & Rosen, C.L. (2002). Overview of current management of sleep disturbances in children: II–behavioral interventions. *Current Therapeutic Research, 63*(Suppl.B), B38-B52.

Patton, G.C. (1992). Eating disorders: Antecedents, evolution and course. *Annals of Medicine, 24*, 281-285.

Pollard, J.W. (2001). Don't go there: Impulse control in stage-specific short-term counseling. *Journal of College Student Psychotherapy, 16*(1/2) 65-84.

Richert, G.Z., & Bergland, C. (1992). Treatment choices: Rehabilitation services used by patients with multiple personality disorder. *The American Journal of Occupational Therapy, 46*, 634-638.

Rockwell, L.E. (1990). Frames of reference and modalities used by occupational therapists in the treatment of patients with eating disorders. *Occupational Therapy in Mental Health, 10*, 47-64.

Ross, C.A. (1997). *Dissociative identity disorder: Clinical features and treatment of treatment of multiple personality disorder.* New York: John Wiley & Sons.

Saxe, G.N., Chawla, N., & Van der Kolk, B. (2002). Self-destructive behavior in patients with dissociative disorders. *Suicide and Life-Threatening Behavior, 32*, 313-320.

Smith, Y.L.S., Cohen, L., & Cohen-Kettenis, P.T. (2002). Postoperative psychological functioning of adolescent transsexuals: A Rorschach study. *Archives of Sexual Behavior, 31*, 255-261.

Spiegel, D., & Cardena, E. (1991). Disintegrated experience: The dissociative disorders revisited. *Journal of Abnormal Psychology, 100*, 366-378.

Treur, T., Fabian, Z., & Furedi, J. (2001). Internet addiction associated with features of impulse control disorder: Is it a real psychiatric disorder? *Journal of Affective Disorders, 66*, 283.

Waid, K.M. (1993). An occupational therapy perspective in the treatment of multiple personality disorder. *The American Journal of Occupational Therapy, 47*, 872-876.

Waller, G. (1992). Sexual abuse and bulimic symptoms in eating disorders: Do family interaction and self-esteem explain the links? *International Journal of Eating Disorders, 12*, 235-240.

Ward, J.D. (1999). Psychosocial dysfunction in adults. In M.E. Neistadt & E.B. Crepeau (Eds.), *Willard and Spackman's occupational therapy* (9th ed., pp. 716-740). Philadelphia: Lippincott, Williams, & Wilkins.

White, J.H., & Litovitz, G. (1998). A comparison of in-patient and out-patient women with eating disorders. *Archives of Psychiatric Nursing, 12*, 181-194.

Chapter 11

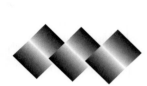

Psychopharmacology

Darrell Hulisz, PharmD
and Phillip J. Fischer, MD

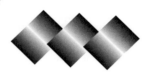

INTRODUCTION

For more than four decades, research on mental disorders has followed several parallel tracks. One track has led to a literal explosion of information about brain function and behavior. Beginning in the late 1950s, dramatic improvement in understanding of medication for mental disorders has led to theories and research about the possible biological contributions to emergence of these illnesses. This illness model has led to a change in the way mental health professionals and the general public have come to understand psychiatric disorders. The idea that these illnesses are solely due to personal weakness or improper parenting has given way to the biopsychosocial approach to diagnosis and treatment.

Research diagnostic criteria were developed and used in multidisciplinary field trials leading to the APA's DSM-IV-TR (2000). The careful application of this diagnostic system based on observable symptoms and behaviors not only serves to improve the specificity of treatment but has led to advances in epidemiologic research. This, in turn, has somewhat decreased the degree of stigma psychiatric patients experience and will hopefully influence society to consider mental illness as equivalent to physical illness in health care reform efforts.

While psychotropic medications are effective for a variety of psychiatric diseases, they should never be perceived as a singular solution to the complex problems related to human emotion and behavior, and the administration of psychopharmacologic agents should never be done in cavalier fashion. Many of the medications discussed here have serious, even potentially life-threatening, side effects. Thus, the physician must carefully consider both the potential risks and benefits of medication use before prescribing any psychotropic agent.

Occupational therapists have a number of roles to play in the monitoring and management of psychopharmacological interventions. First, occupational therapists may be in the best position to provide the prescribing physician with accurate information about positive and negative effects, information that can be vital in efforts to titrate dose and determine the most effective medication. Second, therapists need to be able to communicate with patients, family, and other professionals, recognizing the limits of their role but also providing essential information, encouraging clients to take medications as recommended, and assisting them to negotiate problems with the physician. Third, therapists might need to assist clients with medication management, setting up reminder systems (e.g., pill organizers, alarm clock reminders), figuring out how to open medication bottles, or managing transportation to get to a drug store to get a prescription filled. These roles are described in greater detail at the end of the chapter.

Many psychotropic medications affect performance beyond their effect on psychological status. They can, for example, affect memory and recall, fine and gross motor skills, reaction time, and concentration. In designing activity programs with clients, it is important for therapists to keep these effects in mind so that suitable adjustments can be made.

There are many unanswered questions and many clinical and social controversies around the use of psychotropic medications. Some of these concerns (e.g., about the possibility that Ritalin is being prescribed excessively to treat ADHD) have been mentioned in previous chapters. For some cultural groups, use of herbal remedies may be perceived as preferable to use of prescription medications. New controversies will undoubtedly emerge as new information becomes available or as cultural beliefs about psychiatric illness change.

The purpose of this chapter is to introduce some general principles for using psychopharmacology so that all members of the multidisciplinary treatment team can reinforce gains, recognize adverse drug reactions, and communicate problems that interfere with the patient's maximal functioning.

HISTORY

Throughout history mankind has been searching for ways to reduce the pain and suffering of psychic distress. Each culture has had its armamentarium of treatments. Ancient peoples bored holes in the skull (i.e., trephination) to let out evil spirits. The use of alcohol to reduce dysphoria, herbal remedies, opiates, cocaine, marijuana, coffee, tobacco, and many other plant-derived psychotropic agents have been used as remedies. The effects of some of these compounds have been studied, and many found their way into Western medicine.

The discoveries of the antimanic effect of lithium and of chlorpromazine's (Thorazine) antipsychotic properties signaled the beginning of modern psychopharmacology (Healy, 2002). In the ensuing 40 years, many new drugs have been developed that have improved the quality of life for patients afflicted with a variety of psychiatric disorders. The discovery and development of these compounds started with unexpected clinical findings of efficacy. Research has improved the understanding of basic psychopharmacology and drug side effects, leading to the ongoing development of better drugs and suggesting biologic theories of causation for some psychiatric illnesses.

Chlorpromazine (Thorazine) was synthesized as an antihistamine in 1952 and was found to produce an easily arousable sedation that was useful as a preanesthetic (Davis, 1985). The observation that it produced behavioral changes led to experimental trials of the drug in psychotic patients. Many of these "hopeless cases" experienced dramatic improvement. Since that time, the further development of newer antipsychotic drugs has permitted many individuals to function outside of psychiatric hospitals instead of being institutionalized for life.

The first two major classes of antidepressants—tricyclic antidepressants (TCA) and monoamine oxidase inhibitors (MAOI)—were also discovered accidentally. Imipramine (Tofranil), the first of the tricyclic antidepressants, was discovered while researchers were looking for a better chlorpromazine-like drug (Davis, 1985). It was found that although imipramine was ineffective in schizophrenics, it did produce improvement in depressed patients. The first MAOI, ipronozid, was used to treat tuberculosis and was observed to produce an elevated mood at the same time.

Many of the psychotropic drugs were discovered by chance when they were given experimentally or were given for one condition and were observed to be helpful in a different disorder. In 1949, Cade, an Australian state hospital superintendent, tried lithium experimentally and found that it reduced mania. The history of the development of antidepressant and antipsychotic drugs highlights the fact that major scientific discoveries can evolve as consequences of clinical investigation rather than deductions from animal models (Davis, 1985). More recently, however, the development of new drugs has been due to specific engineering for selective actions, leading to increasing more effective and "cleaner" agents.

GENERAL PRINCIPLES OF PSYCHOPHARMACOTHERAPY

When considering, initiating, and maintaining drug treatment of major mental disorders, the following principles should be followed:

1. A thorough diagnostic assessment is the foundation of treatment. When a patient presents with symptoms, the clinician's goal is to formulate these problems based upon objective and subjective signs and symptoms, keeping in mind that multiple causes can produce very similar syndromes

2. Pharmacotherapy alone is generally insufficient to complete recovery. While drug therapy may be the cornerstone of recovery, there is always a need for educational and psychosocial interventions, as well as psychotherapy

3. The phase of an illness, whether acute or chronic, is of critical importance in terms of the initial treatment as well as treatment duration. Some patients may need short-term care, while others may need lifetime maintenance therapy and/or prophylaxis

4. The risk-to-benefit ratio (i.e., the extent to which the drug is likely to have detrimental side effects as compared with the extent to which it will improve the situation) must always be considered. Physical conditions must be kept in mind. The presence of medical conditions, pregnancy, addictive disorders, etc., must be evaluated so that the treatment is not worse then the disease. Another important consideration is cost; a treatment the patient cannot afford will not be useful

5. Prior personal and family history of a good or bad response to a specific treatment modality usually provides guidance for treatment

6. It is important to target specific symptoms that serve as markers for the underlying psychopathology and monitor their presence or absence over an entire course of treatment. Certain symptoms may respond differently at different times. For example, the neurovegetative symptoms of depression, lethargy, and depressed appetite may improve weeks before the mood actually improves

7. It is necessary to monitor for the development of adverse effects throughout the entire course of treatment, often using the laboratory to ensure safety and optimal efficacy.

ROLE OF LABORATORY TESTING IN DIAGNOSIS AND MEDICATION USE

Regardless of the type of medication, practitioners are increasingly better able to make decisions because of expanding knowledge about drug actions. When psychotropic medications were first discovered, they were used largely on a trial-and-error basis. However, laboratory tests are now routinely being used to rule in or out other medical conditions that can mimic or complicate psychiatric illnesses. Laboratory results are used to aid in diagnosis and to monitor the safety and efficacy of drug treatment. The ability to monitor blood levels of psychotropic drugs can help determine if the proper dosage is being prescribed to get the patient to a therapeutic level and also to validate medication adherence or rule out drug toxicity. This has taken some of the guesswork out of prescribing.

In the past, a psychiatrist might select an antidepressant, for example, and adjust the dose based on clinical response, side effects, and published data on the acceptable dosage range. This sometimes led to improper dosing and subsequent treatment failure. For example, under earlier guidelines, the dosage range for the antidepressant imipramine (Tofranil) was considered to be between 50 mg to 350 mg per day. It was thought that at doses below 50 mg per day, there would be no response and more than 350 mg per day was thought to be toxic and unlikely to yield further significant improvement. The practice was to start the drug at a low dose and increase it every few days until one of three outcomes was observed, namely:

1. A clear and clinical improvement was noted, in which case the drug would be maintained at this level for 3 to 9 months

2. Intolerable side effects occurred, in which case the drug would be discontinued and another drug tried

3. The dose was increased to what was believed to be the maximum allowed. If there was not improvement in 4 to 6 weeks, another drug was tried. Sometimes, what might have been considered treatment-resistant depression was really the result of under-treatment.

Now it is possible to tailor treatment with more precision. It is known that therapeutic blood levels can be seen at what were previously thought to be extremely low doses (e.g., 25 mg to 50 mg of imipramine) with good clinical improvement. In principle, it is always best to use the lowest effective dose possible, especially in children, the elderly, and individuals with medical illnesses. However, using laboratory results to guide dosage, the clinician now has the flexibility to extend the upper limits of dosage, turning many "failed drug trials" into positive outcomes and in shorter time.

The laboratory can also be used to detect medication noncompliance and drug abuse and to monitor blood levels for relapse prevention. In addition to blood and urine parameters, there are several other diagnostic tools available to the clinician today, including EEG and polysomnography, CT scan, magnetic resonance imaging (MRI), position emission tomography (PET scan), topical brain mapping, and psychological tests (psychometrics) (McKim, 2003). The laboratory, then, is an increasingly vital part of modern psychiatric treatment. As refinements and new technology develop, it will be even more important.

The psychotropic drugs to be discussed in this chapter have proved efficacy as well as the potential to cause serious adverse effects. When prescribing any medication, a careful judgment has to be based on consideration of the risk-versus-benefit ratio, the degree to which any benefits exceed the potential for negative side effects.

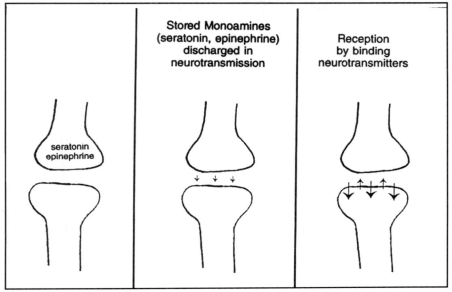

Figure 11-1. (A) Presynaptic neuron. (B) Postsynaptic neuron. (C) Reception by binding neurotransmitters.

ANTIDEPRESSANTS

Pathophysiology of Depressive Illness

Before discussing specific agents, it is important to have an overview of what is believed about "biological" depression. As a diagnosis, depression implies an underlying chemical imbalance of the CNS. One commonly accepted hypothesis today is that a functional deficiency or dysregulation of central neurotransmitters (norepinephrine and serotonin) is important in depressive illness (Grilly, 2002). These two substances, also called monoamines, are contained in vesicles and stored in the presynaptic neuron (Figure 11-1A). These monoamines are discharged into the interneural space (synaptic cleft) and become carriers of impulse transmission to the postsynaptic neuron (Figure 11-1B) (Hackett & Cassem, 1978). Transmission occurs when these monoamines bind to the postsynaptic neuron. The binding is brief and the molecule is released back into the synaptic cleft to be reabsorbed or metabolized (Figure 11-1C). For norepinephrine, about 50% of that stored comes from reuptake. Destruction of the unstored monoamine occurs within the cell by the monoamine oxidase enzymes and in the extracellular space by the enzymes called methyltransferases.

The complexity of the electrochemical processes necessary for normal brain function makes the possibility of dysfunction readily understandable. Failure to terminate the action of a released neurotransmitter would be likely to prolong, inhibit, or exaggerate its action. Likewise, the production and release of excess monoamines or excessive sensitivity of the receptor site at the action of these neurotransmitters would produce an exaggerated effect at the cellular level, which might be seen as a clinical abnormality. Deficient synthesis or release of neurotransmitters, or decreased sensitivity of the receptor site, also would likely produce a physiologic abnormality that again could be manifested clinically in abnormalities of thought process, mood, or behavior (McKim, 2003). Most antidepressant drugs likely work at the level of neurotransmission to "normalize" transmission of both noradrenergic and serotonergic impulses (Frazer, 1997).

Tricyclic Antidepressants

TCAs, such as amitriptyline (Elavil), imipramine (Tofranil), and doxepin (Sinequan, Adapin) were, for many years, the mainstay of the pharmacological treatment of depression. There are a variety of tricyclic drugs that are more or less equally effective in the treatment of depression (Table 11-1). These compounds probably work by blocking neuronal reuptake of norepinephrine and serotonin. The TCAs mainly differ in the extent and severity of their side effects. To varying degrees, all available TCAs block acetylcholine and consequently inhibit the parasympathetic nervous system. This cholinergic blockade by TCAs is responsible for commonly reported side effects that include blurred vision, dry mouth, reduced sweating, constipation, urinary retention, and tachycardia (Grilly, 2002). For some patients, these side effects are extremely unpleasant and make the drug unsuitable. Patients with cardiac diseases or other medical problems that would make them vulnerable to anticholinergic drugs should be treated cautiously with TCAs.

Sedation is a common side effect associated with TCAs. This effect may be inconvenient or unpleasant and may interfere with the activities of daily living, especially early in therapy. However, this sedative side effect can be beneficial, since insomnia and anxiety are frequently among the most troublesome symptoms of depression. Usually, the sedation lessens over   a 2 to 4 week period as the patient "adjusts" to the medication. Interestingly, this same 2 to 4 week period is when the patient receiving a proper dose notices a subjective sense of improvement.

It should be kept in mind that TCAs may interact with a variety of other medications. The sedative effect of TCAs may be increased when they are used with a variety of CNS depressant drugs. Alcohol should be avoided since its effects will be increased and because alcohol, a CNS depressant, can worsen depression itself. Patients should be cautioned about driving or working around hazardous machinery until a functional assessment can be made. The selection of the least sedative TCA is prudent in the patient who must be alert during the day. Frequently, giving the medication as a single evening dose can minimize this problem. Although the sedative effect is usually transient, a trial of a different class of drug may be needed to identify the drug with the least sedative side effects. TCAs interfere with the antihypertensive effect of centrally-acting blood pressure medications, such as clonidine (Stahl, 2000). If a TCA is indicated, the antihypertensive drug can be changed in cooperation with the patient's primary care specialist.

TCAs can produce orthostatic (postural) hypotension (i.e., the transient and precipitous lowering of blood pressure as the patient arises from a supine to standing position). This can lead to blackouts, which can further lead to falls and serious injury. Postural hypotension associated with TCAs is thought to be secondary to blockade of alpha adrenergic receptors. The elderly are particularly prone to this side effect, which can lead to devastating injuries, particularly fractured hips and wrists. Therefore, it is extremely important to discuss this and the other side effects with the patient and, if possible, with a significant family member or friend. Therapists should also be alert to this effect in clients taking TCAs, standing nearby when the client rises from a bed or chair and helping the client learn to rise slowly and with a sturdy object nearby to provide support.

Table 11-1

Summary of Antidepressant Drugs Currently Used in the United States

Class	Generic Name	Trade Name	Tablet	Capsule	Solution	Comments, Advantages/ Disadvantages
Dopamine-reuptake blocking compounds	Bupropion	Wellbutrin Wellbutrin SR Zyban	75 and 100 mg 100 and 150 mg 150 mg			Contraindicated in patients with seizure, bulimia, anorexia Low incidence of sexual dysfunction
SSRIs	Citalopram	Celexa	20 and 40 mg		10 mg/5 mL	Solution is alcohol- and sugar-free and has a peppermint taste CYP2D6 inhibitor (weak)
	Escitalopram	Lexapro	5, 10, and 20 mg			S isomer of citalopram Possibly less side effects
	Fluvoxamine	Luvox	25, 50, and 100 mg			Contraindicated with pimozide, thioridazine, mesoridazine, CYPA-12, 2C19, and 3A3/4 inhibitors
Serotonin/norepinephrine reuptake inhibitors	Venlafaxine	Effexor	25, 37.5, 50, 75, and 100 mg			High-dose is useful to treat refractory depression
		Effexor XR		37.5, 75, and 150 mg		

(continued)

Table 11-1 (Continued)

Class	Generic Name	Trade Name	Tablet	Capsule	Solution	Comments, Advantages/ Disadvantages
5HT2 antagonist properties	Nefazodone	Serzone	50,100, 150, 200, and 250 mg			Contraindicated with carbamapine pimozide, astemizole, cisapride, and terfenadine Caution with traizolam and alpra-zolam Low incidence of sexual dysfunc-tion
	Trazodone	Desyrel	50, 100, 150, and 300 mg			
Noradrenergic	Mirtazapine antagonist	Remeron	15, 30, and 45 mg Oral disinte-grating: 15, 30, and 45 mg			Dose>15mg/d is less sedating Low incidence of sexual dysfunc-tion

---

Table 11-2
Summary of Antidepressant Side Effects

- Dry mouth
- Aggravation of narrow-angle glaucoma
- Constipation
- Sedation
- Heart block
- Paralytic ileus
- Hallucinations, delusions in latent psychosis
- Loss of accommodation (blurred vision)
- Skin rash
- Bone marrow depression
- Black tongue
- Nausea
- Orthostatic hypotension
- Vomiting
- Palpitations
- Tachycardia
- Urinary retention
- Agitation
- Myocardial infarction
- Peculiar taste
- Galactorrhea
- Gynecomastia
- Edema
- Diarrhea
- Fainting

The anticholinergic effects of tricyclic drugs can be additive with anticholinergic effects of other agents that medical patients may be receiving (e.g., antiparkinsonian drugs) (McKim, 2003). TCAs can also produce or worsen cardiac arrhythmias. Therefore, it is a good idea to obtain baseline and follow-up EKGs, especially in the elderly.

Some patients receiving TCAs may become confused or agitated. This effect is linked either to their anticholinergic effect or to the ability of these drugs to uncover a previously unrecognized psychotic disturbance.

Larger doses of tricyclic drugs may cause toxic psychosis with auditory and visual hallucinations. Visual hallucinations are assumed to be organically based until proven otherwise, so drugs must be considered as a possible cause. Some patients with an unrecognized underlying bipolar disorder may experience a "manic switch" or acute manic psychosis after treatment for depressive illness with tricyclic drugs. Occasional confusion and less well-defined memory deficits have been associated with TCAs. Table 11-2 summarizes the side effects.

Clinical Effects

In normal persons, tricyclic drugs produce slight sedation; however, in severely depressed psychotic patients, they produce improvement in behavior and lessening of depression, often 3 to 10 days after the start of treatment. Using the drug doubles the chance of recovery after 3 to 4 weeks of treatment (Furukawa, McGuire, & Barbui, 2002). Patients who do not respond after receiving an adequate dose of the drug for 3 weeks probably will not respond at all, and the degree of response in the first week predicts the ultimate therapeutic response. One important consideration for therapists is the suicide risk posed during the first several weeks of administration. Since therapeutic blood-levels have not yet been reached and because these drugs can be lethal at relatively low doses, attention to suicidal intent during this phase is crucial. A particular risk is the period in which the patient is beginning to experience more energy, but not yet a lift in mood, since this is a time when action on a suicidal impulse is most likely.

Monoamine Oxidase Inhibitors

This group of psychoactive agents is frequently effective in the treatment of severe endogenous depression, panic disorders, and in the atypical depression associated with BPD (Krishnan, 1998). These agents are divided into two categories: hydrazines and non-hydrazines. The hydrazines include isocarboxazid and phenelzine (Nardil). The only non-hydrazine in use is tranylcypromine (Parnate). The structural difference is clinically important. Tranylcypromine has somewhat stimulant amphetamine-like qualities that often produce clinical improvement in about 10 days. Tranylcypromine, however, has a greater degree of side effects, particularly of the cardiovascular system. The hydrazines are effective within 3 to 4 weeks and have a lower incidence of side effects.

MAOIs inhibit many enzyme systems. They elevate body levels of epinephrine, norepinephrine, 5HT, and dopamine by irreversibly binding to the degradation enzymes of these substances. This process increases the body's available biogenic amines. It is hypothesized that this CNS effect is responsible for the antidepressant activity. However, the MAOIs can produce many serious side effects and should be prescribed only by experienced practitioners (Krishnan, 1998).

Cardiovascular side effects of the MAOIs, including orthostatic hypotension, tachycardia, and palpitations, can be life-threatening. When orthostatic hypotension occurs, it is important to get the client immediately to a sitting or, even better, lying position. The patient can then be instructed to remember to rise slowly close to a stationary object that can provide support. In cardiac patients, these MAOIs can eliminate or delay the onset of angina pectoris by blocking the response of the cardiovascular system to exercise (Gumnick & Nemeroff, 2000), promoting conditions that predispose to myocardial infarction. The most worrisome cardiovascular side effect is hypertension (Krishnan, 1998). This can occur at therapeutic doses, but usually occurs when high doses of the MAOIs are taken, when the drug is combined with a TCAs or sympathomimetic agents (such as cough and cold preparations), or when tyramine (found in a variety of foods) is consumed. The hypertension is caused by the release of catecholamines in the peripheral nervous system. A severe, atypical headache is usually the first sign and may foretell an impending hypertensive crisis that can lead to a cerebrovascular accident (stroke) and death.

Eating foods with a high tyramine content is a major concern. Tyramine is a fermentation by-product, so foods with aged protein should be avoided. Aged cheeses, meats, and fish; most alcoholic beverages, especially beer and red wine; and overripe fruits and vegetables should be avoided. Consumption of chocolate and coffee should be limited.

MAOIs and many pharmacologic agents are synergistic and can result in hypertensive crisis. These include amphetamines, ephedrine, procaine, epinephrine, methyldopa, meperidine (Demerol), and pseudoephedrine, which is found in many over-the-counter cold preparations. Patients must be informed to check with their psychiatrist before taking any other medication while on MAOIs. Therapists should be alert to patient mention of other medications, including herbal preparations that the patient may not perceive as a drug.

TCAs should be discontinued at least 7 days before a trial of MAOIs and vice versa. SSRIs, such as fluoxetine (Prozac), should be discontinued 5 to 6 weeks before starting a MAOI. MAOIs and TCAs are occasionally combined for severe, treatment-resistant depressions under special and controlled circumstances. Fortunately, hypertensive reaction is very rare and can be reversed with prompt administration of an antidote, phentolamine. These drugs can precipitate hypomania or mania. The overall side effect profile is similar to the TCAs and is summarized in Table 11-1. Overall, the MAOIs are safe and effective in experienced hands, with proper precautions, and in patients able and willing to comply with restrictions.

> ## Table 11-3
> ### *Common Side Effects of SSRI*
>
> - Nausea
> - Anorexia
> - Insomnia
> - Nervousness
> - Tremor
>
> - Diarrhea
> - Drowsiness
> - Dry mouth
> - Loss of libido
> - Sexual dysfunction

Selective Serotonin Inhibitors

Over the past 15 years there has been increasing evidence that serotonin neurotransmission is decreased in depression. Fluoxetine (Prozac) and other SSRI antidepressants (see Table 11-1) selectively inhibit neuronal uptake of serotonin. SSRIs are now the most prescribed antidepressant class because of their relative safety, and the fact that the main effect of the drug is more pronounced than any side effects noted, leading to high levels of patient acceptance (Sampson, 2001). In addition to their antidepressant effects, SSRIs such as paroxetine have shown promising results in the treatment of OCD, panic disorder, social anxiety disorder (i.e., social phobia), generalized anxiety disorder (GAD), and PTSD (Wagstaff, Cheer, Matheson, Ormrod, & Goa, 2002). SSRIs are also employed in the treatment of premenstrual dysphoria and eating disorders.

Fluoxetine has very little anticholinergic activity and, thus, a low incidence of drowsiness, dry mouth, cognitive impairment, constipation, and weight gain. The most common side effects are transient nausea, nervousness, and insomnia (Sampson, 2001). In comparison studies, fluoxetine is as effective as the TCAs (Williams et al., 2000).

Sertraline (Zoloft) was put on the U.S. market in 1992. It is effective in patients with moderate to severe depression, with or without melancholia, with low or high anxiety, with or without insomnia, with psychomotor agitation or psychomotor retardation. The dosage range is 50 mg to 200 mg per day (Tollefson & Rosenbaum, 1998).

Paroxetine (Paxil) became available in 1993. It has also been shown to be superior to placebo and equally effective to other SSRIs, TCAs, and MAOIs. Dosage range is 20 mg to 50 mg per day.

Venlafaxine (Effexor) is a novel compound with demonstrated antidepressant properties that has a neuropharmacologic profile distinct from that of other agents. It significantly inhibits the uptake of serotonin and epinephrine, and to a lesser extent, dopamine. The dosage range is 75 mg to 375 mg per day in two or three divided doses. It may have a more rapid onset of action than other antidepressants and is well-tolerated. The main side effects are nausea, somnolence, dizziness, dry mouth, sweating, and headaches. The side effects are generally mild and transient. The risk of suicide by overdose is very small.

In general, all of the SSRIs are effective, well-tolerated, and represent a major breakthrough in treating depression and OCD. They can be administered once a day, which increases the compliance rate. Also, it is generally believed that overdosing on these medications is much less likely to produce fatality than TCAs or MAOIs. The most common side effects of SSRIs are shown in Table 11-3. These are usually mild and transient, often clearing in 10 to 14 days.

Table 11-4
Central Serotonin Syndrome

Gastrointestinal	Neurological
• Abdominal cramping • Bloating • Diarrhea	• Tremulousness • Myoclonus • Dysarthria • Uncoordination • Severe headache

Cardiovascular	Psychiatric
• Tachycardia • Hypotension • Hypertension • Cardiovascular collapse (death)	• Hypomania • Racing thoughts • Pressure speech • Confusion • Disorientation

Other

• Diaphoresis
• Elevated temperature
• Hyperthermia
• Hyperreflexes

A rare consequence of SSRI administration is "serotonin syndrome." This syndrome is characterized by gastrointestinal, neurological, cardiovascular, and psychiatric symptoms (Sternback, 1991) (Table 11-4). Another under-reported but often troubling side effect of the SSRIs is their impact on sexual functioning. A substantial percentage of patients report decreased or absent libido, and many more report difficulty achieving orgasm. This problem can lead to poor medication compliance, and therapists should be alert for patient reports that should be passed along to the prescribing physician.

Bupropion (Wellbutrin) is the only marketed aminoketone antidepressant. It is not an SSRI, an MAOI, or a TCA but does produce down-regulation of postsynaptic beta-nora-drenergic receptors (Grilly, 2002). Bupropion is chemically unrelated to other antidepressant agents. The exact neurochemical mechanism of the antidepressant effect is unknown. The advantages of bupropion are that it is nonsedating, has low incidence of weight gain, little effect on sexual function, little effect on EKG, and low toxicity with overdose. The adverse effects most frequently observed are agitation, dry mouth, insomnia, nausea, constipation, overstimulation, low seizure threshold, and tremor. It is not recommended for use in anyone with a seizure potential nor in those with a history of bulimia or anorexia nervosa. Bupropion is also a favored antidepressant in bipolar disease and is used as an adjunct in smoking cessation (Goldberg, 2000).

Table 11-5
Antianxiety Drugs

Class	Chemical Name	Trade Name	Dosage
Benzodiazepine	Chlordiazepoxide	Librium	10 to 100 mg/d
	Diazepam	Valium	2 to 40 mg/d
	Oxazepam	Serax	15 to 90 mg/d
	Flurazepam	Dalmane	15 to 30 mg/d
	Alprazolam	Xanax	0.1254 mg/d
	Clorazepate	Tranxene	15 to 60 mg/d
Antihistamines	Cyclizine	Maverzine	
	Hydroxyzine	Atarax, Vistaril	75 to 400 mg/d
	Diphenhydramine	Benadryl	25 to 100 mg/d
Barbiturates		Amytal	
		Seconal	
		Nembutal	
Carbamate	Meprobamate		400 mg

ANTIANXIETY AGENTS

Anxiety is a universal response to stress and is necessary for effective functioning and coping. It is experienced as a state of tension accompanied by feelings of dread and potential danger. However, in some individuals, the symptom complex is so severe that the patient is immobilized and dysfunctional. The decision whether to medicate for anxiety is complex. Clearly, medication is one modality that should be integrated into a more comprehensive plan.

Antianxiety drugs (anxiolytics) produce symptomatic relief of anxiety (Ballenger, 1998). Even if the anxiety is adaptive, an anxiolytic may improve the patient's ability to cope or enhance the effectiveness of other types of treatment. Anxiolytics are useful in only a few situations and always in the context of an ongoing relationship between the patient, the prescribing physician, and the interdisciplinary treatment team. Generally, they should be used for short-term administration. Major types of anxiolytics are listed in Table 11-5.

Benzodiazepines

The currently marketed benzodiazepines are listed in Table 11-5. Extensive use of benzodiazepines has been associated with considerable controversy. Critics of benzodiazepines cite two properties of the drugs that make them susceptible to abuse: they produce euphoria and generally have a rapid onset of action. Others argue that abuse and habituation is relatively infrequent and limited primarily to those with histories of substance abuse (Ballenger, 1998). The negative publicity surrounding the benzodiazepines has produced a number of problems, foremost among them a hesitancy to prescribe the medications in cases in which their ben-

Table 11-6

Therapeutic Effects of Benzodiazepines

- Anxiety reduction
- Sedation
- Anticonvulsant activity
- Muscle relaxation
- Antistress effect
- Anesthesia
- Amnesia
- Antipanic activity
- Antidepressant
- Alcohol withdrawal

efits clearly outweigh their potential harm. Sensationalized accounts of diazepam (Valium) abuse have served to deflect attention from the therapeutically useful role benzodiazepines can play. They have also obscured awareness of some important liabilities associated with the class as a whole, some of which are more prevalent and clinically significant than abuse.

The widespread use of benzodiazepines derives from their therapeutic usefulness for a broad range of indications (Table 11-6). Most reviews emphasize their effectiveness as antianxiety agents. Specific effects include reduction in worry, shakiness, physiologic symptoms, and panic attacks (Grilly, 2002). They appear to be more effective in people suffering from severe anxiety and appear to have little impact on those with low anxiety levels. Benzodiazepines are especially useful for the early treatment of panic disorder. Therapeutic effects are generally achieved within the first week of treatment. Another benzodiazepine, clonazepam (Klonopin), which is normally used as an anticonvulsant, has been found to be an effective antipanic drug. In addition to diazepam and clonazepam, lorazepam (Ativan) has also proven effective in treating panic disorder (Davidson, 1998).

Benzodiazepines block stress-induced increases in corticosteroid concentration and plasma catecholamines (Stahl, 2000). Therefore, these drugs are often used for patients with hyperadrenergic states, such as alcohol withdrawal. Since these agents attach to the same receptor sites in the brain as alcohol, these agents can be substituted and then tapered off over a 5 to 7 day period.

All of the benzodiazepines produce similar pharmacologic effects (Stahl, 2000). The differences among the drugs involve pharmacokinetics, such as rates of absorption, elimination of half-life, pathways of metabolism and lipid solubility; factors that contribute to the overall effect by influencing the onset and duration of action. The single most important difference is elimination half-life. Slowly eliminated drugs accumulate and lead to an increased risk of accidents and cognitive impairment. Problems of accumulation are even more challenging in the elderly because of slowed metabolic activity of the liver and kidneys, which is part of the normal aging process. Short half-life drugs also have special risks, such as a more intense withdrawal syndrome, as well as rebound anxiety.

Although comparatively safe, benzodiazepines can produce a wide array of adverse effects (Grilly, 2002). Psychomotor impairment may be the most lethal of all benzodiazepine-related side effects (Table 11-7). Impairment of driving skills puts drivers at considerably greater risk of involvement in a serious accident as compared with those not taking benzodiazepines. Global cognitive impairment in the elderly is a significant problem, with long half-life anxiolytics and hypnotics accounting for the greatest incidence. The onset of impairment is often insidious, with signs of cognitive impairment becoming evident after years of treatment. Thinking ability improves once the drug is discontinued. These adverse effects are of particular import to therapists who may be considering engaging clients in the use of sharp tools or in activities that require cognitive alertness.

Table 11-7
Side Effects of Benzodiazepines

- Sedation
- Psychomotor impairment
- Depression
- Amnesia
- Dependence

- Impaired concentration
- Weakness
- Impaired sexual function
- Agitation (rare)

Benzodiazepines can induce amnesia, which is usually an unwanted effect when these agents are used as anxiolytics. However, it is a beneficial effect when used in anesthesia, as it helps the patient forget the more traumatic aspects of diagnostic and surgical procedures.

Other side effects include treatment-emergent depression and paradoxical aggression or mania (Grilly, 2002). Benzodiazepines can cause breathing impairment and, thus, should be used with caution in patients with chronic obstructive lung disease.

Approximately 40% of those who use benzodiazepines for 6 months or more exhibit withdrawal symptoms upon discontinuation. Some may develop dependence after only 6 weeks. Nevertheless, many patients who have been taking benzodiazepines for years do not experience withdrawal symptoms (Ballenger, 1998).

Some commonly reported withdrawal symptoms are anxiety and insomnia. Withdrawal symptoms also include tinnitus (i.e., ringing in the ears), involuntary movements, perceptual changes (i.e., increased sensitivity to environmental stimuli), confusion, and depersonalization (Stahl, 2000).

Abrupt discontinuation of high dose therapy with diazepam produces the most severe withdrawal syndrome with disorientation, delirium, seizures, and psychotic reactions. General strategies for minimizing the clinical impact of withdrawal include stopping the drug as soon as the reason for taking it has ceased and avoidance of abrupt withdrawal by tapering the dose gradually (Stahl, 2000).

Buspirone (Buspar) is an anxiolytic agent distinct from the benzodiazepines. It appears to be about as effective as benzodiazepines in the treatment of generalized anxiety disorder. However, it does not appear to be useful for treating panic disorder. Buspirone has a low incidence of sedation, psychomotor impairment, interaction with alcohol, and dependency, and it does not impair memory (Ninan, Cole, & Yonkers, 1998). Buspirone does not cause breathing impairment nor does it block benzodiazepine withdrawal symptoms. The major limitations of buspirone include decreased efficacy in patients recently treated with benzodiazepines, the need for multiple doses, and a lag period of 1 to 2 weeks for full anxiolytic effects to appear. These latter features limit patient acceptance.

Propranolol and Related Drugs

Anxiety is characterized by a number of autonomic symptoms, such as palpitations, rapid heartbeat, tremor, tingling, cold sweats, and chest tightness. These symptoms could, in part, be caused by the secretion of epinephrine during stress. Many of the symptoms can be blocked by a beta adrenergic receptor antagonist. Propranolol (Inderal), as well as other beta blockers, have been used for general anxiety and for anxiety-provoking situations, such as public speaking (i.e., performance anxiety). Ongoing research has verified their usefulness in situational anxiety and less impressive results in panic disorders. These drugs are generally prescribed for a variety of medical conditions such as hypertension and angina pectoris. Their side effects include hypotension and depression. They are contraindicated in asthma and cardiac conditions for which slowing of the heart would be detrimental.

Overall, psychopharmacologic treatment of anxiety is still relatively problematic (Sramek, Zarotsky, & Cutler, 2002). However, a number of newer drugs, including newer serotonin 5-HT1A receptor agonists, cholecystokinin receptor antagonists, neurokinin receptor antagonists, and several others, show promise. While research is ongoing, and none of these interventions is yet ready for use, there is hope that in the not too distant future, pharmacologic interventions for anxiety will be significantly improved.

SEDATIVES/HYPNOTICS

Drugs used to facilitate sleep are known as hypnotics. They are CNS depressants that, in large doses, can produce anesthesia and death. Most of the hypnotic agents effectively induce and maintain sleep the first few days, but this effect diminishes after several days. These agents should only be used for very brief periods because of their addiction and abuse potential. The side effects include hangover, memory impairment, and paradoxical combativeness. Zolpidem (Ambien) and zaleplon (Sonata) are newer nonbenzodiazepine sedative/hypnotic drugs approved for the short-term treatment of insomnia. They have less potential for abuse and addiction than benzodiazepines (Israel & Kramer, 2002).

PSYCHOSTIMULANTS

Psychostimulants have been studied for the treatment of hyperactivity and ADD since 1936. These agents are moderately to significantly effective in 75% of affected children and adults (Tables 11-8 and 11-9). They have also been used to augment therapy in patients with treatment-resistant depression, especially in elderly and severely medically compromised patients. They are also sometimes used to improve the quality of life in the terminally ill. These drugs may help such patients stay awake and alert to interact with their loved ones.

Psychostimulants are controlled substances that can only be prescribed in limited quantities and for the specific indication of ADHD, narcolepsy, and treatment-resistant depression. They cannot legally be prescribed for weight control or enhance work-related performance. In children with ADHD, a paradoxical "calming" effect is actually a response to the improvement in attention, concentration, and overall cognitive functioning (Smucker & Hedayat, 2001). These effects can be demonstrated in nearly anyone who takes these medications in low to moderate doses. At higher doses, the drugs can cause distractibility and increased psychomotor activity (see Table 11-9). When used appropriately, these agents are safe, well-tolerated, and have a much lower addiction potential than is generally believed. The idea that "speed kills" is due to the street abuse of amphetamines.

The main drawbacks and side effects of these drugs are jitteriness, palpitations, insomnia, sexual dysfunction, rebound depression, and dependence (Grilly, 2002). Florid psychosis, resembling acute paranoid psychosis, can be precipitated or unmasked by these drugs. Anorexia is the most troublesome side effect but can be managed by giving the drug after meals. Tolerance to anorexia and insomnia usually develops after a few weeks. Increased

Table 11-8

Psychostimulants Used to Treat ADHD in Children and Adults

Generic Name	Trade Name	Elimination Half-Life	Time to Peak Plasma Concentration	Daily Dose Range (mg/kg/day)	Daily Dose Range (mg/day)
Methylphenidate	Ritalin	2 to 3 hours	1 to 3 hours	0.3 to 2	5 to 90
	Concerta	2 to 4 hours	6 to 8 hours		18 to 54
	Metadate CD	2 to 4 hours	6 to 8 hours		20 to 60
	Metadate ER	2 to 4 hours	6 to 8 hours		5 to 90
	Methylin	2 to 4 hours	6 to 8 hours		5 to 90
	Methylin ER	2 to 4 hours	6 to 8 hours		5 to 9
	Ritalin LA	2 to 4 hours	6 to 8 hours		20 to 60
	Ritalin-SR	2 to 4 hours	6 to 8 hours		5 to 90
Pemoline	Cylert	Children: 7 to 8.6 hours Adults: 12 hours	2 to 4 hours	0.5 to 3	37.5 to 112.5
Dextroamphetamine	Dexedrine	Adults: 10 to 13 hours	Immediate release: 3 hours Sustained release: 8 hours	0.1 to 0.5	2.5 to 40
Amphetamine and dextroamphetamine	Adderall	Children: D-amphetamine: 9 hours; L-amphetamine: 11 hours Adults: D-amphetamine: 10 hours; L-amphetamine: 13 hours	3 hours		2.5 to 40
	Adderall XR		7 hours		5 to 30
Dexmethylphenidate	Focalin	2.2 hours	1 to 1.5 hours		5 to 20

Table 11-9

Summary of Psychostimulant Adverse Effects

Common and Time Limited	Less Common, More Serious
• Anorexia • Weight loss • Irritability • Abdominal pain	• Increased blood pressure • Tachycardia • Precipitation of tic-like movement disorder • Nightmares • Hepatotoxicity • Psychotic symptoms • Rash

motor activity, abdominal pain, tearfulness, social withdrawal, and tachycardia are frequently encountered. The seizure threshold may be lowered. Habituation to CNS stimulants in children has not been reported and, as stated previously, there is no evidence suggesting that these drugs predispose to later addictive diseases.

Methylphenidate (Ritalin) is the most widely used and best studied medication for ADHD. It is generally given in divided doses, since the elimination half-life is short. A sustained release preparation is also available, but its pharmacokinetic profile is inconsistent (i.e., its effect may wax and wane over the course of a single dose) (Szymanski & Zolotor, 2001).

Pemoline (Cylert) has a longer half-life that further increases with long-term administration. It can be given once a day and is generally reserved for cases in which the effects of methylphenidate do not persist long enough for optimal control of hyperactivity and distractibility. Because of a long onset of action, it is believed that it has less abuse potential then methylphenidate or dextroamphetamine, but it has not been shown to be as effective as methylphenidate or amphetamines (Szymanski & Zolotor, 2001).

Amphetamines also have a longer half-life than methylphenidate but not as long as pemoline. Because of the rapid onset of action and longer half-life, proponents think that amphetamines are better agents for the treatment of ADHD. They are clearly useful alternatives, since up to 20% of children who respond poorly to one psychostimulant will respond well to another.

Newer sustained release formulations of methylphenidate have been marketed (e.g., Concerta, Metadate CD). These preparations allow for once or twice daily administration and are summarized in Table 11-8.

In summary, these agents are very effective in the treatment of ADHD, narcolepsy, and depression. They are relatively safe and well-tolerated. Research has shown improvement in task and off task behavior, increase in positive social behavior, improved parent-child and teacher-child relationships, leading to improved self-esteem (Smucker & Hedayat, 2001). Therapists have an important role in monitoring the effectiveness of specific drugs administered, as well as assisting in the identification of the optimal dose.

ANTIPSYCHOTIC DRUGS

Psychoses are among the least understood and most devastating illnesses to affect mankind. Psychotic illnesses cause serious disruption in the lives of individuals and their loved ones and have a major impact on society by incapacitating significant numbers of people. The discovery of chlorpromazine (Thorazine) 50 years ago was an important milestone in the treatment of psychotic illness. Since chlorpromazine became available in clinical practice, there have been significant advances in understanding the mechanisms and etiologies of psychosis. It is unlikely that a single cause will explain what appears to be a varied group of illnesses. This section will discuss the drugs useful in treating schizophrenia, bipolar disorder, and other psychotic illnesses.

To avoid confusion, these drugs are best referred to as antipsychotic drugs. They have also been called "neuroleptics" and "major tranquilizers." There are now about 20 antipsychotic drugs on the market, divided among five distinct chemical classes. Only eight or nine of these products are in widespread clinical use. These antipsychotic drugs appear to act by blocking dopamine, suggesting the possibility that in schizophrenia, the underlying disease mechanism may involve an abnormality of dopamine release or receptor sensitivity (Carlsson, 2001).

The clinical use of antipsychotic drugs is primarily directed toward disturbed psychomotor behavior, abnormal affect, psychotic perceptual disturbances (i.e., hallucinations), delusional thinking, catatonic behavior, autistic withdrawal, and others (Ho & Andreasen, 2001).

Unfortunately, all available therapeutic agents in this class produce some degree of extrapyramidal effects (EPS) (e.g., tremor, shuffling gait) that must be managed when these drugs are administered. The connection between the beneficial effects and the side effects has become better understood as dopamine receptor blockage has been recognized as the most likely mechanism of antipsychotic drug action. Newer medications, described in the section following, show promise of providing benefits for many individuals, with fewer side effects.

Most experts agree that the various agents do not differ in their antipsychotic effects if equivalent doses are given. Although there is little evidence that any of these drugs is clearly superior to another in antipsychotic effect, they do have different side effect profiles. Since specific side effects may be more or less problematic for particular patients, this is one basis for the choice of a particular drug. Although there are no clear indications for specific antipsychotic drugs, clinicians observe that patients who fail to respond to one antipsychotic drug may respond to another, even though it belongs to the same chemical group.

As plasma levels of antipsychotics reveal, there are extreme individual variations in absorption, metabolism, and excretion of psychoactive drugs, which may explain why a certain person may respond to one drug but not another (Ho & Andreasen, 2001). However, it is important to give a particular drug an adequate clinical trial, as these drugs must be given in a generally accepted dosage range and over a certain time period to confirm effectiveness.

Therapy with antipsychotic drugs can be divided into three phases. The initial phase of treatment is generally aimed at providing behavioral control and reducing agitation, fear, delusions, and hallucinations. This can take from hours to weeks (Kane, 2001).

The next phase of antipsychotic therapy involves stabilization and gradual reduction of the medication dosage to receive the best possible control using the lowest possible dose, thereby reducing the patient's vulnerability to drug side effects.

The third phase of treatment of the psychotic patient may be referred to as maintenance therapy and involves long-term continuous administration of the lowest possible dose of effective medication to prevent recurrence of the illness. Clearly, a great deal of emotional support to patients and their families, rehabilitation services, and community networking are essential to maximize the patient's recovery and reintegration. Specific psychotherapeutic intervention is beyond the scope of this chapter. It has been repeatedly shown, however, that psychotherapeutic interventions in the absence of adequate drug treatment of psychotic disorders lead to suboptimal outcomes.

In the schizophrenic patient, treatment is generally best accomplished by starting and continuing treatment with a single antipsychotic agent, provided the patient can tolerate this medication without incapacitating side effects. If side effects do develop, they can usually be managed by adjusting the dosage, adding an antiparkinsonism medication, or changing to a different medication.

In the treatment of the acutely manic patient, treatment is usually initiated with an antipsychotic drug in conjunction with lithium carbonate. The antipsychotics can usually be withdrawn gradually and the patient maintained on lithium.

Treatment of the psychotically depressed patient is usually initiated by using antipsychotic drugs to manage the delusions, along with an antidepressant to manage the affective aspects of the disorder. The patient with psychosis should generally receive maintenance medication consisting either of antidepressant drugs alone or in combination with antipsychotic drugs or lithium. The duration for maintenance therapy varies. About 70% of psychotically depressed patients who respond to pharmacologic treatment are off all medication within 1 year. The majority of schizophrenic patients may require maintenance medication for many years, possibly for life (Kane, 2001).

Side Effects

The side effects of antipsychotic drugs can be classified as follows: autonomic effects, EPS, other CNS effects, behavioral toxicity, allergic reactions, agranulocytosis, skin and eye effects, and endocrine effects.

Autonomic side effects include dry mouth, blurred vision, skin flushing, constipation, paralytic ileus, mental confusion, and postural hypotension. Dry mouth is one of the most often complained about side effects and can be managed by advising the patient to rinse the mouth frequently with water. The use of sugarless chewing gum can be helpful. Regular sugared gum and candy should be avoided because the sugar added to the dry mouth can predispose to fungal infections and dental caries. Patients usually develop tolerance to blurred vision, which is often problematic only in the first few weeks of treatment. The blurred vision can be managed with reassurance that this is temporary and by the use of magnifying lenses or reading glasses.

Orthostatic hypotension may occur in the first few days of treatment. The main danger of this is that patients may fall and injure themselves. Instructing the patient to arise slowly from a lying to standing position is important. Support hose may help by preventing blood pooling in the lower extremities.

The most dramatic and the most theoretically important group of side effects shown by all of the antipsychotic drug agents are the extrapyramidal reactions (EPD) (Kane, 2001). These side effects are classified into three categories: parkinsonian syndrome, dystonias, and akathisia. The parkinsonian syndrome consists of a mask-like face, tremor at rest, rigidity, shuffling gait, and motor retardation (i.e., bradykinesia). This syndrome is symptomatically identical to idiopathic parkinsonism (i.e., Parkinson's disease). The dystonias consist of a broad range of bizarre movements of the tongue, face, and neck. The tongue may protrude and partially obstruct the airway. The patient's eyes may roll upward (i.e., oculogyric crisis). Akathisia is a motor restlessness in which the patient has a great urge to move about and may not be able to sit or stand still.

These side effects are fairly common, vary in intensity, and are easily reversible. They are very distressing to the patient and if not properly managed, can lead to medication non-compliance, compromising the patient's chances for recovery (Stanilla & Simpson, 1998). Therapists may be able to assist in managing some of the distressing effects and in finding ways to engage clients in activities that distract them from their discomfort until side effects diminish.

Younger patients tend to experience dystonic reactions more often than middle-aged patients, possibly because they have higher levels of dopamine. The acute dystonias typically occur early in the course of treatment even with small doses of antipsychotic drugs. They usually resolve within minutes of intramuscular administration of one of the antiparkinsonian drugs, such as benztropine (Cogentin), diphenhydramine (Benadryl), or trihexyphenidyl (Artane). Amantadine (Symmetrel) is helpful with parkinsonian symptoms and akathisia.

There is controversy in psychiatry about whether one should administer an antiparkinsonian medication to all patients being treated with antipsychotic drugs or give it only if side effects occur. Common practice is to coadminister antiparkinsonian drugs and then attempt to discontinue them gradually after about 3 months.

A rare syndrome, described as the neuroleptic malignant syndrome (NMS), characterized by muscular rigidity, hyperthermia, altered consciousness, and autonomic dysregulation has been recognized (Kane, 2001). This is a potentially fatal complication that must be diagnosed and treated early. Discontinuance of the drug combined with supportive measures, such as lowering body temperature, using muscle relaxants such as dantrolene, IV fluids, and possibly, emergency electroconvulsive therapy, are life saving. Antipsychotics can usually be safely restarted if needed when the crisis is over. There is little evidence implicating one class of antipsychotic drug over another. There may be a greater likelihood of NMS when multiple psychotropic drugs are used together.

Tardive dyskinesia (TD) is an extrapyramidal syndrome that emerges relatively late in the course of antipsychotic treatment. Long-term, high-dose treatment increases the incidence of TD. TD may also appear days or weeks after antipsychotics are discontinued. This syndrome is sometimes irreversible, and no consistently effective treatment has been identified. TD presents with facial grimaces, buccolingual movements such as lip smacking, lateral jaw movements, flicking of the tongue, jerking movements of the arms (i.e., chorea), and athetoid movements of the arms and fingers. Neck and trunk movements can also be found. Symptoms are absent during sleep. The overall incidence of TD is correlated with length of exposure to the drug and total lifetime dose (Simpson & Pi, 2001). TD is particularly problematic because, unlike other side effects, it does not disappear over time, nor does it necessarily disappear when the drug is discontinued.

As with all forms of treatment, careful decisions have to be made considering the risks of a drug versus its potential benefits. Psychosis is a frightening, debilitating affliction and usually renders patients dysfunctional. The antipsychotic drugs, despite their liabilities, have helped hundreds of thousands to live outside of psychiatric institutions. In conjunction with psychotherapies and social and occupational rehabilitation, patients can lead relatively normal lives. The various antipsychotic drugs and their side effects are shown in Table 11-10.

Table 11-10

Antipsychotic Drugs

Class	Generic Name	Trade Name	Side Effects of All Antipsychotics
Aliphatic	Chlorpromazine Triflupromazine	Thorazine Vesprin	Bizarre dreams Blood dyscrasias Blurred vision Breast engorgement and lactation
Piperazine	Prochlorperazine Perphenazine Trifluoperazine Fluphenazine Acetophenazine Butaperazine Carphenazine	Compazine Trifalon Stelazine Prolixin Permitil Tindal Repoise Proketazine	Confusion Constipation Cutaneous flushing Delayed ejaculation Deposits in the cornea and lens Dermatitis Drooling
Piperidine	Thioridazine Mescridazine Piperacetazine	Mellaril Berentil Quide	Dry mouth and throat Dyskinesias Jaundice Mask-like face
Butyrophenone	Haloperidol Pimozide	Haldol Orap	Mental confusion Miosis Motor retardation
Thioxanthene	Chlorprothixene Thiothixene	Taractan Navane	Myariasis Orthostatic hypotension Paralytic ileus
Dibenzoxazepine	Loxapine	Loxitane	Parkinsonian syndrome Photosensitivity
Dihydroindolone	Molindone	Moban	Rigidity Sedation Shuffling gait Tardive dyskinesia Tremor at rest Uncoordination Urinary retention Weight gain

Atypical Antipsychotic Agents

Until very recently, clinicians have had low expectations and little reason for optimism in the treatment of a significant proportion of the population with schizophrenia. Given the limitations of available treatments, the best one could hope for in the management of many patients with schizophrenia was to dampen some of the positive symptoms (hallucinations and delusions) of psychosis and to bring about some marginal increase in level of functioning. There is increasing evidence that new, atypical antipsychotic agents can ameliorate both positive and negative symptoms (e.g., anhedonia, flat affect) of schizophrenia in heretofore treatment-resistant patients and can also improve patient's vocational, social, and cognitive functioning (Kane, Gunduz, & Malhotra, 2001). The next section will discuss newer, atypical antipsychotic agents, such as clozapine and risperidone (Table 11-11).

The commercial reintroduction of Clozaril to the U.S. market in 1989 was heralded as the first truly major advance in antipsychotic drugs since the introduction of chlorpromazine (Thorazine) 35 years earlier (Kane et al., 2001). This hope was based on a possibly greater efficacy in treatment-resistant schizophrenic patients, a markedly reduced tendency to produce EPS, and improvement in the "negative symptoms" of schizophrenia.

The pharmacology of clozapine is complex, in part because of the multiplicity of its neurotransmitter interactions. The large number of competing hypotheses demonstrates the varied pharmacology and a lack of understanding of the exact neurochemical mechanisms underlying schizophrenia and EPS.

Clozapine causes several major side effects and complications. It is more likely than many other antipsychotics to lower the seizure threshold, causing a 14% risk of seizures at doses greater than 600 mg per day. This necessitates the coadministration of anticonvulsant drugs in some cases. It has also been observed that occasional cataplectic episodes in which a sudden loss of muscle tone during wakefulness results in a fall. Orthostatic hypotension is perhaps the most serious adverse reaction, accompanied by respiratory depression. Agranulocytosis, an acute lowering in number of white blood cells (WBCs), is the most clinically significant side effect. The approximate incidence rate for agranulocytosis following clozapine use is 0.8%, with a few deaths attributable to this adverse reaction in Europe (Meltzer & Fatemi, 1998). The problem has been well-handled by a special patient management system in which the patient must have weekly monitoring of WBCs before being provided with medication for the following week. While this causes some inconvenience and increases the cost of treatment, it is well worth the effort since this medication is prescribed for patients with treatment-resistant schizophrenia, 30% of whom realize the significant clinical benefit. Other occasionally troublesome side effects include sedation, weight gain, and hypersalivation.

The clozapine dose is initiated at 25 mg per day and is increased by 25 mg every 2 to 3 days to an effective level. The dose range is 200 mg to 900 mg per day with a mean of 500 mg per day. Blood levels often help to determine appropriate dosing requirements.

Risperidone (Risperdal) is the second "atypical" antipsychotic to be approved in this country (Marder, 2001). Risperidone appears to be well-tolerated in patients taking up to 10 mg per day, with sedation being reported more frequently at higher doses. This drug produces less EPS than standard antipsychotic drugs. The most common adverse side effects reported are agitation, anxiety, insomnia, EPS, headache, nausea, sedation, and tachycardia. Unlike clozapine, risperidone is not associated with agranulocytosis and to date there have been no reported cases of tardive dyskinesia.

Risperidone was released in February 1994, and no specific drug interactions have been reported. Because risperidone is metabolized in the liver, the potential exists for interactions with other drugs metabolized in this way (i.e., beta-blockers, SSRIs, carbamazepine, phenobarbital, and benzodiazepines).

Risperidone should be administered starting with 1 mg twice daily gradually increasing to 6 mg per day, the dose at which most patients respond. This gradually minimizes potential orthostatic hypotension during the initial titration period. Nonresponders may need up to 16 mg per day. The safety and efficacy of doses greater than 16 mg per day has not been evaluated.

Table 11-11
Atypical Antipsychotic Drugs

Generic Name	Trade Name	Side Effects
Olanzapine	Zyprexa	Headache Somnolence Insomnia Agitation Nervousness Hostility Dizziness Potential for weight gain Lipid abnormalities Diabetes
Clozapine	Clozaril	1% incidence of agranulocytosis, so a weekly CBC is required Tachycardia Orthostasis Drowsiness Dizziness Constipation Weight gain Diarrhea Sialorrhea Urinary incontinence
Quetiapine	Seroquel	Headache Somnolence Weight gain
Risperidone	Risperdal	Dysphagia Esophageal dysmotility Insomnia Agitation Anxiety Headache
Ziprasidone	Geodon	QTc prolongation (dose-related) Somnolence

Lithium

Lithium has been extensively studied for a variety of clinical conditions (Grilly, 2002). Its widest and best known application is in the treatment of mania and bipolar disorders. The main use of lithium today is for prophylaxis in recurrent affective disorders. It has been shown to be highly effective in preventing both depressive and manic episodes of affective disorder and schizoaffective disorders. The prophylactic effect does not differ in unipolar and bipolar patients. Lithium prevents, or at least reduces, the intensity and duration of affective episodes in the majority of these patients. A patient with an atypical affective or cyclic psychosis responding to prophylactic lithium treatment should be maintained on it. Other indications, such as therapy for schizophrenia, alcoholism, and some types of personality disorders, are less clearly established. Its use as adjunctive therapy for depression is becoming more popular as is its use in treatment of resistant migraine headaches, thyrotoxicosis, and premenstrual syndrome.

Because of its slower effect and lack of sedation, lithium alone often cannot adequately control acute manic symptoms. Therefore, lithium and antipsychotic drugs are often combined during acute phases of the disorder (Mitchell & Malhi, 2002).

Numerous trials have shown that the prophylactic effect of lithium in affective disorders is obtained in only 70% to 80% of cases. Because of this and also the fact that a significant number of patients are lithium intolerant, other bipolar drugs are being tried, particularly the anticonvulsants carbamazepine (Tegretol) and sodium valproate (Depakote).

Lithium is contraindicated in patients with severe cardiovascular disease, in diseases in which dietary sodium is restricted, in Addison's disease, and the first 4 months of pregnancy. Women on lithium should be counseled against breastfeeding. The use of lithium with diuretics is a relative contraindication since urinary sodium loss and volume depletion can produce toxic lithium blood levels. Lithium is contraindicated in certain kidney diseases.

Side-effects occurring in the initial period of lithium therapy tend to disappear with continued treatment. They include polydipsia (i.e., excessive thirst), polyuria (i.e., excessive urination), fine hand tremor, and diarrhea. Less, often found side effects include nausea, sedation, dizziness, fatigue, and abdominal discomfort. Side effects occurring days or weeks later include edema, weight gain, and myxedema (hypothyroidism). It is rarely necessary to discontinue lithium because of its side effects.

Lithium produces a generally benign lowering in the concentration of circulatory thyroid hormones. In most cases, the effects of lithium on thyroid function do not require treatment. If necessary, thyroid supplementation may be administered. Underlying thyroid disorder is not a contraindication to lithium therapy per se.

Lithium produces two distinct categories of renal effects. The most frequent and benign effect is a nephrogenic diabetes insipidus. The other more serious effect is damage to kidney morphology (structure) (Bowden, 1998). Several contradictory studies raise doubt whether these lesions are due to lithium alone. With appropriate patient selection, careful renal evaluation, and close clinical and lab follow-up, the risk of kidney disease is remote.

The effects of lithium on the CNS range from commonly observed mild effects to irreversible life-threatening brain damage in rare instances of severe toxicity. The neurotoxic reaction is characterized by symptoms of organic brain syndrome, such as disorientation, confusion, dysarthria (i.e., slurred speech), ataxia, reduced concentration, somnolence, lethargy, and extrapyramidal signs (Bowden, 1998). Although neurotoxicity has been reported with lithium alone, the extreme neurotoxic syndrome is more often associated with the combination of lithium and an antiseptic drug.

Prior to lithium therapy, a general medical workup should be done, including physical examination, EKG, complete blood count, kidney function tests, urinalysis, and thyroid functions. Renal and thyroid functions should be rechecked at least once a year. Treatment is usually started at a dose expected to produce plasma levels within the therapeutic range. After 1 week of continued treatment with a constant dose, the blood level is checked and dosage is adjusted accordingly until effective serum levels of 0.5 to 0.8 mg/L are attained. In manic states, higher levels may be necessary. Once the lithium level is established, it should be checked monthly the first half year and then every 3 months thereafter.

Lithium is available as lithium carbonate (Eskalith, Lithonate, Lithane) in capsules and liquid (as citrate). It is also available in sustained release form (Lithobid, Eskalith CR) in various doses (300 mg, 450 mg) and as lithium citrate, lithium acetate, and lithium sulfate. The sustained release forms may be preferable because they might avoid peaks in blood levels and are apt to cause fewer side effects. These medications are administered in divided doses, two or three times per day, although single doses may be as effective with fewer renal effects (Bowden, 1998).

Alternative Treatment Strategies for Mood Disorders

While lithium has been a major advance in the treatment of bipolar affective disorder and other mood disorders, there are some factors that limit its usefulness, including slow onset of action, inadequate response (20% to 40%), intolerance to the drug, adverse effects on the thyroid and kidney, tremor, edema, and weight gain. Furthermore, certain subgroups of mood disordered patients may be less likely to benefit from lithium, including rapid cyclers (5% to 20% of all bipolar patients); dysphoric, mixed, or complex mania (up to 40% of all episodes); severe episodes with psychosis; schizoaffective disorder; the elderly manic patient; patients with coexistent alcohol or substance abuse; personality disorders; and/or mental retardation (McKim, 2003).

As a result, there has been significant research to develop alternative treatments for these patients (Janicak, Newman, & Davis, 1992). One such strategy is the use of ECT, which is the only truly bimodal therapy in that it is equally effective for both the acute depressed and manic phases of mood disorders. A full discussion of ECT is outside the scope of this chapter. However, it is worth noting that for some patients, it is the only effective intervention. It is also worth noting that current practices for ECT differ significantly from those found in many early reports of the practice. Patients are sedated during the procedure, and the typical course of ECT rarely exceeds eight treatments.

Among the drugs that have taken a prominent position in the treatment of mood disorders are the anticonvulsants carbamazepine (Tegretol) and valproic acid (Depakote) (Stahl, 2000).

Carbamazepine (Tegretol) is labeled for the management of temporal lobe epilepsy and paroxysmal pain disorders (tic douloureux). Tegretol has a chemical structure similar to imipramine. Research has shown it to be a potential alternative treatment for acute mania when lithium has been unsuccessful. Its spectrum of efficacy appears similar to that of lithium, and it may be superior in mixes of dysphoric mania, rapid cyclers, and more severe episodes (Bowden, 1998). If carbamazepine is considered in mania, the pretreatment evaluation should include the assessment of baseline hematological and hepatic functions, since these two organ systems may be affected by this agent. Carbamazepine has also been tried with variable results in the management of aggression and in chronic self-injurious, self-mutilating behaviors.

The most serious adverse effect is aplastic anemia, occurring in 1 out of 125,000 patients (Bowden, 1998). Agranulocytosis is more rare, usually occurring within 2 to 3 months of treatment, but it may occur at any time. In addition to monitoring blood counts at appropriate intervals, patients should be instructed to look for signs and symptoms of hematological dysfunction, such as fever, sore throat, and malaise, and to report such symptoms to their physician immediately. Carbamazepine may also adversely affect the liver, so liver function should be monitored every 6 to 12 months. Other side effects are listed in Table 11-12 (Joffe, Post, Roy-Byrne, & Uhde, 1985).

Table 11-12

Anticonvulsants: Adverse Side Effects

Carbamazepine (Teqdetol)	Valproic Acid (Depakote)
• Nausea, anorexia, and vomiting	• Nausea, anorexia, and vomiting
• Sedation	• Sedation
• Ataxia and clumsiness	• Tremor
• Dizziness	• Weight gain or loss
• Blurred vision and diplopia	• Transient abpecia
• Inappropriate antidiuretic hormone secretion	• Edema
• Lethargy	• Impaired task performance
• Impaired task performance	• Hyperactivity
• Irritability	• Aggression
• Dyssomnia	• Depression
• Depression	• Psychosis
• Confusion	• Liver failure
• Blood dyscrasias	

Reports on the benefit of valproic acid in various formulations date to the mid-1960s. The first work concentrated on maintenance therapy of manic depressive disease with patients stabilized on valproate for up to 10 years. A few researchers studied the drug in acute mania and found it to be beneficial. It has a rapid onset of action, reaching peak plasma levels in 1 to 4 hours and the half-life ranges from 6 to 16 hours (McElroy, Keck, Pope, Hudson, & Morris, 1991).

Valproic acid appears to be at least comparable to lithium and carbamazepine for the acute mania phase of bipolar disorder (McElroy et al., 1991). Similarly, like lithium and carbamazepine, it does not appear to be as beneficial for the depressive phase of the illness. The drug appears to be especially useful in patients with mixed states and rapid cyclers (Calabrese, Woyshville, Kimmel, & Rapport, 1993).

Starting doses are 250 mg to 500 mg twice per day with doses titrated to blood levels in the range of 50 mg/mL to 120 mg/mL. The average dose to reach these levels is 750 mg to 1250 mg daily. The most serious adverse effect of valproic acid involves the liver. There have been a few deaths due to liver failure in patients receiving more than one anticonvulsant. There are no reports of death due to liver failure in adults receiving valproic acid monotherapy. Baseline liver function tests, repeat testing in the first few weeks, and testing every 3 to 6 months thereafter is necessary. Signs and symptoms of hepatotoxicity may include decreased appetite, gastrointestinal distress (e.g., nausea, vomiting, abdominal pain), dependent edema, malaise, and easy bruising. See Table 11-12 for the common adverse effects.

Lamotrigine (Lamictal) is another anticonvulsant that has demonstrated efficacy in the management of bipolar disease (Calabrese et al., 1999). Other anticonvulsants, such as gabapentin (Neurontin) and topiramate (Topamax), are also occasionally used as alternatives to lithium, carbamazepine, or valproate in treating bipolar affective disorder. These newer anticonvulsants may be added to augment primary pharmacotherapy and are generally reserved for patients who do not tolerate conventional therapy.

Calcium Channel Blockers

The calcium antagonists (calcium channel blockers) have been used mainly for the treatment of heart disorders such as arrhythmias, hypertension, and angina. These calcium ion inhibitors, such as verapamil (Calan), exert their effects by modulating an influx of calcium across the cell membrane, thus interfering with calcium dependent functions. More recently, based partly on the common effects of lithium and this class of drugs, they have been studied as a potential treatment for psychiatric illnesses ranging from mania, rapid cycling, and aggression (Dubovsky, 1998).

Verapamil is administered orally in doses ranging from 80 mg twice daily to 160 mg three times daily. The drug is well-tolerated and no specific laboratory monitoring is needed. The most common adverse effects are hypotension and bradycardia, which are usually easily managed with dose adjustments.

THE ROLE OF THE OCCUPATIONAL THERAPIST IN MEDICATION MANAGEMENT

Occupational therapists have several essential roles in the medical management of clients. As members of the interdisciplinary treatment team, occupational therapists are responsible for monitoring the functional status of clients. They are in a position to report to the physician and others what functional impairment the client may have and to indicate how that changes over time. Since an important goal of medication is to improve function, observations and formal assessment completed by the occupational therapist provide vital information about the effectiveness of the selected medication and its dosage.

In addition, the therapist must know what medication the client is taking and its side effects. For example, several medications cause postural hypotension, which can lead to falls. Therapists must be alert to the potential for clients to fall while engaged in activity and must implement appropriate preventive measures. Other medications cause drowsiness; clients should not use heavy machinery under these circumstances. Still other medications may lead to adverse reactions to sunlight; clients should be kept out of the sun while taking such medications. Recognition of the risk of suicide during initiation of some psychotropic medications, most notably the tricyclic antidepressants, is essential as well.

It is also important to keep in mind that unpleasant side effects can lead to poor follow-through on the part of the client. If the therapist has reason to believe that the client is not taking medication as prescribed, this information must be conveyed to the physician. This has become an increasingly important role for nonphysicians, since treatment is provided much more often in community rather than in-patient settings, putting clients more in charge of their own medication management. It may also be helpful for therapists to encourage patients during the first several weeks following initiation of a medication, when side effects might be most pronounced, and to assist patients to find ways to manage the side effects.

Cultural factors can also affect patient cooperation with medication plans. Some cultural groups believe that an illness is present only when symptoms are active. Individuals with this belief might be inclined to stop medication as soon as symptoms improve, even when the medication might be indicated as a long-term mechanism for avoiding relapse. In addition, some cultural groups believe in the efficacy of various herbal and folk remedies. These remedies might actually be of value, but there is the potential for problematic interaction with prescribed medications. The patient may not tell the psychiatrist about other remedies being used, and the therapist can assist by conveying the information.

Thus, the therapist must be informed about what kinds of pharmacologic interventions are being undertaken and report both main effects noted and undue side effects. Therapists should guard against giving medical advice, but should be sure to direct client questions to the physician. In addition, therapists should convey their own concerns about the medication to the physician. Because the physician may not have regular opportunities to observe the client while engaged in activity, such information can be essential to effective medical management.

Many psychotropic medications alter function in ways that affect the ability to accomplish needed or desired activities. Antidepressant medications, particularly the TCAs, may be sedating, leading to poor concentration and slowed cognition. The benzodiazepines can affect fine motor function in subtle ways, causing problems with activities requiring fine coordination. Energy, motivation, attention, ability to learn new material, motor function, and an array of other skills may be affected, each of which can alter performance ability. Therapists must be alert to these effects and assist clients in finding ways to manage them.

Medication management itself can become a complex task for some clients. They may be taking a number of different medications on different schedules. Monitoring time, manipulating medicine bottles, getting prescriptions filled and refilled, paying for medication, and monitoring side effects and main effects are all activities that clients must master. Therapists can use these tasks as a way to deal with other issues, as well, including organization, communication, transportation, and money management.

In sum, while the physician is the professional responsible for prescribing psychotropic medication, occupational therapists and other health care providers play an important role in the success of the medications. Because knowledge of psychotropic medication is changing rapidly, therapists have an obligation to inform themselves regularly of advances in practice.

REFERENCES

American Psychiatric Association. (2000). *The diagnostic and statistical manual of mental disorders* (4th ed., text revision). Washington, DC: Author.

Ballenger, J.C. (1998). Benzodiazepine. In A.F. Schatzberg & C.B. Nemeroff (Eds.), *American Psychiatric Press textbook of psychopharmacology* (2nd ed., pp. 271-286). Washington, DC: American Psychiatric Press.

Bowden, C.L. (1998). Treatment of bipolar disorder. In A.F. Schatzberg & C.B. Nemeroff (Eds.), *American Psychiatric Press textbook of psychopharmacology* (2nd ed., pp. 733-746). Washington, DC: American Psychiatric Press.

Calabrese, J.R., Bowden C.L., Sachs, G.S., Ascher, J.A., Monaghan, E., & Rudd, G.D. (1999). A double-blind, placebo-controlled study of lamotrigine monotherapy in patients with bipolar I depression. *Journal of Clinical Psychiatry, 60,* 79-88.

Calabrese, J.R., Woyshville, M.D., Kimmel, S.E., & Rapport, D.J. (1993). Mixed states and rapid cyclic bipolar disorder and their treatment with divalproex sodium. *Psychiatric Annals, 23*(2), 70-78.

Carlsson, A. (2001). Neurotransmitters: Dopamine and beyond. In A. Breier, F. Bymaster, P. Tran, & M. Lewis (Eds.), *Current issues in the psychopharmacology of schizophrenia* (pp. 3-11). Philadelphia: Lippincott, Williams & Wilkins.

Davidson, J.R.T. (1998). Long-term treatment of panic disorder. *Journal of Clinical Psychiatry, 59*(suppl 8), 17-21.

Davis, J. (1985). Antipsychotic drugs. In H. Kaplan & B. Saddock (Eds.), *Comprehensive textbook of psychiatry,* IV (pp. 1481-1537). Baltimore: Williams and Wilkins.

Dubovsky, S.L. (1998). Calcium channel antagonists as novel agents for the treatment of bipolar disorder. In A.F. Schatzberg & C.B. Nemeroff (Eds.), *American Psychiatric Press textbook of psychopharmacology* (2nd ed., pp. 455-472). Washington, DC: American Psychiatric Press.

Frazer, A. (1997). Pharmacology of antidepressants. *Journal of Clinical Psychopharmacology, 17*(suppl 1), 2S-18S.

Furukawa, T.A., McGuire, H., & Barbui, C. (2002). Meta-analysis of effects and side effects of low dosage tricyclic antidepressants in depression: Systematic review. *British Medical Journal, 325.* Retrieved December 13, 2002, from http://www.bmj.com.

Goldberg, J.F. (2000). New drugs in psychiatry. *Emergency Medicine Clinics of North America, 18,* 211-31.

Grilly, D.M. (2002). *Drugs and human behavior* (4th ed.). Boston: Allyn and Bacon.

Gumnick, J.F., & Nemeroff, C.B. (2000). Problems with currently available antidepressants. *Journal of Clinical Psychiatry, 61*(suppl). 5-15.

Hackett, T., & Cassem, N. (Eds.). (1978). *Massachusetts General Hospital handbook of general psychiatry.* St. Louis: C.V. Mosby.

Healy, D. (2002). *The creation of psychopharmacology.* Cambridge, MA: Harvard University Press.

Ho, B., & Andreasen, N.C. (2001). Positive symptoms, negative symptoms and beyond. In A. Breier, F. Bymaster, P. Tran, & M. Lewis (Eds.), *Current issues in the psychopharmacology of schizophrenia* (pp. 407-416). Philadelphia: Lippincott, Williams & Wilkins.

Israel, A.G., & Kramer, J.A. (2002). Safety of zaelplon in the treatment of insomnia. *The Annals of Pharmacotherapy, 36,* 852-859.

Janicak, P.G., Newman, R.H., & Davis, J.M. (1992). Advances in the treatment of mania and related disorders: A reappraisal. *Psychiatric Annals, 22*(2), 92-103.

Joffe, R.T., Post, R.M., Roy-Byrne, P.P., & Uhde, T.W. (1985). Hematological effects of carbamazepine in patients with affective illness. *American Journal of Psychiatry, 142,* 1196-1199.

Kane, J.M. (2001). Long-term therapeutic management in schizophrenia. In A. Breier, F. Bymaster, P. Tran, & M. Lewis (Eds.), *Current issues in the psychopharmacology of schizophrenia* (pp. 430-446). Philadelphia: Lippincott, Williams & Wilkins.

Kane, J.M., Gunduz, H., & Malhotra, A.K. (2001). Clozapine. In A. Breier, F. Bymaster, P. Tran, & M. Lewis (Eds.), *Current issues in the psychopharmacology of schizophrenia* (pp. 209-223). Philadelphia: Lippincott, Williams & Wilkins.

Krishnan, K.R.R. (1998). Monoamine oxidase inhibitors. In A.F. Schatzberg & C.B. Nemeroff (Eds.), *American Psychiatric Press textbook of psychopharmacology* (2nd ed., pp. 239-250). Washington, DC: American Psychiatric Press.

Marder, S.R. (2001). Risperidone. In A. Breier, F. Bymaster, P. Tran, & M. Lewis (Eds.), *Current issues in the psychopharmacology of schizophrenia* (pp. 243-251). Philadelphia: Lippincott, Williams & Wilkins.

McElroy, S.L., Keck, P.E., Pope, H.S., Hudson, J.I., & Morris, D. (1991). Correlates of antimanic response to valproate. *Psychopharmacology Bulletin, 27,* 127-133.

McKim, W.A. (2003). *Drugs and behavior: An introduction to behavioral pharmacology.* Upper Saddle River, NJ: Prentice Hall.

Meltzer, H.Y., & Fatemi, S.H. (1998). Treatment of schizophrenia. In A.F. Schatzberg & C.B. Nemeroff (Eds.), *American Psychiatric Press textbook of psychopharmacology* (2nd ed., pp. 747-774). Washington, DC: American Psychiatric Press.

Mitchell, P.B., & Malhi, G.S. (2002). The expanding pharmacopoeia for bipolar disorder. *Annual Review of Medicine, 53,* 173-188.

Ninan, P.T., Cole, J.O., & Yonkers, K.A. (1998). Nonbenzodiazepine anxiolytics. In A.F. Schatzberg & C.B. Nemeroff (Eds.), *American Psychiatric Press textbook of psychopharmacology* (2nd ed., pp. 287-300). Washington, DC: American Psychiatric Press.

Sampson, S.M. (2001). Treating depression with selective serotonin reuptake inhibitors: A practical approach. *Mayo Clinic Proceedings, 76,* 739-744.

Simpson, G.M., & Pi, E.H. (2001). Management of suboptimal treatment response. In A. Breier, F. Bymaster, P. Tran, & M. Lewis (Eds.), *Current issues in the psychopharmacology of schizophrenia* (pp. 447-458). Philadelphia: Lippincott, Williams & Wilkins.

Smucker, W.D., & Hedayat, M. (2001). Evaluation and treatment of ADHD. *American Family Physician, 64,* 817-829.

Sramek, J.J., Zarotsky, V., & Cutler, N.R. (2002). Generalized anxiety disorder: Treatment options. *Drugs, 62*, 1635-1648.

Stahl, S.M. (2000). *Essential psychopharmacology: Neuroscientific basis and practical applications* (2nd ed.). Cambridge, England: Cambridge University Press.

Stanilla, J.K., & Simpson, G.M. (1998). Treatment of extrapyramidal side effects. In A.F. Schatzberg & C.B. Nemeroff (Eds.), *American Psychiatric Press textbook of psychopharmacology* (2nd ed., pp. 349-378). Washington, DC: American Psychiatric Press.

Sternback, H. (1991). The serotonin syndrome. *American Journal of Psychiatry, 148*, 705-713.

Szymanski, M.L., & Zolotor, A. (2001). Attention-deficit/hyperactivity disorder: Management. *American Family Physician, 64*, 1355-1362.

Tollefson, G.D., & Rosenbaum, J.F. (1998). Selective serotonin reuptake inhibitors. In A.F. Schatzberg & C.B. Nemeroff (Eds.), *American Psychiatric Press textbook of psychopharmacology* (2nd ed., pp. 219-238). Washington, DC: American Psychiatric Press.

Wagstaff, A.J., Cheer, S.M., Matheson, A.J., Ormrod, D., & Goa, K.L (2002). Spotlight on paroxetine in psychiatric disorders in adults. *CNS Drugs 2002, 16*(6), 425-34.

Williams, J.W., Jr., Mulrow, C.D., Chiquette, E., Noel, P.H., Aguilar, C., & Cornell, J. (2000). A systematic review of newer pharmacotherapies for depression in adults: Evidence report summary. *Annals of Internal Medicine, 132*, 743-756.

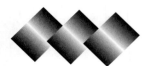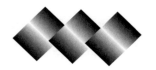

Glossary

activities of daily living (ADLs): The most basic self-care needs, including feeding, hygiene and grooming, toileting, and dressing.

activity therapies: Therapies in which doing rather than talking is the primary mode of intervention.

affect: "A pattern of observable behaviors that is the expression of a subjectively experienced feeling state (emotion)" (APA, 2000, p. 819); may be abnormally flat, labile, or inappropriate.

agraphia: An inability to write, caused by impairment of CNS processing (i.e., not by paralysis).

akathisia: Motor restlessness.

amok: "A dissociative episode characterized by a period of brooding followed by an outburst of violent, aggressive, or homicidal behavior directed at people and objects" (APA, 2000, p. 899). Original reports are from Malaysia.

anhedonia: An inability to experience pleasure.

aphasia: A communication deficit that may be expressive (i.e., the inability to effectively express a thought) or receptive (i.e., the inability to process what is being said). Occurs at the CNS level.

ataxia: Poor balance and awkward movement that results from CNS processing deficits.

avolition: Absence of interest or will to undertake activities.

behaviorism: A theory of behavior and intervention that holds that behavior is learned, that behaviors which are reinforced tend to recur, those that are not, to disappear.

biofeedback: Provision of visual or auditory cues about physical processes (e.g., heart rate, muscle tension). May allow the individual to gain control of these processes.

bradykinesia: Motor retardation.

catatonia: Motor abnormality usually characterized by immobility or rigidity in which no organic base has been identified.

codependence: A condition in which substance dependence is subtly supported by the codependent who meets some need through the continued dependence of the individual.

cognitive therapy: An approach to intervention that holds that emotional disturbance is the result of faulty belief systems.

compulsion: Repetitive, purposeful behavior undertaken to diminish obsessive thoughts; usually recognized as not genuinely helpful, but feels out of control to the individual.

confabulation: Fabrication of facts that the individual can't remember. The individual is not aware that he or she is fabricating; thus, he or she is not intentionally lying.

defense mechanisms: Patterns of thinking or behavior that are mediated at an unconscious level to provide psychic protection to an individual (e.g., projection, denial).

delusion: A fixed, firmly held belief system that is not in keeping with external reality.

desensitization: A technique employed by behaviorists to diminish fear and anxiety related to a stimulus, usually by pairing the stimulus with an incompatible response (e.g., relaxation).

dissociation: "A disruption in the usually integrated functions of consciousness, memory, identity, or perception of the environment" (APA, 2000, p. 822).

double depression: A diagnosis of major depressive episode superimposed on a diagnosis of dysthymia.

dual diagnosis: Presence of more than one DSM diagnosis at the same time, most often a combination of a substance use disorder and some other condition, but may include any situation in which comorbidity exists.

dyskinesia: "Distortion of voluntary movements with involuntary muscular activity" (APA, 2000, p. 822).

dyssomnia: Sleep disorder.

echolalia: Repetitive verbalization that does not fit the situation.

echopraxia: Repetitive movement that does not fit the situation.

educational approaches: Interventions that make use of factual learning/teaching to change behaviors.

encopresis: inability to control bowel function.

enuresis: Inability to control urine, usually bed-wetting.

environmental approaches: Interventions based on changing the environment (e.g., changing support systems, modifying job, home).

environmental press: The demands of the environment for particular levels of performance by the individual.

extinction: A behavioral approach to discouraging a particular behavior by ignoring it and reinforcing other more acceptable behaviors.

family therapy: Intervention into the entire family system, based on the theory that individual psychological difficulties are symptomatic of family disorder.

flight of ideas: Rapid continuous speech with rapid, unclear shifts from subject to subject.

gender dysphoria: "A persistent aversion toward some or all of those physical characteristics or social roles that connote one's own biological sex" (APA, 2000, p. 823).

group therapy: Any intervention directed toward groups of individuals rather than an individual alone.

habilitation: Enabling for the first time, for someone who never acquired a particular skill as in the case of mental retardation.

hallucination: A sensory experience that does not match external reality.

hyperactivity: Extreme activity, distractibility.

hypersomnia: Excessive sleeping.

instrumental activities of daily living (IADLs): Self-care activities that are higher order than ADL; includes cooking, shopping, budgeting, home repair, etc.

loose associations: Thoughts shift with little or no apparent logic.

mainstreaming: The idea that individuals should, as much as possible, be in the least restrictive environment. Most often applies to educational settings, and having retarded children and others with dysfunction be placed in regular classrooms where possible.

meta-analysis: A type of research in which previous research studies are examined to determine outcome trends.

milieu therapy: Treatment in which the environment is designed to provide specific levels of press and feedback.

nervios: A hispanic idiom for "nerves," used to describe a variety of psychological symptoms in individuals of those cultural groups.

neurotic: An analytic concept that reflects psychodynamic conflicts that cause an individual difficulty. The individual remains in contact with reality.

neurotransmitters: Chemical substances that convey new impulses at the synapses (gaps between nerve cells).

obsession: An irresistible thought pattern, usually anxiety-provoking, that incudes on normal thought processes.

panic attack: A state of extreme anxiety, usually including sweating, shortness of breath, chest pains, and fear. May come on unpredictably or as a result of a particular stimulus.

paranoia: A thought pattern that reflects a belief that others are persecuting or attempting to harm one, in the absence of a realistic basis for such fears.

parasomnia: Abnormal sleep behavior, including sleepwalking and bruxing (i.e., grinding the teeth).

perseveration: An inability to shift from thought to thought; persistence of an idea even when the subject changes.

phobia: Fear of a particular stimulus (e.g., heights, snakes). The stimulus provokes both anxiety and avoidance of the stimulus.

pica: Compulsive eating of non-nutritive substances like dirt.

polydrug abuse: Abuse of several psychoactive drugs (e.g. alcohol and cocaine).

pribloktoq: "An abrupt dissociative episode accompanied by extreme excitement of up to 30 minutes' duration and frequently followed by convulsive seizures and coma lasting up to 12 hours. This is observed primarily in arctic and subarctic Eskimo communities" (APA, 2000, p. 901).

prodromal: A preliminary phase of an illness that warns of upcoming major/primary symptoms.

psychoanalysis: A verbal therapy based on analytic theories of intrapsychic conflict.

psychodynamic: Any therapy that examines intrapsychic conflicts.

psychotic: A psychological state characterized by hallucinations and delusion (i.e., a loss of contact with reality).

psychotropic medications: Drugs that act to relieve psychological symptoms.

rational emotive therapy: A form of cognitive therapy. Intervention is designed to provide clients with cognitive understanding and control of emotions.

reality orientation: A therapeutic intervention often used with demented patients. Includes both group techniques to remind the patient of facts, and patterned environment, which provides memory cues.

reality therapy: A form of therapy designed to provide individuals with experience of reasonable consequences of actions.

rehabilitation: Helping individuals regain skills and abilities that have been lost as a result of illness or disorder.

reinforcement: A desired outcome or behavior. In behavior therapy, reinforcement is provided to encourage specific activities.

relaxation: An technique that increases relaxation, including biofeedback or systematic relaxation exercises.

reliability: The predictability of an outcome, regardless of observer. In diagnosis, it refers to the probability that several therapists will apply the same label to a given individual.

rumination: Repetitive chewing of food regurgitated after ingestion.

self-concept: The view one has of one's self.

self-esteem: The value one places on the attributes that comprise one's self-concept.

self-help: Various methods by which individuals attempt to remedy their difficulties without making use of formal care providers. Examples include Alcoholics Anonymous and several organizations of former mental patients.

sensory-integration: The ability of the CNS to process sensory information; also refers to a therapeutic intervention that uses strong kinesthetic and proprioceptive stimulation to attempt to better organize the CNS.

sensory-motor: Therapeutic interventions that make use of both motor and sensory input in an effort to better organize the CNS.

sensory stimulation: A therapeutic intervention that makes use of patterned sensory input.

sheltered living: Living arrangements, such as group homes, that provide structure and supervision for individuals who do not require institutionalization but are not fully capable of independent living.

social skills training: A cognitive/behavioral approach to teaching skills basic to social interaction.

standard error: The possible range in which a person's "true" score on a test might fall; a number that recognizes the amount by which a score might vary on different days or in different situations.

***susto*:** "A folk illness prevalent among some Latinos in the United States... attributed to a frightening event that causes the soul to leave the body and results in unhappiness and sickness" (APA, 2000, p. 903).

systematic desensitization: A behavioral procedure that uses relaxation paired with an anxiety provoking stimulus in an attempt to reduce the anxiety response.

tachycardia: Racing heartbeat.

tardive dyskinesia: An extra-pyramidal syndrome that is a long-term consequence of use of antipsychotic medications.

teratogenic: Substances that harm the developing fetus, causing birth defects.

therapeutic community: A structured in-patient environment that is designed to provide rehabilitative experiences.

thought form: The pattern or flow of ideas; the way in which thoughts take form.

token economy: A structured in-patient environment in which behavioral principles are employed. Some form of token is used for reinforcement/reward of desired behaviors.

verbal therapies: Any therapy in which talk/discussion is the primary mode of intervention.

waxy rigidity: A symptom of catatonia in which an individual will assume any position in which he or she is placed and remain there until moved again.

***zar*:** A term used in some African and Middle Eastern cultures to suggest possession by spirits.

REFERENCE

American Psychiatric Association. (2000). *Diagnostic and statistical manual of mental disorders* (4th ed., text revision). Washington, DC: Author.

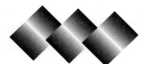 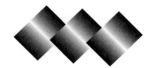

DSM-IV-TR Classification

NOS = Not Otherwise Specified

An X appearing in a diagnostic code indicates that a specific code number is required.

An ellipsis (…) is used in the names of certain disorders to indicate that the name of a specific mental disorder or general medical condition should be inserted when recording the name (e.g., 293.0 Delirium Due to Hypothyroidism).

Numbers in parentheses are page numbers.

If criteria are currently met, one of the following severity specifiers may be noted after the diagnosis:
- Mild
- Moderate
- Severe

If criteria are no longer met, one of the following specifiers may be noted:
- In Partial Remission
- In Full Remission
- Prior History

DISORDERS USUALLY FIRST DIAGNOSED IN INFANCY, CHILDHOOD, OR ADOLESCENCE (37)

Mental Retardation (39)

Note: These are coded on Axis II.

317	Mild Mental Retardation (41)	
318.0	Moderate Mental Retardation (41)	
318.1	Severe Mental Retardation (41)	

318.2   Profound Mental Retardation (41)
319   Mental Retardation, Severity Unspecified (42)

Learning Disorders (46)

315.00   Reading Disorder (48)
315.1   Mathematics Disorder (50)
315.2   Disorder of Written Expression (51)
315.9   Learning Disorder NOS (53)

Motor Skills Disorder

315.4   Developmental Coordination Disorder (53)

Communication Disorders (55)

315.31   Expressive Language Disorder (55)
315.31   Mixed Receptive-Expressive Language Disorder (58)
315.39   Phonological Disorder (61)
307.0   Stuttering (63)
307.9   Communication Disorder NOS (65)

Pervasive Developmental Disorders (65)

299.00   Autistic Disorder (66)
399.80   Rett's Disorder (71)
299.10   Childhood Disintegrative Disorder (73)
299.80   Asperger's Disorder (75)
299.80   Pervasive Developmental Disorder NOS (77)

Attention-Deficit and Disruptive Behavior Disorders (78)

314.xx   Attention-Deficit/Hyperactivity Disorder (78)
.01   Combined Type
.00   Predominantly Inattentive Type
.01   Predominantly Hyperactive-Impulsive Type
314.9   Attention-Deficit/Hyperactivity Disorder NOS (85)
312.8   Conduct Disorder (85)
Specify type: Childhood-Onset Type/Adolescent-Onset Type
313.81   Oppositional Defiant Disorder (91)
312.9   Disruptive Behavior Disorder NOS (94)

Feeding and Eating Disorders of Infancy or Early Childhood (94)

307.52   Pica (95)
307.53   Rumination Disorder (96)
307.59   Feeding Disorder of Infancy or Early Childhood (98)

Tic Disorders (100)

307.23   Tourette's Disorder (101)
307.22   Chronic Motor or Vocal Tic Disorder (103
307.21   Transient Tic Disorder (104)
Specify if: Single Episode/Recurrent
307.20   Tic Disorder NOS (105)

Elimination Disorders (106)

----.--   Encopresis (106)
787.6   With Constipation and Overflow Incontinence
307.7   Without Constipation and Overflow Incontinence
307.6   Enuresis (Not Due to a General Medical Condition) (108)
Specify type: Nocturnal Only/Diurnal Only/Nocturnal and Diurnal

Other Disorders of Infancy, Childhood, or Adolescence

309.21   Separation Anxiety Disorder (110)
Specify if: Early Onset
313.23   Selective Mutism (114)
313.89   Reactive Attachment Disorder of Infancy or Early Childhood (116)
Specify type: Inhibited Type/Disinhibited Type
307.3   Stereotypic Movement Disorder (118)
Specify if: With Self-Injurious Behavior
313.9   Disorder of Infancy, Childhood, or Adolescence NOS (121)

DELIRIUM, DEMENTIA, AND AMNESTIC
AND OTHER COGNITIVE DISORDERS (123)

Delirium (124)

293.0   Delirium Due to... [Indicate the General Medical Condition] (127)
----.--   Substance Intoxication Delirium (129) (refer to Substance-Related Disorders
            for substance-specific codes)
----.--   Substance Withdrawal Delirium (129) (refer to Substance-Related Disorders
            for substance-specific codes)
----.--   Delirium Due to Multiple Etiologies (code each of the specific etiologies) (132)
780.09   Delirium NOS (133)

Dementia (133)

290.xx	Dementia of the Alzheimer's Type, With Early Onset (also code 331.0 Alzheimer's disease on Axis III) (139)
.10	Uncomplicated
.11	With Delirium
.12	With Delusions
.13	With Depressed Mood

Specify if: With Behavioral Disturbance

290.xx	Dementia of the Alzheimer's Type, With Late Onset (also code 331.0 Alzheimer's disease on Axis III) (139)
.0	Uncomplicated
.3	With Delirium
.20	With Delusions
.21	With Depressed Mood

Specify if: With Behavioral Disturbance

290.xx	Vascular Dementia (143)
.40	Uncomplicated
.41	With Delirium
.42	With Delusions
.43	With Depressed Mood

Specify if: With Behavioral Disturbance

294.9	Dementia Due to HIV Disease (also code 043.1 HIV infection affecting central nervous system on Axis III) (148)
294.1	Dementia Due to Parkinson's Disease (also code 332.0 Parkinson's disease on Axis III) (148)
294.1	Dementia Due to Huntington's Disease (also code 333.4 Huntington's disease on Axis III) (149)
290.10	Dementia Due to Pick's Disease (also code 331.1 Pick's disease on Axis III) (149)
290.10	Due to Creutzfeldt-Jakob Disease (also code 046.1 Creutzfeldt-Jakob disease on Axis III) (150)
294.1	Dementia Due to...[Indicate the General Medical Condition not listed above] (also code the general medical condition on Axis III) (151)
----.--	Substance-Induced Persisting Dementia (refer to Substance-Related Disorders for substance-specific codes) (152)
----.--	Dementia Due to Multiple Etiologies (code each of the specific etiologies) (154)
294.8	Dementia NOS (155)

Amnestic Disorders (156)

294.0	Amnestic Disorder Due to... [Indicate the General Medical Condition] (158)
294.1	Dementia Due to Head Trauma (also code 854.00 head injury on Axis III) (148)

Specify if: Transient/Chronic

----.--	Substance-Induced Persisting Amnestic Disorder (refer to Substance-Related Disorders for substance-specific codes) (161)
294.8	Amnestic Disorder NOS (163)

Other Cognitive Disorders (163)

294.9	Cognitive Disorder NOS (163)

MENTAL DISORDERS DUE TO A GENERAL MEDICAL CONDITION NOT ELSEWHERE CLASSIFIED (165)

293.89   Catatonic Disorder Due to… [Indicate the General Medical Condition] (169)
310.1   Personality Change Due to… [Indicate the General Medical Condition] (171)
Specify type: Labile Type/Disinhibited Type/Aggressive Type/Apathetic Type/Paranoid Type/Other Type/Combined Type/Unspecified Type
293.9   Mental Disorder NOS Due to… [Indicate the General Medical Condition] (174)

SUBSTANCE-RELATED DISORDERS (175)

The following specifiers may be applied to Substance Dependence:
  • With Physiological Dependence/Without Physiological Dependence
  • Early Full Remission/Early Partial Remission/Sustained Full Remission/Sustained Partial Remission On Agonist Therapy/In a Controlled Environment
The following specifiers apply to Substance-Induced Disorders as noted:
  • With Onset During Intoxication/With Onset During Withdrawal

Alcohol-Related Disorders (194)

Alcohol Use Disorders

303.90   Alcohol Dependence (195)
305.00   Alcohol Abuse (196)

Alcohol-Induced Disorders

303.00   Alcohol Intoxication (196)
291.8   Alcohol Withdrawal (197)
Specify if: With Perceptual Disturbances
291.0   Alcohol Intoxication Delirium (129)
291.0   Alcohol Withdrawal Delirium (129)
291.2   Alcohol-Induced Persisting Dementia (152)
291.1   Alcohol-Induced Persisting Amnestic Disorder (161)
291.x   Alcohol-Induced Psychotic Disorder (310)
.5   With Delusions
.3   With Hallucinations
291.8   Alcohol-Induced Mood Disorder (370)

291.8   Alcohol-Induced Anxiety Disorder (439)
291.8   Alcohol-Induced Sexual Dysfunction (519)
291.8   Alcohol-Induced Sleep Disorder (601)
291.9   Alcohol-Related Disorder NOS (204)

Amphetamine- (or Amphetamine-Like) Related Disorders (204)

Amphetamine Use Disorders

304.40   Amphetamine Dependence (206)
305.70   Amphetamine Abuse (206)

Amphetamine-Induced Disorders

292.89   Amphetamine Intoxication (207)
Specify if: With Perceptual Disturbances
292.0   Amphetamine Withdrawal (208)
292.81   Amphetamine Intoxication Delirium (129)
292.xx   Amphetamine-Induced Psychotic Disorder (310)
.11   With Delusions
.12   With Hallucinations
292.84   Amphetamine-Induced Mood Disorder, (370)
292.89   Amphetamine-Induced Anxiety Disorder (439)
292.89   Amphetamine-Induced Sexual Dysfunction (519)
292.89   Amphetamine-Induced Sleep Disorder (601)
292.9   Amphetamine-Related Disorder NOS (211)

Caffeine-Related Disorders (212)

Caffeine-Induced Disorders

305.90   Caffeine Intoxication (212)
292.89   Caffeine-Induced Anxiety Disorder (439)
292.89   Caffeine-Induced Sleep Disorder (601)
292.9   Caffeine-Related Disorder NOS (215)

Cannabis-Related Disorders (215)

Cannabis Use Disorders

304.30   Cannabis Dependence (216)
305.20   Cannabis Abuse (217)

Cannabis-Induced Disorders

292.89   Cannabis Intoxication (217)
Specify if: With Perceptual Disturbances

292.81   Cannabis Intoxication Delirium (129)
292.xx   Cannabis-Induced Psychotic Disorder (310)
.11   With Delusions
.12   With Hallucinations
292.89   Cannabis-Induced Anxiety Disorder (439)
292.9   Cannabis-Related Disorder NOS (221)

Cocaine-Related Disorders (221)

Cocaine Use Disorders

304.20   Cocaine Dependence (222)
305.60   Cocaine Abuse (223)

Cocaine-Induced Disorders

292.89   Cocaine Intoxication (223)
Specify if: With Perceptual Disturbances
292.0   Cocaine Withdrawal (225)
292.81   Cocaine Intoxication Delirium (129)
292.xx   Cocaine-Induced Psychotic Disorder (310)
.11   With Delusions
.12   With Hallucinations
292.84   Cocaine-Induced Mood Disorder (370)
292.89   Cocaine-Induced Anxiety Disorder (439)
292.89   Cocaine-Induced Sexual Dysfunction (519)
292.89   Cocaine-Induced Sleep Disorder (601)
292.9   Cocaine-Related Disorder NOS (229)

Hallucinogen-Related Disorders (229)

Hallucinogen Use Disorders

304.50   Hallucinogen Dependence (230)
305.30   Hallucinogen Abuse (231)

Hallucinogen-Induced Disorders

292.89   Hallucinogen Intoxication (232)
292.89   Hallucinogen Persisting Perception Disorder (Flashbacks) (233)
292.81   Hallucinogen Intoxication Delirium (129)
292.xx   Hallucinogen-Induced Psychotic Disorder (310)
.11   With Delusions
.12   With Hallucinations
292.84   Hallucinogen-Induced Mood Disorder (370)
292.89   Hallucinogen-Induced Anxiety Disorder (439)
292.9   Hallucinogen-Related Disorder NOS (236)

Inhalant-Related Disorders (236)

Inhalant Use Disorders
304.60   Inhalant Dependence (238)
305.90   Inhalant Abuse (238)

Inhalant-Induced Disorders
292.89   Inhalant Intoxication (239)
292.81   Inhalant Intoxication Delirium (129)
292.82   Inhalant-Induced Persisting Dementia (152)
292.xx   Inhalant-Induced Psychotic Disorder (310)
.11   With Delusions
.12   With Hallucinations
292.84   Inhalant-Induced Mood Disorder (370)
292.89   Inhalant-Induced Anxiety Disorder (439)
292.9   Inhalant-Related Disorder NOS (242)

Nicotine-Related Disorders (242)

Nicotine Use Disorder
305.10   Nicotine Dependence (243)

Nicotine-Induced Disorder
292.0   Nicotine Withdrawal (244)
292.9   Nicotine-Related Disorder (NOS) (247)

Opioid-Related Disorders (247)

Opioid Use Disorders
304.00   Opioid Dependence (248)
305.50   Opioid Abuse (249)

Opioid-Induced Disorders
292.89   Opioid Intoxication (249)
Specify if: With Perceptual Disturbances
292.0   Opioid Withdrawal (250)
292.81   Opioid Intoxication Delirium (129)
292.xx   Opioid-Induced Psychotic Disorder (310)
.11   With Delusions
.12   With Hallucinations
292.84   Opioid-Induced Mood Disorder (370)
292.89   Opioid-Induced Sexual Dysfunction (519)

292.89   Opioid-Induced Sleep Disorder (601)
292.9   Opioid-Related Disorder NOS (255)

Phencyclidine (or Phencyclidine-Like)-Related Disorders (255)

Phencyclidine Use Disorders

304.90   Phencyclidine Dependence (256)
305.90   Phencyclidine Abuse (257)

Phencyclidine-Induced Disorders

292.89   Phencyclidine Intoxication (257)
Specify if: With Perceptual Disturbances
292.81   Phencyclidine Intoxication Delirium (129)
292.xx   Phencyclidine-Induced Psychotic Disorder (310)
.11   With Delusions
.12   With Hallucinations
292.84   Phencyclidine-Induced Mood Disorder (370)
292.89   Phencyclidine-Induced Anxiety Disorder (439)
292.9   Phencyclidine-Related Disorder NOS (261)

Sedative-, Hypnotic-, or Anxiolytic-Related Disorders (261)

Sedative-, Hypnotic-, or Anxiolytic-Use Disorders

304.10   Sedative, Hypnotic, or Anxiolytic Dependence (262)
305.40   Sedative, Hypnotic, or Anxiolytic Abuse (263)

Sedative-, Hypnotic-, or Anxiolytic-Induced Disorders

292.89   Sedative, Hypnotic, or Anxiolytic Intoxication (263)
292.0   Sedative, Hypnotic, or Anxiolytic Withdrawal (264)
Specify if: With Perceptual Disturbances
292.81   Sedative, Hypnotic, or Anxiolytic Intoxication Delirium (129)
292.81   Sedative, Hypnotic, or Anxiolytic Withdrawal Delirium (129)
292.82   Sedative-, Hypnotic-, or Anxiolytic-Induced Persisting Dementia (152)
292.83   Sedative-, Hypnotic-, or Anxiolytic-Induced Persisting Amnestic Disorder (161)
292.xx   Sedative-, Hypnotic-, or Anxiolytic-Induced Psychotic Disorder (310)
.11   With Delusions
.12   With Hallucinations
292.84   Sedative-, Hypnotic-, or Anxiolytic-Induced Mood Disorder (370)
292.89   Sedative-, Hypnotic-, or Anxiolytic-Induced Anxiety Disorder (439)
292.89   Sedative-, Hypnotic-, or Anxiolytic-Induced Sexual Dysfunction (519)
292.89   Sedative-, Hypnotic-, or Anxiolytic- Induced Sleep Disorder (601)
292.9   Sedative-, Hypnotic-, or Anxiolytic-Related Disorder NOS (269)

Polysubstance-Related Disorder

304.80   Polysubstance Dependence (270)

Other (or Unknown) Substance-Related Disorders (270)

Other (or Unknown) Substance Use Disorders

304.90   Other (or Unknown) Substance Dependence (176)
305.90   Other (or Unknown) Substance Abuse (182)

Other (or Unknown) Substance-Induced Disorders

292.89   Other (or Unknown) Substance Intoxication (183)
Specify if: With Perceptual Disturbances
292.0   Other (or Unknown) Substance-Withdrawal (184)
Specify if: With Perceptual Disturbances
292.81   Other (or Unknown) Substance-Induced Delirium (129)
292.82   Other (or Unknown) Substance-Induced Persisting Dementia (152)
292.83   Other (or Unknown) Substance-Induced Persisting Amnestic Disorder (161)
292.xx   Other (or Unknown) Substance-Induced Psychotic Disorder (310)
.11   With Delusions
.12   With Hallucinations
292.84   Other (or Unknown) Substance-Induced Mood Disorder (370)
292.89   Other (or Unknown) Substance-Induced Anxiety Disorder (439)
292.89   Other (or Unknown) Substance-Induced Sexual Dysfunction (519)
292.89   Other (or Unknown) Substance-Induced Sleep Disorder (601)
292.9   Other (or Unknown) Substance-Related Disorder NOS (272)

SCHIZOPHRENIA AND OTHER PSYCHOTIC DISORDERS (273)

295.xx   Schizophrenia (274)
The following Classification of Longitudinal Course applies to all subtypes of Schizophrenia:
   • Episodic With Interepisode Residual Symptoms (specify if: With Prominent
     Negative Symptoms)/Episodic With No Interepisode Residual Symptoms/
     Continuous (specify if: With Prominent Negative Symptoms)
   • Single Episode in Partial Remission (specify if: With Prominent Negative
     Symptoms)/Single Episode In Full Remission
   • Other or Unspecified Pattern
.30   Paranoid Type (287)
.10   Disorganized Type (287)
.20   Catatonic Type (288)
.90   Undifferentiated Type (289)
.60   Residual Type (289)
295.40   Schizophreniform Disorder (290)
Specify if: Without Good Prognostic Features/With Good Prognostic Features

295.70   Schizoaffective Disorder (292)
Specify type: Bipolar Type/Depressive Type
297.1   Delusional Disorder (296)
Specify type: Erotomanic Type/Grandiose Type/Jealous Type/Persecutory Type/Somatic Type/Mixed Type/Unspecified Type
298.8   Brief Psychotic Disorder (302)
Specify if: With Marked Stressor(s)/Without Marked Stressor(s)/With Postpartum Onset
297.3   Shared Psychotic Disorder (305)
293.xx   Psychotic Disorder Due to…[Indicate the General Medical Condition] (306)
.81   With Delusions
.82   With Hallucinations
----.--   Substance-Induced Psychotic Disorder (refer to Substance-Related Disorders for substance-specific codes) (310)
Specify if: With Onset During Intoxication/With Onset During Withdrawal
298.9   Psychotic Disorder NOS (315)

MOOD DISORDERS (317)

Code current state of Major Depressive Disorder or Bipolar I Disorder in fifth digit:
- 1 = Mild
- 2 = Moderate
- 3 = Severe Without Psychotic Features
- 4 = Severe With Psychotic Features

Specify: Mood-Congruent Psychotic Features/Mood-Incongruent Psychotic Features
- 5 = In Partial Remission
- 6 = In Full Remission
- 0 = Unspecified

The following specifiers apply (for current or most recent episode) to Mood Disorders as noted:
- Severity/Psychotic/Remission
- Specifiers/Chronic/With Catatonic Features/With Melancholic Features/ With Atypical Features/With Postpartum Onset

The following specifiers apply to Mood Disorders as noted:
- With or Without Full Interepisode Recovery/With Seasonal Pattern/With Rapid Cycling

Depressive Disorders

296.xx   Major Depressive Disorder (339)
.2x   Single Episode
.3x   Recurrent
300.4   Dysthymic Disorder (345)
Specify if: Early Onset/Late Onset
Specify: With Atypical Features
311   Depressive Disorder NOS (350)

Bipolar Disorders

296.xx	Bipolar I Disorder, (350)
.0x	Single Manic Episode

Specify if: Mixed

.40	Most Recent Episode Hypomanic
.4x	Most Recent Episode Manic
.6x	Most Recent Episode Mixed
.5x	Most Recent Episode Depressed
.7	Most Recent Episode Unspecified
296.89	Bipolar II Disorder a,b,c,d,e,f,g,h,i (359)

Specify (current or most recent episode): Hypomanic/Depressed

301.13	Cyclothymic Disorder (363)
296.80	Bipolar Disorder NOS (366)
293.83	Mood Disorder Due to...[Indicate the General Medical Condition] (366)

Specify type: With Depressive Features/With Major Depressive-Like Episode/With Manic Features/With Mixed Features

----.--	Substance-Induced Mood Disorder (refer to Substance-Related Disorders for substance-specific codes) (370)

Specify type: With Depressive Features/With Manic Features/With Mixed Features
Specify if: With Onset During Intoxication/With Onset During Withdrawal

296.90	Mood Disorder NOS (375)

ANXIETY DISORDERS (393)

300.01	Panic Disorder Without Agoraphobia (397)
300.21	Panic Disorder With Agoraphobia (397)
300.22	Agoraphobia Without History of Panic Disorder (403)
300.29	Specific Phobia (405)

Specify type: Animal Type/Natural Environment Type/Blood-Injection-Injury Type/ Situational Type/Other Type

300.23	Social Phobia (411)

Specify if: Generalized

300.3	Obsessive-Compulsive Disorder (417)

Specify if: With Poor Insight

309.81	Post-traumatic Stress Disorder (424)

Specify if: Acute/Chronic
Specify if: With Delayed Onset

308.3	Acute Stress Disorder (429)
300.02	Generalized Anxiety Disorder (432)
293.89	Anxiety Disorder Due to...[Indicate the General Medical Condition] (436)

Specify if: With Generalized Anxiety/With Panic Attacks/With Obsessive-Compulsive Symptoms

----.--	Substance-Induced Anxiety Disorder (refer to Substance-Related Disorders for substance-specific codes) (439)

Specify if: With Generalized Anxiety/With Panic Attacks/With Obsessive-Compulsive Symptoms/With Phobic Symptoms/With Phobic Symptoms
Specify if: With Onset During Intoxication/With Onset During Withdrawal

300.00	Anxiety Disorder NOS (444)

SOMATOFORM DISORDERS (445)

300.81   Somatization Disorder (446)
300.81   Undifferentiated Somatoform Disorder (450)
300.11   Conversion Disorder (452)
Specify type: With Motor Symptom or Deficit/With Sensory Symptom or Deficit/With Seizures or Convulsions/With Mixed Presentation
307.xx   Pain Disorder (458)
.80   Associated With Psychological Factors
.89   Associated With Both Psychological Factors and a General Medical Condition
Specify if: Acute/Chronic
300.7   Hypochondriasis (462)
Specify if: With Poor Insight
300.7   Body Dysmorphic Disorder (466)
300.81   Somatoform Disorder NOS (468)

FACTITIOUS DISORDERS (471)

300.xx   Factitious Disorder (471)
.16   With Predominantly Psychological Signs and Symptoms
.19   With Predominantly Physical Signs and Symptoms
.19   With Combined Psychological and Physical Signs and Symptoms
300.19   Factitious Disorder NOS (475)

DISSOCIATIVE DISORDERS (477)

300.12   Dissociative Amnesia (478)
300.13   Dissociative Fugue (481)
300.14   Dissociative Identify Disorder (484)
300.6   Depersonalization Disorder (488)
300.15   Dissociative Disorder NOS (490)

SEXUAL AND GENDER IDENTITY DISORDERS (493)

Sexual Dysfunctions (493)

The following specifiers apply to all primary Sexual Dysfunctions:
- Lifelong Type/Acquired Type Generalized Type/Situational Type Due to Psychological Factors/Due to Combined Factors

Sexual Desire Disorders

302.71   Hypoactive Sexual Desire Disorder (496)
302.79   Sexual Aversion Disorder (499)

Sexual Arousal Disorders

302.72   Female Sexual Arousal Disorder (500)
302.72   Male Erectile Disorder (502)

Orgasmic Disorders

302.73   Female Orgasmic Disorder (505)
302.74   Male Orgasmic Disorder (507)
302.75   Premature Ejaculation (509)

Sexual Pain Disorders

302.76   Dyspareunia (Not Due to a General Medical Condition) (511)
306.51   Vaginismus (Not Due to a General Medical Condition) (513)

Sexual Dysfunction Due to a General Medical Condition (515)

625.8   Female Hypoactive Sexual Desire Disorder Due to... [Indicate the General Medical Condition] (515)
608.89   Male Hypoactive Sexual Desire Disorder Due to... [Indicate the General Medical Condition] (515)
607.84   Male Erectile Disorder Due to... [Indicate the General Medical Condition] (515)
625.0   Female Dyspareunia Due to... [Indicate the General Medical Condition] (515)
608.89   Male Dyspareunia Due to... [Indicate the General Medical Condition] (515)
625.8   Other Female Sexual Dysfunction Due to... [Indicate the General Medical Condition] (515)
608.89   Other Male Sexual Dysfunction Due to... [Indicate the General Medical Condition] (515)
----.--   Substance-Induced Sexual Dysfunction (refer to Substance-Related Disorders for substance-specific codes) (519)
Specify if: With Impaired Desire/With Impaired Arousal/With Impaired Orgasm/With Sexual Pain
Specify if: With Onset During Intoxication
302.70   Sexual Dysfunction NOS (522)

Paraphilias (522)

302.4   Exhibitionism (525)
302.81   Fetishism (526)
302.89   Frotteurism (527)
302.2   Pedophilia (527)
Specify if: Sexually Attracted to Males/Sexually Attracted to Females/Sexually Attracted to Both
Specify if: Limited to Incest
Specify type: Exclusive Type/Nonexclusive Type
302.83   Sexual Masochism (529)

302.84   Sexual Sadism (530)
302.3   Transvestic Fetishism (530)
Specify if: With Gender Dysphoria
302.82   Voyeurism (532)
302.9   Paraphilia NOS (532)

Gender Identity Disorders (532)

302.xx   Gender Identity Disorder (532)
.6   in Children
.85   in Adolescents or Adults
Specify if: Sexually Attracted to Males/Sexually Attracted to Females/Sexually Attracted to Both/Sexually Attracted to Neither
302.6   Gender Identity Disorder NOS (538)
302.9   Sexual Disorder NOS (538)

EATING DISORDERS (539)

307.1   Anorexia Nervosa (539)
Specify type: Restricting Type; Binge-Eating/Purging Type
307.51   Bulimia Nervosa (545)
Specify type: Purging Type/Nonpurging Type
307.50   Eating Disorder NOS (550)

SLEEP DISORDERS (551)

Primary Sleep Disorders (553)

Dyssomnias (553)

307.42   Primary Insomnia (553)
307.44   Primary Hypersomnia (557)
Specify if: Recurrent
347   Narcolepsy (562)
780.59   Breathing-Related Sleep Disorder (567)
307.45   Circadian Rhythm Sleep Disorder (573)
Specify type: Delayed Sleep Phase Type/Jet Lag Type/Shift Work Type/Unspecified Type
307.47   Dyssomnia NOS (579)

Parasomnias (579)

307.47   Nightmare Disorder (580)
307.46   Sleep Terror Disorder (583)

307.46	Sleepwalking Disorder (587)
307.47	Parasomnia NOS (592)

Sleep Disorders Related to Another Mental Disorder (592)

307.42	Insomnia Related to… [Indicate the Axis I or Axis II Disorder] (592)
307.44	Hypersomnia Related to… [Indicate the Axis I or Axis II Disorder] (592)

Other Sleep Disorders

780.xx	Sleep Disorder Due to… [Indicate the General Medical Condition] (597)
.52	Insomnia Type
.54	Hypersomnia Type
.59	Parasomnia Type
.59	Mixed Type
----.--	Substance-Induced Sleep Disorder (refer to Substance-Related Disorders for substance-specific codes) (601)

Specify type: Insomnia Type/Hypersomnia Type/Parasomnia Type/Mixed Type
Specify if: With Onset During Intoxication/With Onset During Withdrawal

IMPULSE-CONTROL DISORDERS NOT ELSEWHERE CLASSIFIED (609)

312.34	Intermittent Explosive Disorder (609)
312.32	Kleptomania (612)
312.33	Pyromania (614)
312.31	Pathological Gambling (615)
312.39	Trichotillomania (618)
312.30	Impulse-Control Disorder NOS (621)

ADJUSTMENT DISORDERS (623)

309.xx	Adjustment Disorder (623)
.0	With Depressed Mood
.24	With Anxiety
.28	With Mixed Anxiety and Depressed Mood
.3	With Disturbance of Conduct
.4	With Mixed Disturbance of Emotions and Conduct
.9	Unspecified

Specify if: Acute/Chronic

PERSONALITY DISORDERS (629)

Note: These are coded on Axis II.

301.0	Paranoid Personality Disorder (634)
301.20	Schizoid Personality Disorder (638)
301.22	Schizotypal Personality Disorder (641)
301.7	Antisocial Personality Disorder (645)
301.83	Borderline Personality Disorder (650)
301.50	Histrionic Personality Disorder (655)
301.81	Narcissistic Personality Disorder (658)
301.82	Avoidant Personality Disorder (662)
301.6	Dependent Personality Disorder (665)
301.4	Obsessive-Compulsive Personality Disorder (669)
301.9	Personality Disorder NOS (673)

OTHER CONDITIONS THAT MAY BE A FOCUS OF CLINICAL ATTENTION (675)

Psychological Factors Affecting Medical Condition (675)

316   ...[Specified Psychological Factor] Affecting... [Indicate the General Medical Condition] (675)

Choose name based on nature of factors:

- Mental Disorder Affecting Medical Condition
- Psychological Symptoms Affecting Medical Condition
- Personality Traits or Coping Style Affecting Medical Condition
- Maladaptive Health Behaviors Affecting Medical Condition
- Stress-Related Physiological Response Affecting Medical Condition
- Other or Unspecified Psychological Factors Affecting Medical Condition

Medication-Induced Movement Disorder (678)

332.1	Neuroleptic-Induced Parkinsonism (679)
333.92	Neuroleptic Malignant Syndrome (679)
333.7	Neuroleptic-Induced Acute Dystonia (679)
333.99	Neuroleptic-Induced Acute Akathisia (679)
333.82	Neuroleptic-Induced Tardive Dyskinesia (679)
333.1	Medication-Induced Postural Tremor (680)
333.90	Medication-Induced Movement Disorder NOS (680)

Other Medication-Induced Disorder

995.2   Adverse Effects of Medication NOS (680)

Relational Problems (680)

V61.9   Relational Problem Related to a Mental Disorder or General Medical Condition (681)
V61.20   Parent-Child Relational Problem (681)
V61.1   Partner Relational Problem (681)
V61.8   Sibling Relational Problem (681)
V62.81   Relational Problem NOS (681)

Problems Related to Abuse or Neglect (682)

V61.21   Physical Abuse of Child (682) (code 995.5 if focus of attention is on victim)
V61.21   Sexual Abuse of Child (682) (code 995.5 if focus of attention is on victim)
V61.21   Neglect of Child (682) (code 995.5 if focus of attention is on victim)
V61.1   Physical Abuse of Adult (682) (code 995.81 if focus of attention is on victim)
V61.1   Sexual Abuse of Adult (682) (code 995.81 if focus of attention is on victim)

Additional Conditions That may be a Focus of Clinical Attention (683)

V15.81   Noncompliance With Treatment (683)
V65.2   Malingering (683)
V71.01   Adult Antisocial Behavior (683)
V71.02   Child or Adolescent Antisocial Behavior (684)
V62.89   Borderline Intellectual Functioning (684) *Note: This is coded on Axis II*
780.9   Age-Related Cognitive Decline (684)
V62.82   Bereavement (684)
V62.3   Academic Problem (685)
V62.2   Occupational Problem (685)
313.82   Identity Problem (685)
V62.89   Religious or Spiritual Problem (685)
V62.4   Acculturation Problem (685)
V62.89   Phase of Life Problem (685)

ADDITIONAL CODES

300.9   Unspecified Mental Disorder (nonpsychotic) (687)
V71.09   No Diagnosis or Condition on Axis I (687)
799.9   Diagnosis or Condition Deferred on Axis I (687)
V71.09   No Diagnosis on Axis II (687)
799.9   Diagnosis Deferred on Axis II (687)

MULTIAXIAL SYSTEM

Axis I   Clinical Disorders/Other Conditions That May Be a Focus of Clinical Attention

Axis II   Personality Disorders Mental Retardation

Axis III   General Medical Conditions

Axis IV   Psychosocial and Environmental Problems

Axis V   Global Assessment of Functioning

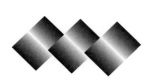

An Overview of the International Classification of Function

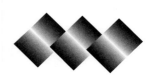

	Part 1: Functioning and Disability		Part 2: Contextual Factors	
Components	Body Functions and Structures	Activities and Participation	Environmental Factors	Personal Factors
Domains	Body functions Body structures	Life areas (tasks, actions)	External influences on functioning and disability	Internal influences on functioning and disability
Constructs	Change in body functions (physiological) Change in body structures (anatomical)	Capacity Executing tasks in a standard environment Performance Executing tasks in the current environment	Facilitating or hindering impact of features of the physical, social, and attitudinal world	Impact of attributes of the person
Positive aspect	Functional and structural integrity	Activities Participation	Facilitators	not applicable
	Functioning			
Negative aspect	Impairment	Activity limitation Participation restriction	Barriers / hindrances	not applicable
	Disability			

Reprinted with permission from World Health Organization. (2001). *International classification of function.* Geneva: Author.

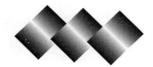 # Index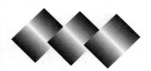

abuse
> drug. *See* substance-related disorders
> post-traumatic stress disorder after, 133–136
> problems related to, 230

academic skills disorders, 41–43, 214
activities of daily living, defined, 207
activity therapies, defined, 207
ADHD (attention-deficit hyperactivity disorder), 49–52, 56
adjustment disorders, 169, 228
adolescents. *See* children, adolescents, and infants
affect, defined, 207
agoraphobia, 128, 129–130, 137
agraphia, defined, 207
AIDS dementia complex, 70
akathisia, defined, 207
alcohol use and abuse, 78–82
> dementia in, 70
> DSM-IV-TR classification, 217–218
> etiology, 79–80
> function, 81–82
> incidence, 80
> prognosis, 80
> treatment, 81–82

Allen's cognitive approach, 20, 22
Alzheimer's disease
> diagnosis, 67
> etiology, 67–68
> function, 69–71, 73
> incidence, 67
> prognosis, 68
> stages, 69
> symptoms, 73
> treatment, 69–71
> types, 68

Americans with Disabilities Act, 25
aminoketone antidepressants, 186
amnesia, dissociative, 165
amnestic disorder, 72, 74, 216
amok, defined, 207

amphetamines, 191, 192
    abuse of, 82–83, 218
anhedonia, defined, 207
anorexia nervosa, 166–169
Anthony rehabilitation model, 22, 23
antianxiety agents, 187–190, 221
anticonvulsants, 200–201
antidepressants, 179–186
    in current use, 181
    depression pathophysiology and, 179–180
    dopamine-reuptake blockers, 181
    noradrenergic, 182
    selective serotonin receptor inhibitors, 181, 185–186
    serotonin/norepinephrine receptor inhibitors, 181
    tricyclic, 180, 182–183
antihistamines, 187
antipsychotic drugs, 193–202
    anticonvulsants, 200–201
    atypical, 196–198
    calcium channel blockers, 202
    lithium, 198–200
    side effects, 194–196
antisocial personality disorder, 145–146
anxiety disorders, 127–139
    agoraphobia, 129–130, 137
    DSM-IV-TR classification, 224
    generalized, 136
    obsessive-compulsive disorder, 132–133, 137
    panic attack, 127
    panic disorder, 128–129, 137
    post-traumatic stress disorder, 133–137
    separation, 54–55, 57, 161–162
    specific phobia, 130–131, 137
anxiolytics, 187–190
    abuse of, 221
aphasia, defined, 207
Asperger's syndrome, 48–49
ataxia, defined, 207
attention-deficit hyperactivity disorder, 49–52, 56
    diagnosis, 50
    DSM-IV-TR classification, 214
    etiology, 50
    function, 51–52
    incidence, 50
    occupational therapy, 52
    prognosis, 51
    symptoms, 49–50
    treatment, 51–52, 190–192
autism, 45–48, 56
    etiology, 45
    function, 46–47
    incidence, 45–46
    occupational therapy, 47–48
    prognosis, 46
    treatment, 46–47

avoidant personality disorder, 150
avolition, defined, 207

barbiturates, 187
behavior disorders, disruptive, 49–55, 214
behaviorism, defined, 207
biofeedback, defined, 207
bipolar disorder, 118–121, 198–200, 224
body dysmorphic disorder, 162–163
borderline personality disorder, 146–148
bradykinesia, defined, 207
bulimia nervosa, 166–169

caffeine abuse, 87–88, 218
CAGE questionnaire, for substance abuse, 90
calcium channel blockers, 202
cannabis, 86, 218–219
carbamates, 187
catatonia, defined, 207
catatonic schizophrenia, 96–97
central serotonin syndrome, 186
children, adolescents, and infants, disorders of, 35–63
    Asperger's syndrome, 48–49
    attention-deficit hyperactivity disorder, 49–52, 56, 190–192, 214
    autism, 45–48, 56
    communication disorders, 44, 214
    conduct disorder, 52–54, 57
    disruptive behavior disorders, 49–55, 214
    DSM-IV-TR classification, 213–215
    eating, 160, 214
    elimination, 161, 215
    learning disorders, 41–44, 214
    mental retardation, 36–41, 56, 213–215
    motor skills disorder, 43–44
    not otherwise classified, 161–162
    oppositional defiant disorder, 54
    pervasive developmental disorders, 45–49, 214
    selective mutism, 161–162
    separation anxiety disorder, 54–55, 57, 161–162
    stereotypic movement, 161–162
cigarette smoking, 87, 220
classification
    DSM-IV-TR, 213–231
    function, 19–20, Appendix B
    mental retardation, 38
"club drugs," 82–83
cocaine abuse, 82–83, 219
codependence, defined, 207
codes, for DSM-IV-TR, 213–231
cognitive disorders. *See also* dementia
    amnestic disorders, 72, 74
    delirium, 65–66, 73, 215
    occupational therapy, 71–72
cognitive therapy, defined, 207

communication disorders, 44, 214
compulsion, defined, 207
conduct disorder, 52–54, 57
confabulation, defined, 207
consultation, 25
conversion disorder, 162–163
crack cocaine, 82–83, 219
criminal behavior, in antisocial personality disorder, 145–146
cultural considerations in, 27
cyclothymia, 119–121

defense mechanisms, defined, 208
delirium, 65–66
    DSM-IV-TR classification, 215
    function, 73
    symptoms, 73
delusion, defined, 208
delusional disorder, 104
dementia, 66–72
    differential diagnosis, 67
    DSM-IV-TR classification, 216
    etiology, 66–68
    function, 69–71, 73
    incidence, 66–68
    occupational therapy, 71–72
    prognosis, 68
    symptoms, 73
    treatment, 69–71
densensitization, defined, 208
dependent personality disorder, 150–151
depersonalization disorder, 165
depression
    in bipolar disorder, 118–121, 224
    in cyclothymia, 119–120, 121
    depressive disorders, 116–117, 223
    in DSM from version I through IV-TR, 9–12
    dysthymia, 117, 121
    major depressive episode, 109–114, 121
    pathophysiology, 179–180
    in schizophrenia, 99
    treatment. *See* antidepressants
depressive dementia, 67, 68, 70
developmental coordination disorder (motor skills disorder), 43–44
diagnosis, dual
    defined, 208
    in substance abuse, 88–89
Diagnostic and Statistical Manual of Mental Disorders, Fourth edition, Text Revision. See DSM-IV-TR
disorganized schizophrenia, 97
disruptive behavior disorders, 49–55, 214
dissociation, defined, 208
dissociative disorders, 165, 225
dopamine-reuptake blockers, 181
double depression, defined, 208
drug(s). *See also* psychopharmacology; specific drugs
    abuse of. *See* substance-related disorders

DSM-IV-TR
  axes in, 8–9
  classification, 213–231
  as DSM-IV revision, 5
  format, 8–9
  history, 1–5
DSM-V, development, 6–7
dual diagnosis
  defined, 208
  in substance abuse, 88–89
dyskinesia, defined, 208
dyssomnia, 168–169, 227
  defined, 208
dysthymia, 117, 121
dysthymic disorder, in DSM from version I through IV-TR, 9–12

eating disorders, 160, 166–169
  DSM-IV-TR classification, 227
  etiology, 167
  function, 168
  incidence, 167
  of infancy or early childhood, 160, 214
  occupational therapy, 168
  prognosis, 167
  treatment, 168
  types, 166–167
echolalia, defined, 208
echopraxia, defined, 208
ecstasy abuse, 82–83
educational approaches, defined, 208
elimination disorders, 161, 215
encopresis, 161
  defined, 208
enuresis, 161
  defined, 208
environmental approaches, defined, 208
environmental press, defined, 208
erotomanic delusions, 104
expressive language disorder, 44
extinction, defined, 208

factitious disorders, 164, 225
family therapy
  defined, 208
  for schizophrenia, 101
feeding disorders, of infancy and early childhood, 160, 214
fetishism, 165–166
flight of ideas, defined, 208
folie a deux, defined, 105
fragile X syndrome, 49

gambling, pathological, 169
Ganser syndrome, 66–67
gender dysphoria, defined, 208

gender identity disorders, 165–166, 227
generalized anxiety disorder, 136
grandiosity
    in delusion disorder, 104
    in narcissistic personality disorder, 149–150
group therapy, defined, 208

habilitation, defined, 208
hallucination, defined, 208
hallucinogens, 83–84, 219
hashish, 86
heroin abuse, 84–86
histrionic personality disorder, 148–149
human immunodeficiency virus infection, dementia in, 70
hydrocarbon inhalation, 87, 220
hyperactivity
    in ADHD, 49–52, 56, 190–192
    defined, 208
hypersomnia, 168–169
    defined, 208
hypnotics, 190
    abuse of, 221
hypochondriasis, 162–163, 170
hypomanic episode, 116
hysterical dementia, 70

identity disorders
    gender, 165–166, 227
    multiple personality, 165, 225
impulse control disorders, not elsewhere classified, 169, 228
incoordination (motor skills disorder), 43–44
infants. *See* children, adolescents, and infants
inhalant abuse, 87, 220
instrumental activities of daily living, defined, 208
intelligence, subaverage. *See* mental retardation
intermittent explosive disorder, 169
International Classification of Diseases, 1
International Classification of Function, Appendix B
International Classification of Functioning, Disability, and Health, 19–20
intoxication, 73

Jakob-Creutzfeldt disease, dementia in, 68
jealousy, in delusion disorder, 104

Kielhofner's Model of Human Occupation, 20, 22, 23
kleptomania, 169
Korsakoff's syndrome, 72

laboratory testing, in medication use, 178
language disorders, 44
learning disorders, 41–44, 214
lithium, 198–200
loose associations, defined, 208

mainstreaming, defined, 208
major depressive episode, 109–114
    diagnosis, 109–110
    etiology, 111
    function, 112
    incidence, 111
    occupational therapy, 113–114
    prognosis, 111–112
    symptoms, 110
    treatment, 112–113
manic episode, 114–116
marijuana, 86
masochism, 165–166
mathematics disorder, 41–43
medical conditions
    mental disorders in, 162, 217, 229
    sexual dysfunction due to, 226
medications. *See* psychopharmacology; substance-related disorders
memory disorder, 72, 74, 216
mental disorders
    in medical conditions, 162, 217, 229
    occupational therapy and, 20–26
mental retardation, 36–41, 56
    classification, 38
    DSM-IV-TR classification, 213–214
    etiology, 36–37
    function, 38–40
    incidence, 37
    occupational therapy, 40–41
    prognosis, 37–38
    treatment, 38–40
meta-analysis, defined, 208
milieu therapy, defined, 209
mixed expressive-receptive language disorder, 44
Model of Human Occupation (Kielhofner), 20, 22, 23
monoamine oxidase inhibitors, 184
mood disorders, 109–124
    bipolar disorders, 118–121, 198–200, 224
    depressive disorders, 116–117, 223
    DSM-IV-TR classification, 223–224
    dysthymia, 117
    hypomanic episode, 116
    major depressive episode, 109–114, 223
    manic episode, 114–116
    suicide, 120–122
    treatment, 200–201
motor skills disorder, 43–44
motor tic disorder, 160–161
movement disorders
    medication-induced, 229–230
    stereotypic, 161–162
multi-infarct dementia, 67, 68, 70
multiaxial system, 231
multiple personality disorder (now dissociative identity disorder), 165, 225
Munchausen syndrome, 164

narcissistic personality disorder, 149–150
narcotic (opioid) abuse, 84–86, 220–221
neglect, problems related to, 230
nervios, defined, 209
neuroleptic malignant syndrome, 195
neurotic, defined, 209
neurotransmitters
    defined, 209
    in depression, 179–180
nicotine use, 87, 220

obsession, defined, 209
obsessive-compulsive disorder, 132–133, 137
obsessive-compulsive personality disorder, 151–152
Occupational Adaptation model, 22, 23
occupational therapy
    accountability in, 28
    attention-deficit hyperactivity disorder, 52
    autism, 47–48
    bipolar disorder, 119
    in community settings, 26–27
    conduct disorder, 53–54
    consultation in, 25
    cultural considerations in, 27
    cyclothymia, 120
    dementia, 71–72
    DSM-IV and, 17–33
    eating disorders, 168
    goals, 22, 24
    hypochondriasis, 170
    intervention strategies, 24–25
    learning disorders, 43
    major depressive episode, 113–114
    medication management, 202–203
    mental retardation, 40–41
    motor skills disorder, 44
    personality disorder, 152–153
    post-traumatic stress disorder, 136
    process, 22
    psychiatric theories of dysfunction, 17–20
    psychopharmacology, 175–176, 202–203
    schizophrenia, 102–104
    separation anxiety disorder, 55
    substance-related disorders, 89–90
    in team approach, 27
    transsexualism, 170
    trends affecting, 26–28
    view of mental disorder, 20–26
    websites, 28–30
Occupational Therapy Practice Framework; Domain and Process, 20–21
opioid abuse, 84–86, 220–221
oppositional defiant disorder, 54

pain, somatoform, 162–163
panic attack, 127
    defined, 209
panic disorder, 128–129, 137
paranoia, defined, 209
paranoid personality disorder, 142–143
paranoid schizophrenia, 98, 100–101
paraphilias, 165–166, 226–227
parasomnia, 168–169, 227–228
    defined, 209
Parkinson's disease, dementia in, 68
PCP (phencyclidine), 83–84, 221
pedophilia, 165–166
persecutory delusions, 104
perseveration, defined, 209
Personal Environment-Occupational Performance model, 20, 22, 23
personality disorders, 141–156
    antisocial, 145–146
    avoidant, 150
    borderline, 146–148
    clusters of, 142, 154–155
    dependent, 150–151
    DSM-IV-TR classification, 229
    histrionic, 148–149
    narcissistic, 149–150
    obsessive-compulsive, 151–152
    occupational therapy, 152–153
    paranoid, 142–143
    schizoid, 143–144
    schizotypal, 144–145
pervasive developmental disorders, 45–49, 214
phencyclidine (PCP), 83–84, 221
phobia
    defined, 209
    specific, 130–131
phonological disorder, 44
pica, defined, 209
Pick's disease, dementia in, 70
polydrug abuse, defined, 209
post-traumatic stress disorder, 133–137
    defined, 133
    etiology, 134
    function, 135
    incidence, 134
    occupational therapy, 136
    prognosis, 135
    treatment, 135
pribloktoq, defined, 209
prodromal, defined, 209
propranolol, 189–190
pseudodementia (Ganser's syndrome), 66–68
psychiatric theories, 17–20
psychoanalysis, defined, 209
psychodynamic, defined, 209

psychopharmacology
    antianxiety agents, 187–190
    antidepressants, 179–186
    antipsychotic drugs, 193–202
    history, 176–177
    hypnotics, 190
    laboratory testing in, 178
    occupational therapy in, 175–176, 202–203
    principles, 177
    sedatives, 78–79, 190, 221
    stimulants, 190–192
psychostimulants, 190–192
psychotic, defined, 209
psychotic disorders. *See also* schizophrenia
    delusional disorder, 104
    schizoaffective disorder, 105
    schizophreniform disorder, 104
    shared, 105
    treatment. *See* antipsychotic drugs
psychotropic medications, defined, 209
PTSD. *See* post-traumatic stress disorder
pyromania, 169

rational emotive therapy, defined, 209
reactive psychosis, 104
reading disorder, 41–43
reality orientation, defined, 209
reality therapy, defined, 209
rehabilitation, defined, 209
rehabilitation model (Anthony), 22, 23
reinforcement, defined, 209
relational problems, 230
relaxation, defined, 209
reliability, defined, 209
residual schizophrenia, 98
Rett syndrome, 49
rumination, defined, 210

sadism, sexual, 165–166
schizoaffective disorder, 105
schizoid personality disorder, 143–144
schizophrenia, 95–104
    defined, 95
    deinstitutionalization, 102
    diagnosis, 18, 96
    DSM-IV-TR classification, 222–223
    etiology, 98–99
    function, 99–102
    incidence, 99
    occupational therapy, 102–104
    phases, 96
    prodrome, 99–100
    prognosis, 99
    symptoms, 95–96

treatment, 99–102, 193–202
types, 96–98
schizophreniform disorder, 104
schizotypal personality disorder, 144–145
school phobia, 131
sedatives, 190
abuse of, 78–79, 221
selective serotonin receptor inhibitors, 181, 185–186
self-concept, defined, 210
self-esteem, defined, 210
self-help, defined, 210
sensory-integration, defined, 210
sensory-motor, defined, 210
sensory stimulation, defined, 210
separation anxiety disorder, 54–55, 57, 161–162
serotonin/norepinephrine receptor inhibitors, 181
sexual disorders, 165–166, 225–227
shared psychotic disorders, 105
sheltered living, defined, 210
sleep disorders, 168–169, 227–228
smoking, 87, 220
social phobia, 131
social skills training, defined, 210
solvent inhalation, 87, 220
somatic delusion disorder, 104
somatization disorder, 162–163
somatoform disorders, 162–163, 225
somatoform pain disorder, 162–163
specific phobia, 130–131, 137
speech disorders, 44
standard error, defined, 210
stimulants, 190–192
stress
adjustment disorders in, 169, 228
post-traumatic stress disorder after, 133–137
stuttering, 44
substance-related disorders, 77–93
alcohol, 78–82, 217–218
amphetamines, 82–83, 218
caffeine, 87–88, 218
cannabis, 86, 218–219
cocaine, 82–83, 219
DSM-IV-TR classification, 217–222
dual diagnosis, 88–90
hallucinogens, 83–84, 219
inhalants, 87, 220
nicotine, 87, 220
occupational therapy, 89–90
opioids, 84–86, 220–221
PCP, 83–84
sedatives, 78–82, 221
treatment, 88–90
from unknown substances, 222
suicide, 120–122

susto, defined, 210
syphilitic dementia, 70
systematic desensitization, defined, 210

tachycardia, defined, 210
tardive dyskinesia, 195
    defined, 210
teratogenic, defined, 210
therapeutic community, defined, 210
thought form, defined, 210
tic disorders, 160–161, 215
token economy, defined, 210
Tourette's syndrome, 160–161
transient tic disorder, 160–161
transsexualism, 165–166, 170
transvestic fetishism, 165–166
trauma, post-traumatic stress disorder after, 133–137
trichotillomania, 169
tricyclic antidepressants, 180, 182–183

vascular dementia, 67
verbal therapies, defined, 210
vocal tic disorder, 160–161

waxy rigidity, defined, 210
websites, 28–30
withdrawal, 73
written expression, disorder of, 41–43

zar, defined, 210

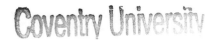